Practical Atlas of Computed Tomography

Published by

Jitendar P Vij

Jaypee Brothers Medical Publishers (P) Ltd

Corporate Office

4838/24 Ansari Road, Daryaganj, **New Delhi** - 110002, India, Phone: +91-11-43574357, Fax: +91-11-43574314

Registered Office

B-3 EMCA House, 23/23B Ansari Road, Daryaganj, **New Delhi** - 110 002, India
Phones: +91-11-23272143, +91-11-23272703, +91-11-23282021
+91-11-23245672, Rel: +91-11-32558559, Fax: +91-11-23276490, +91-11-23245683
e-mail: jaypee@jaypeebrothers.com, Website: www.jaypeebrothers.com

Offices in India

- **Ahmedabad**, Phone: Rel: +91-79-32988717, e-mail: ahmedabad@jaypeebrothers.com
- **Bengaluru**, Phone: Rel: +91-80-32714073, e-mail: bangalore@jaypeebrothers.com
- **Chennai**, Phone: Rel: +91-44-32972089, e-mail: chennai@jaypeebrothers.com
- **Hyderabad**, Phone: Rel:+91-40-32940929, e-mail: hyderabad@jaypeebrothers.com
- **Kochi**, Phone: +91-484-2395740, e-mail: kochi@jaypeebrothers.com
- **Kolkata**, Phone: +91-33-22276415, e-mail: kolkata@jaypeebrothers.com
- **Lucknow**, Phone: +91-522-3040554, e-mail: lucknow@jaypeebrothers.com
- **Mumbai**, Phone: Rel: +91-22-32926896, e-mail: mumbai@jaypeebrothers.com
- **Nagpur**, Phone: Rel: +91-712-3245220, e-mail: nagpur@jaypeebrothers.com

Overseas Offices

- **North America Office, USA,** Ph: 001-636-6279734, e-mail: jaypee@jaypeebrothers.com, anjulav@jaypeebrothers.com
- **Central America Office, Panama City, Panama,** Ph: 001-507-317-0160, e-mail: cservice@jphmedical.com
  Website: www.jphmedical.com
- **Europe Office, UK,** Ph: +44 (0) 2031708910, e-mail: info@jpmedpub.com

Practical Atlas of Computed Tomography

© 2011, Jaypee Brothers Medical Publishers

This book has been published in good faith that the material provided by the authors is original. Every effort is made to ensure accuracy of material, but the publisher, printer and authors will not be held responsible for any inadvertent error (s). In case of any dispute, all legal matters are to be settled under Delhi jurisdiction only.

First Edition: **2011**

ISBN 978-93-80704-92-0

Typeset at JPBMP typesetting unit

Printed at Ajanta Offset & Packagings Ltd., New Delhi

Practical Atlas of
Computed Tomography

(Brig) Hariqbal Singh MD DMRD

Professor and Head
Department of Radiology
Shrimati Kashibai Navale Medical College
Pune, Maharashtra (India)

Sushil Kachewar MD DNB

Assistant Professor
Shrimati Kashibai Navale Medical College
Pune, Maharashtra (India)

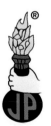

JAYPEE BROTHERS MEDICAL PUBLISHERS (P) LTD

Mumbai • St Louis (USA) • Panama City (Panama) • London (UK) • New Delhi • Ahmedabad
Bengaluru • Chennai • Hyderabad • Kolkata • Kochi • Lucknow • Nagpur

To

Our Loving Children
Amandeep, Jassim, Major Hamitesh Singh
and
Nimeesh Kachewar

Contributors

Abhijit Pawar
Consultant Radiology
Smt Kashibai Navale Medical College
Pune, Maharashtra (India)

Anubhav Khandelwal
Consultant Radiology
Medanta The Medicity
Gurgaon, Haryana (India)

Col RA George
Senior Advisor Radiology
Command Hospital
Pune, Maharashtra (India)

Rajul Rastogi
Head Radiology
Yash Hospital and Research Center
Moradabad, UP (India)

Ravi Varma
Consultant Radiology
Prince Aly Khan Hospital, Mumbai
Maharashtra (India)

Sachin Patil
Head Radiology
Niramaya Hospital, PCMC
Pune, Maharashtra (India)

Sanjay Jain
Head Radiology
Prince Aly Khan Hospital, Mumbai
Maharashtra (India)

Santosh Konde
Consultant Radiology
Smt Kashibai Navale Medical College
Pune, Maharashtra (India)

Shrinivas Desai
Head Radiology
Jaslok Hospital, Mumbai
Maharashtra (India)

Sikandar Shaikh
Consultant PET-CT
Apollo Health City, Hyderabad
Andhra Pradesh (India)

Sushant Bhadane
Consultant Radiology
Smt Kashibai Navale Medical College
Pune, Maharashtra (India)

Priscilla Joshi
Head Radiology
Jehangir Hospital
Pune, Maharashtra (India)

Preface

The value of radiology cannot be measured,
it can only be treasured.

Take it as a fun key.

Images are like a face,
corroborate it with patients' state,
the diagnosis is made.

The treatment is concocted.

Vigor and strength revivify,
all is fine and vivify.

—Hariqbal Singh

The advent of Computed Tomography (CT) has revolutionized the field of medicine. This book provides a large bank of CT images. It includes normal anatomy and a wide range of pathology. With these images in mind, it will help residents, radiologists and practioners to interpret the possible diagnosis during their routine practice. However, they are advised to always correlate with the clinical picture. This book *Practical Atlas of Computed Tomography* also includes a chapter on PET-CT and CT Quiz to make it more interesting to the readers.

This book is meant for radiology residents, radiologists, general practitioners, other specialists, CT technical staff and those who have a special interest in CT imaging. It is meant for medical colleges and institutional libraries, departmental and stand-alone CT scan unit libraries.

Hariqbal Singh
Sushil Kachewar

Acknowledgments

We express our gratitude to Prof MN Navale, Founder President, Sinhgad Technical Educational Society and Dr Arvind V Bhore, Dean, Smt Kashibai Navale Medical College for their kind permission in this endeavor.

Our special thanks to the CT Scan Technicians Mr More Rahul, Mr Demello Thomas, Mr Balasaheb Musmade, Mr Raghvendra Gangoor and Mrs Manjusha Chikale nursing sister and receptionist of the CT unit for their untiring help in retrieving the data.

Dr Anand Kamat, Prashant Naik, Amol Sasane, Rajlaxmi Sharma, Sheetal Dhote, Mrunalini Shah, Amol Nade and Rahul Tupe have genuinely helped in building up this educational entity.

We thank our Artist Sanjay Raut for developing on certain images and Ms Snehal Nikalje, Sunanda Jangalagi and Anna Bansode for their clerical help.

The response from Mr Tarun Duneja (Director-Publishing) and Ms Chetna Malhotra (Senior Manager), M/s Jaypee Brothers Medical Publishers (P) Ltd and their entire team are laudable for their tolerance, with earnest and industrious effort to complete this project.

We are grateful to GOD and mankind who have allowed us to have this wonderful experience.

Contents

SECTION 2

CARDIOVASCULAR SYSTEM AND MEDIASTINUM

SECTION 3

ABDOMEN AND GASTROINTESTINAL SYSTEM

SECTION 4

GENITOURINARY SYSTEM

SECTION 5

MUSCULOSKELETAL SYSTEM

SECTION 6

CENTRAL NERVOUS SYSTEM

SECTION 7

HEAD, NECK AND FACE

SECTION 8

MISCELLANEOUS

SECTION 9

QUIZ

SECTION 10

PET-CT

SECTION 11

RADIATION SAFETY MEASURES

SECTION 12

CT CONTRAST MEDIA

Introduction

CT was invented in 1972 by British engineer Sir Godfrey Newbold Hounsfield in Hayes, United Kingdom at EMI Central Research Laboratories using X-rays. About the same time South Africa born American physicist Allan McLeod Cormack of Tufts University in Massachusetts independently invented a similar process and both shared the 1979 Nobel Prize.

The first clinical CT scan was installed in1974. The initial systems were dedicated only to head scanning due to small gantry, but soon this was overcome and whole body CT systems with larger gantry became available in 1976.

CT Scan

Basic principle is to obtain a tomogram having thickness in millimeters of the region of interest using pencil beam X-radiation. The radiation transmitted through the patient is counted by scintillation detector. This information is analyzed by mathematical algorithms and reconstructed as a tomographic image by the computer so as to provide a peep into the structure being studied.

Developments in CT Technology

A. **Conventional Axial CT:**

Generation of CT scan	Motion of X-ray tube - Detector system	Stationary detectors	X-ray beam type
First	Translate-Rotate	Two detectors	Pencil beam
Second	Translate-Rotate	Multiple detectors up to 30	Narrow fan beam (10°)
Third	Rotate-Rotate	Multiple detectors up to 750	Wide fan beam (50°)
Fourth	Rotate-Fixed	Ring of 1500-4500	Fan beam

B. **Spiral CT:** Spiral CT uses the conventional technology in conjunction with slip ring technology, which simultaneously provides high voltage for X-ray tube, low voltage for control unit and transmits digital data from detector array. Slip ring is a circular instrument with sliding bushes that enables the gantry to rotate continuously while the patient table moves into the gantry simultaneously, thus three dimensional volume rendered image can be obtained. The advantages over the conventional scanner are the reduced scan time, reduced radiation exposure and reduced contrast requirement with superior information.

C. **Electron beam CT (EBCT):** In EBCT both the X-ray source and the detectors are stationary. High energy focused electron beam is magnetically steered on the tungsten target to emit X-rays which pass through the subject on to the detectors and image is acquired. EBCT is particularly used for faster imaging in cardiac studies.

D. **Multislice/Multi-detector CT (MDCT):** Spiral CT uses single row of detectors, resulting in a single slice per gantry rotation. In multislice CT, multiple detector arrays are used resulting in multiple slices per gantry rotation. In addition, fan beam geometry of spiral CT is replaced by cone beam geometry. The major advantages over spiral CT are improved spatial and temporal resolution, reduced image noise, faster and longer anatomic coverage and increased concentration of intravenous contrast.

E. **Dual source CT:** Two X-ray sources are used as against single X-ray source in multislice CT scanner for faster imaging specially for structure like heart.

The enduring continuity of research in CT imaging aims to provide superior resolution, reduced noise, faster imaging, minimize radiations and quantum of contrast medium.

Section 1

Respiratory System

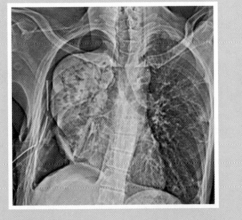
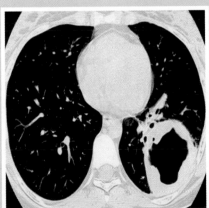
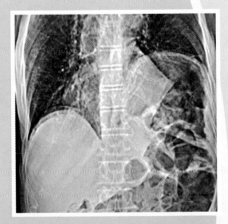

1. NORMAL LUNG

1.1 CT Lungs

Normal Anatomy

Embryologically airway starts developing by fifth week of gestational age in the form of lung buds which grow from ventral aspect of primitive foregut. Trachea and esophagus are also separated by fifth week. Hereafter tracheobronchial tree is formed from fifth to fifteenth week. There are 23-25 airway generations from trachea to bronchiole. A bronchus has cartilage in the wall. Bronchiole is devoid of cartilage.

Interstitium of lung is divided into axial interstitium, parenchymal interstitium and peripheral interstitium. Axial interstitium is made of bronchovascular sheaths and lymphatics. Parenchymal interstitium includes interalveolar septum along alveolar walls. Peripheral interstitium includes sub pleural connective tissue and interlobular septa which encloses the pulmonary veins and lymphatics.

Pulmonary circulation includes primary pulmonary circulation, bronchial circulation and the anastomoses between the two. Primary pulmonary circulation consists of pulmonary arteries and veins that travel down to subsegmental bronchial level and has a diameter same as that of the accompanying airway. Main pulmonary artery arises from the right ventricle.

Bronchial circulation originates from thoracic aorta and supplies through the intercostal arteries which are two in number for each lung.

Segmental Division of Lungs

Right lung has following three lobes:
1. Upper lobe which has an apical, anterior and a posterior segment.
2. Middle lobe has a lateral and a medial segment.
3. Lower lobe has superior segment, medial basal segment, anterior basal segment, lateral basal segment and a posterior basal segment.

Left lung has following two lobes:
1. Upper lobe which has an apico-posterior, anterior, superior lingular and an inferior lingular segment.
2. Lower lobe has superior segment, antero- medial basal segment, lateral basal segment and a posterior basal segment.

Left lung has no middle lobe.

Axial Sections of CT Chest (Figs 1.1A to 1.1L)

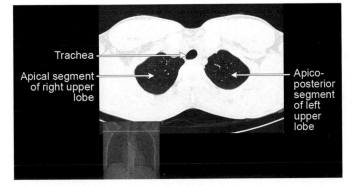

Fig. 1.1A

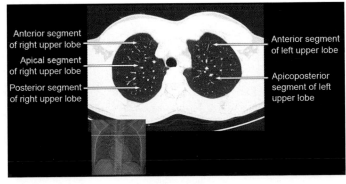

Fig. 1.1B

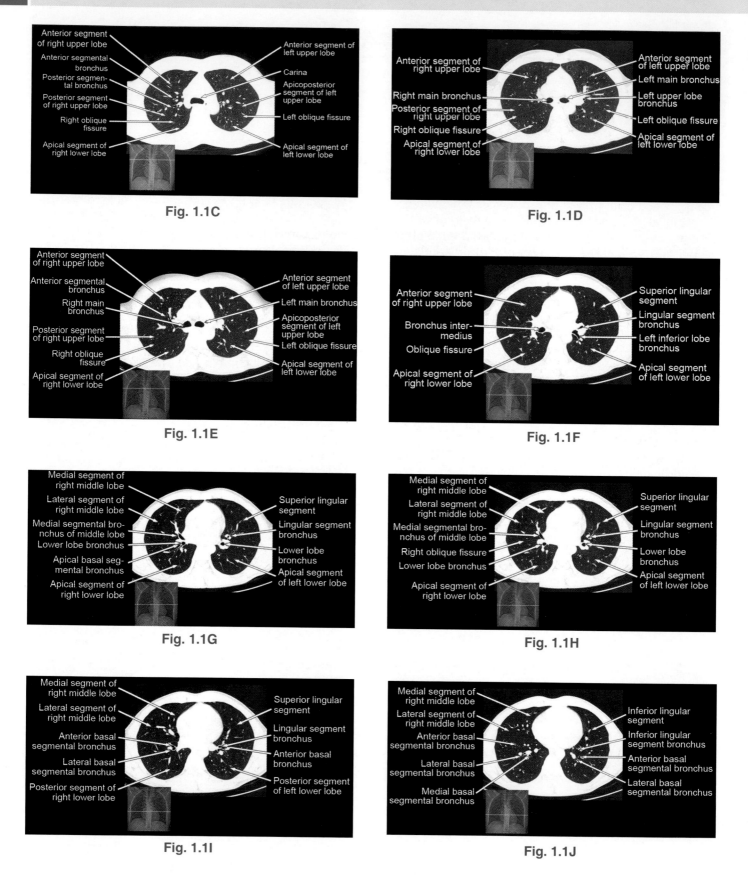

Fig. 1.1C

Fig. 1.1D

Fig. 1.1E

Fig. 1.1F

Fig. 1.1G

Fig. 1.1H

Fig. 1.1I

Fig. 1.1J

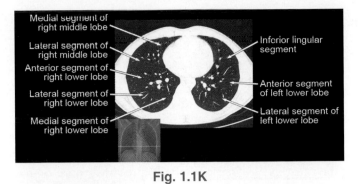

Fig. 1.1K

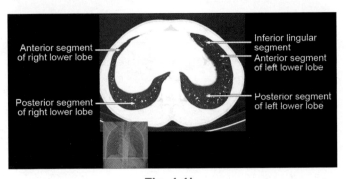

Fig. 1.1L

Figs 1.1A to L: Axial CT sections of chest

2. PULMONARY INFECTIONS

2.1 Consolidation Lung

Consolidation in anterior segment of left upper lobe and lingular segment. Scout image (Fig. 2.1A), Lung window images (Figs 2.1B and C) and mediastinal window (Fig. 2.1D).

Chest CT provides superior anatomic definition of the lungs and airways. Consolidation can be diagnosed on CT chest in a setting of negative or non-diagnostic chest radiographs. It provides more definitive diagnosis of consolidation which significantly alters patient's care.

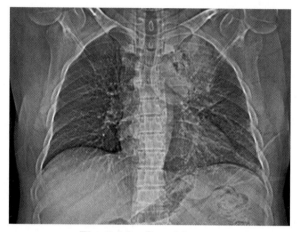

Fig. 2.1A: Scout image

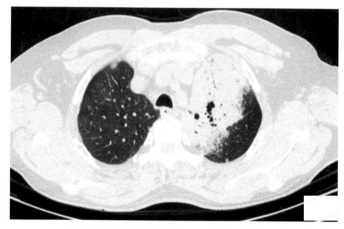

Fig. 2.1B: HRCT chest lung window

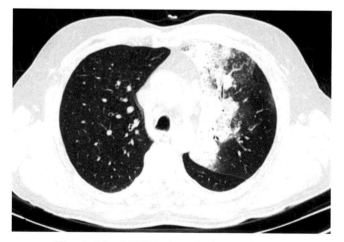

Fig. 2.1C: HRCT chest in lung window

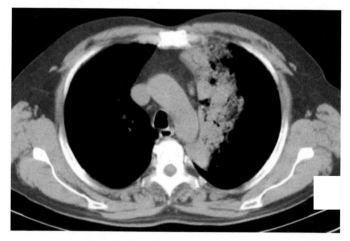

Fig. 2.1D: Mediastinal window

2.2 Consolidation with Pneumothorax

- Scout image show consolidation with pneumothorax (arrow) on right (Fig. 2.2A).
- HRCT Thorax Lung window shows a pneumothorax on right (Fig. 2.2B).
- Lung window shows consolidation with air bronchogram and pneumothorax on right (Fig. 2.2C).
- Mediastinal window shows only consolidation with air bronchogram and no pneumothorax is appreciated (Fig. 2.2D). Hence adequate optimal window settings for specific attenuation structures is important.

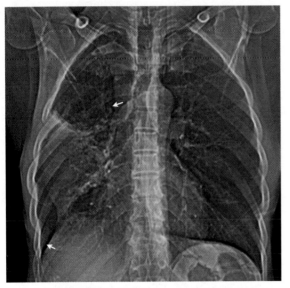

Fig. 2.2A: Scout image showing consolidation in right lower lobe

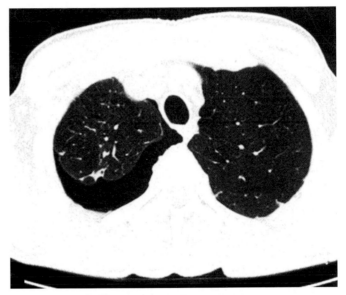

Fig. 2.2B: HRCT chest in lung window

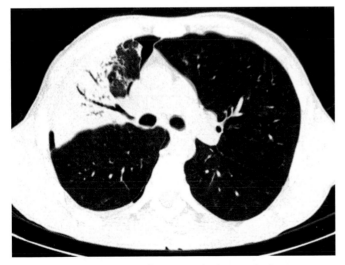

Fig. 2.2C: HRCT chest in lung window

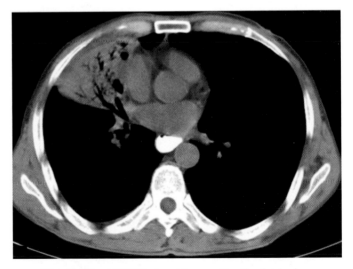

Fig. 2.2D: HRCT chest in mediastinal window

2.3 Consolidation with Synpneumonic Effusion

Right lung shows consolidation with synpneumonic effusion in a 60 years old female with productive cough (Figs 2.3A to D).

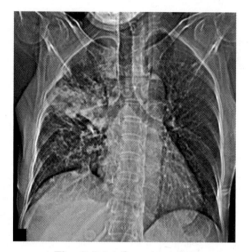

Fig. 2.3A: Scout image

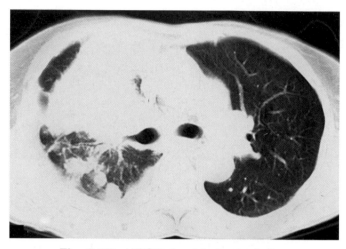

Fig. 2.3B: HRCT chest in lung window

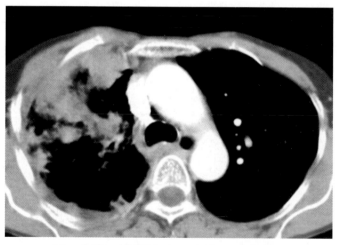

Fig. 2.3C: HRCT chest in lung window

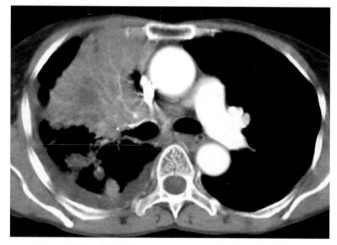

Fig. 2.3D: HRCT chest in mediastinal window

2.4 Pulmonary Koch's

12 years old female presented with history of high grade fever and chills, productive cough and hemoptysis for 7 days. Scout image (Fig. 2.4A), HRCT shows alveolar opacification (tree-in-bud pattern) in left upper lobe (Figs 2.4B and C). Consolidation and areas of breakdown in lingula (Fig. 2.4C). Consolidation in left lower lobe (Figs 2.4C and D) and mediastinal lymphadenopathy (Fig. 2.4E).

HRCT identifies the extent of pulmonary Koch's, especially subtle areas of consolidation, cavitation, bronchogenic and miliary spread.

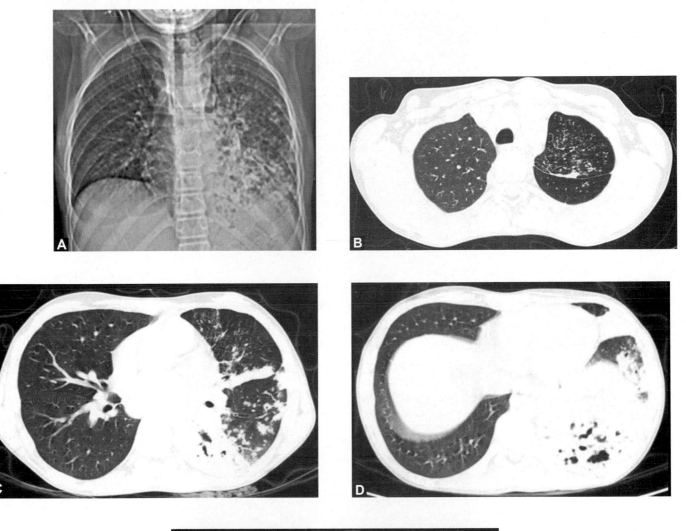

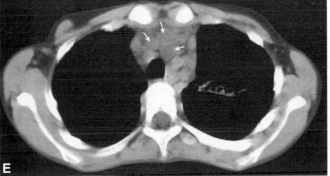

Figs 2.4A to E: CT images in pulmonary Koch's

2.5 Tuberculous Lung Cavity

Atypical location of tubercular cavity in a person who was receiving prolonged treatment with steroids for systemic lupus erythematosis.

- Plain radiograph shows a tubercular cavity in left lung having thick irregular wall (Fig. 2.5A).
- CT confirms the the plain film findings (Fig. 2.5B).

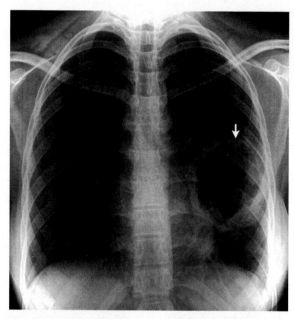

Fig. 2.5A: Pain radiograph shows tubercular cavity in left lung

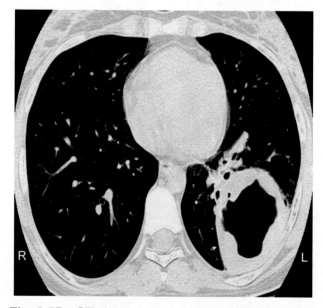

Fig. 2.5B: CT chest delineates the tubercular cavity

2.6 Sequelae to Pulmonary Koch's

60 years female had received treatment for pulmonary Koch's. Now she presented with breathlessness.

HRCT done to look for active disease shows bronchiectatic changes in both lungs along with areas of scarring leading to reduction in functional alveolar volume leading to breathlessness (Figs 2.6A to D).

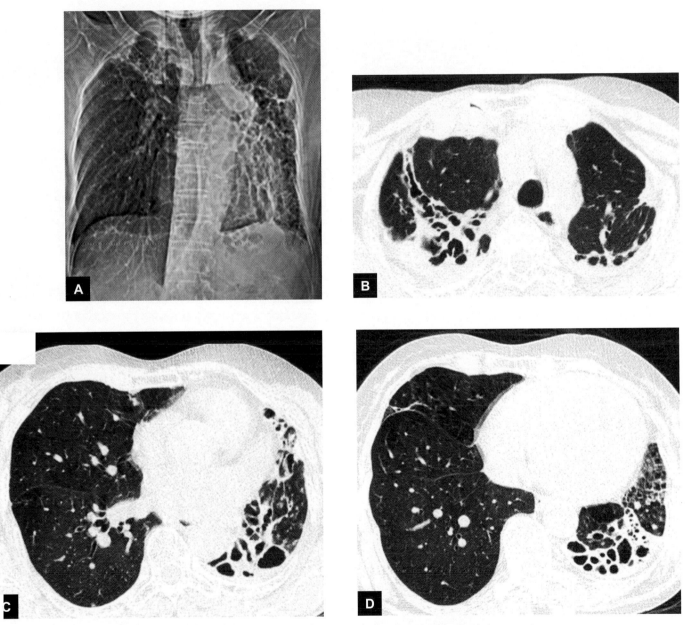

Figs 2.6A to D: HRCT shows bronchiectatic changes in both lungs along with areas of scarring as a sequelae to pulmonary Koch's

2.7 Tubercular Lung Cavity with Paravertebral Cold Abscess

- Scout image (Fig. 2.7A) shows a cavitary lesion in right lung and HRCT (Fig. 2.7B) show that the cavity is thick walled.
- HRCT thorax (mediastinal window) shows the thick walled cavity and the thoracic vertebral body destruction with adjacent paravertebral cold abscess (Fig. 2.7C).
- Post contrast image shows peripheral enhancement in the cold abscess (Fig. 2.7D).

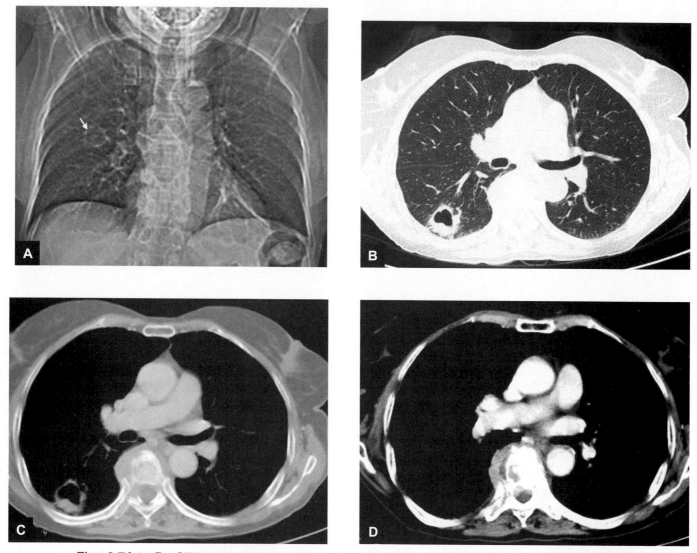

Figs 2.7A to D: CT images showing tubercular lung cavity with paravertebral cold abscess

2.8 Miliary Tuberculosis

- Scout image shows miliary shadows in both lungs (Fig. 2.8A).
- CT Thorax mediastinal window shows pericardial effusion (Fig. 2.8B).
- CT Chest lung window shows bilateral multiple miliary opacities (Figs 2.8C and D).

Miliary tuberculosis infection in the lung results from erosion of the infection into a pulmonary vein. Once the bacteria reach the left side of the heart and enter the systemic circulation, then seed the organs such as the liver and spleen. Alternately the bacteria may enter the lymph node(s), drain into a systemic vein and eventually reach the right side of the heart and seed to the lungs, causing miliary tuberculosis. Chest X-ray shows many tiny nodular lesions 1-5 mm in size distributed throughout the lung fields with the appearance similar to millet seeds, hence the term "miliary" tuberculosis.

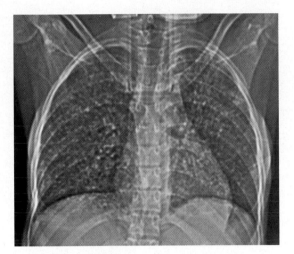

Fig. 2.8A: Scout image shows miliary tuberculosis

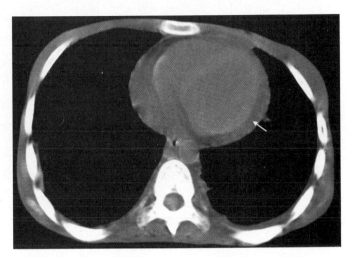

Fig. 2.8B: CT image shows pericardial effusion

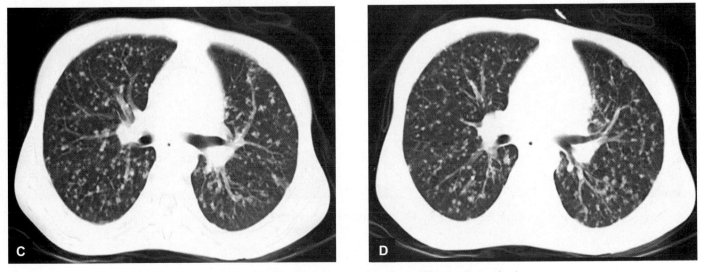

Figs 2.8C and D: CT images showing miliary tuberculosis

2.9 Fungal Ball

Fungal ball in right lower lobe lung cavity.

Radiograph of chest PA view demonstrates a well-defined cavity in right lower zone with fairly well-demarcated opacity seen in it (Fig. 2.9A). On lateral projection it is located in superior segment of right lower lung (Fig. 2.9B). On chest radiograph taken in Trendelenburg (head low) position, opacity within the cavity has moved superiorly. These are typical features of a fungal ball (Fig. 2.9C). CT chest showed a thick-walled cavity in the right lower lobe with a fungal ball inside the cavity (Fig. 2.9D). Fungal ball moved to the dependent position when CT chest was performed in prone position. This fungal ball was caused by *candida albicans* as confirmed by transbronchial biopsy (Fig. 2.9E).

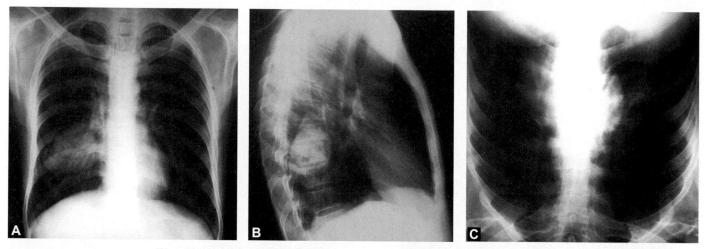

Figs 2.9A to C: Plain radiographs showing fungal ball in right lung

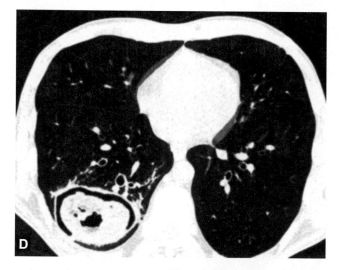
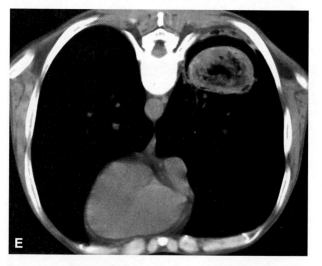

Figs 2.9D and E: CT images show fungal ball in right lung

2.10 Pneumocystis Carinii Pneumonia

- HRCT thorax shows bilateral parahilar and patchy areas of pneumonia presenting as ground glass opacity with pleural effusion (Figs 2.10A and B).

  This was due to *Pneumocystis carinii* as proved on bronchoalveolar lavage aspirate.

  This is commonly seen in immunocompromised patients. This patient was under treatment for leukemia and was admitted with respiratory distress.

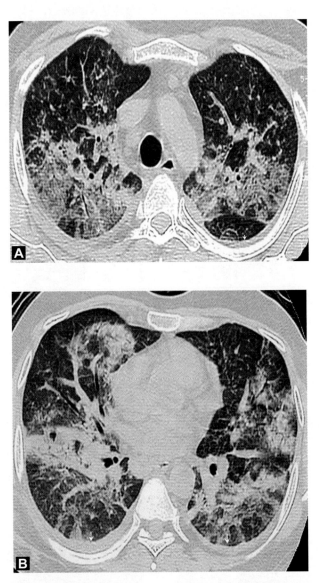

Figs 2.10A and B: CT chest in lung window shows bilateral patchy areas of consolidation

3. TUMORS OF THE LUNG

3.1 Solitary Pulmonary Nodule 1

Solitary pulmonary nodule (SPN) or coin lesion is a mass in the lung smaller than 3 cm in diameter (Fig. 3.1A). It can be an incidental finding and most commonly represents a benign tumor such as a granuloma or hamartoma, but in around 20% of cases it represents a malignancy, specially in smokers and individuals above 40 years of age.

To evaluate SPN one must compare with older X-rays, if available. This is important because doubling time of most malignant SPN's is 1 to 6 months and any nodule that grows more slowly or quickly is likely benign. CT scan is usually considered an essential follow up to the chest X-ray (Figs 3.1B to D).

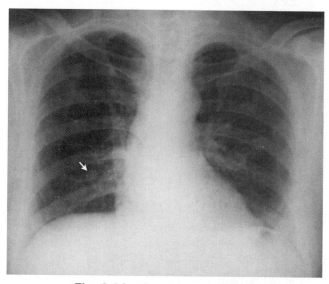

Fig. 3.1A: Scout image shows solitary pulmonary nodule

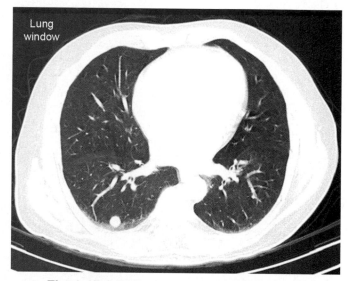

Fig. 3.1B: CT image in lung window shows solitary pulmonary nodule

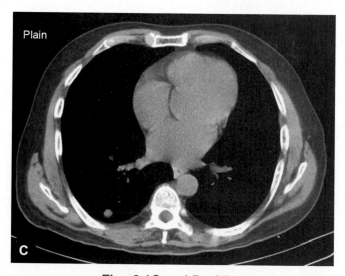

Figs 3.1C and D: CT image in mediastinal window shows solitary pulmonary nodule

3.2 Solitary Pulmonary Nodule 2

* CT thorax shows a heterogeneously enhancing solitary pulmonary nodule in left lung which was proved to be a carcinoma (Fig. 3.2).

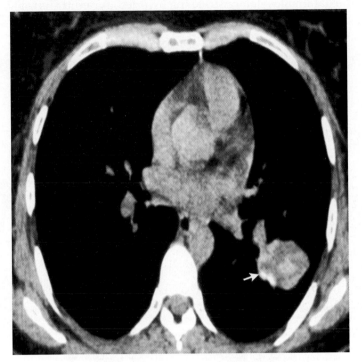

Fig. 3.2: CT chest shows solitary pulmonary nodule

3.3 Bronchogenic Carcinoma 1

Central bronchogenic carcinoma can cause collapse of distal lobe, resulting in the traditional Golden S sign, however a more appropriate nomenclature would be inverted pyramid sign as appreciated in this case.
- Scout image of chest shows right upper lobe collapse consolidation (Fig. 3.3A).
- Post contrast CT shows right upper lobe mass causing collapse consolidation of distal lobe (Fig. 3.3B).
- Coronal reconstructed and axial images demonstrate the inverted pyramid sign (Fig. 3.3C).

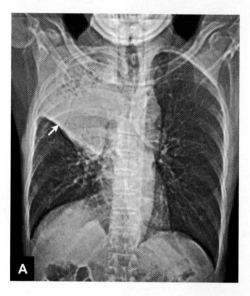
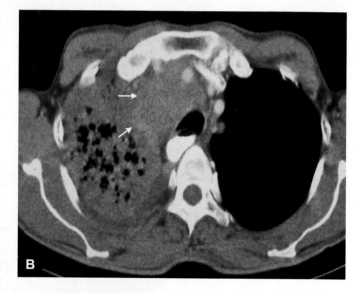

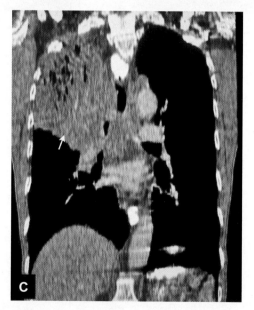

Figs 3.3A to C: CT chest shows the Golden S sign or the inverted pyramid sign

3.4 Bronchogenic Carcinoma 2

Right bronchogenic carcinoma with irregular borders (Fig. 3.4).

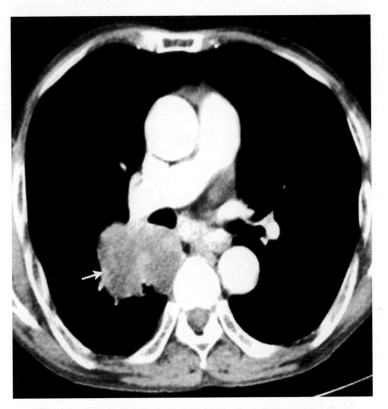

Fig. 3.4: CT chest shows a bronchogenic carcinoma

3.5 Thoracic Neuroblastoma

- Posterior mediastinal mass was diagnosed on incidental chest roentgenograms in a 6 weeks old female infant. CT chest at the level of main bronchi demonstrates posterior mediastinal mass 3 x 3 cm histologically confirmed as neuroblastoma seen lifting the left main bronchus. A small nodule is seen protruding into the left main bronchus (Fig. 3.5A).
- CT scan 3 months later, section at the same level shows marked spontaneous regression of lesion to 8 mm size (Fig. 3.5B).

Some neuroblastoma are known to undergo spontaneous regression or induced differentiation to benign ganglioneuroma.

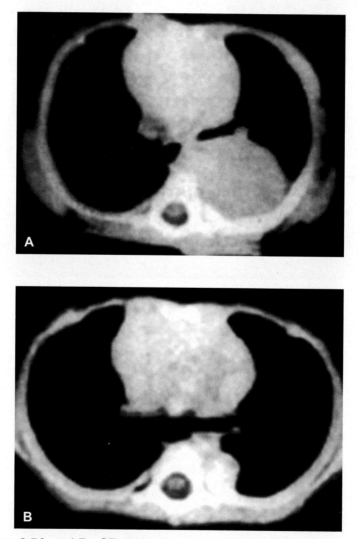

Figs 3.5A and B: CT chest shows a posterior mediastinal mass

3.6 Lymphoma Chest and Abdomen

- CT thorax shows heterogeneously enhancing soft tissues involving pleura, thoracic muscles with destruction of rib in a patient of lymphoma (Fig. 3.6A).
- CT abdomen shows abnormal soft tissues encasing the aorta and large vessels in the same case (Fig. 3.6B).

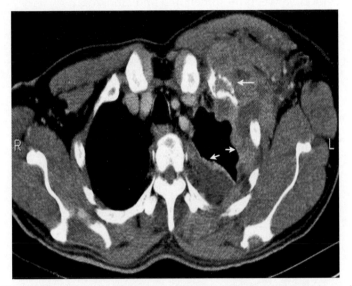

Fig. 3.6A: CT chest shows lymphoma affecting thoracic wall

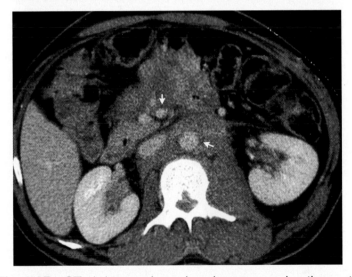

Fig. 3.6B: CT abdomen shows lymphoma encasing the aorta

3.7 Mesothelioma

- Contrast CT chest – mediastinum setting, shows heterogenous enhancement and nodular and thick appearance of pleura. This is diagnostic of pleural mass most commonly mesothelioma (Fig. 3.7A).
- Lung window image shows the pleural thickening and nodularity (Fig. 3.7B).

Mesothelioma is almost always caused by exposure to asbestos. In this disease, malignant cells develop in the mesothelium. There is no association between mesothelioma and smoking.

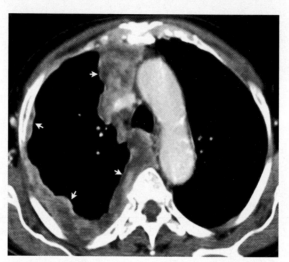

Fig. 3.7A: Contrast CT chest in mediastinum shows mesothelioma

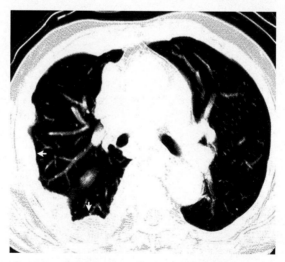

Fig. 3.7B: Contrast CT chest in lung window shows mesothelioma

3.8 Pleural and Pulmonary Metastases

Unknown primary carcinoma with pleural and pulmonary metastases
- Scout image shows left pleural thickening with effusion (Fig. 3.8A).
- CT images show irregular and thick left pleura with effusion (Figs 3.8B and C).
- Lung window images show multiple hyper dense lung metastases, few of which have speculated margins (Figs 3.8D to F).

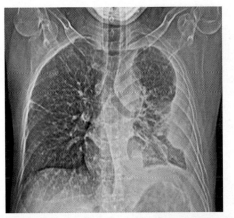

Fig. 3.8A: Scout image shows left pleural effusion

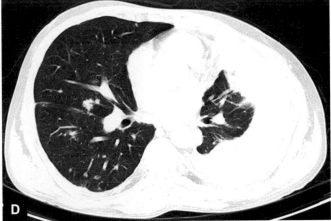

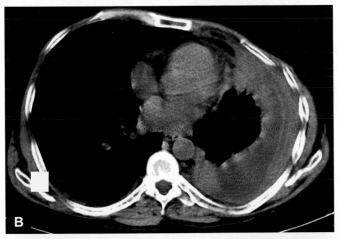

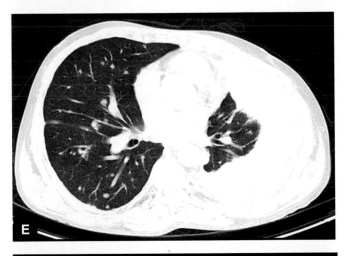

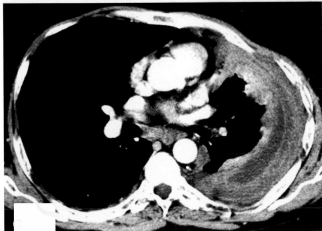

Figs 3.8B and C: CT image in mediastinal window shows pleural effusion and thickening

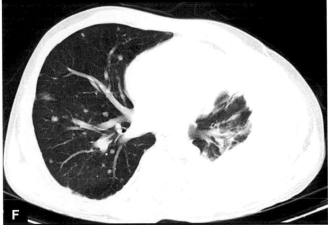

Figs 3.8D to F: CT images in lung window show pulmonary metastases

3.9 Pleural Malignancy

- Contrast CT chest shows thick irregular pleura with intense enhancement on right side and pleural effusion. It was diagnosed as pleural malignancy (Fig. 3.9).

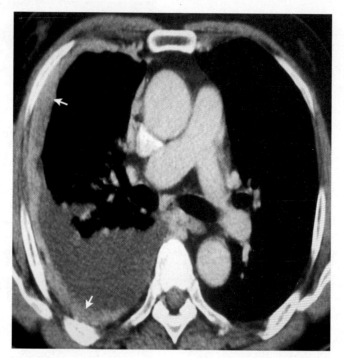

Fig. 3.9: Contrast CT chest shows pleural malignancy

4. THE PLEURA

4.1 Hydropneumothorax 1

- Scout image of CT thorax shows left loculated hydropneumothorax (Fig. 4.1A).
- CT chest of the same patient shows air-fluid level in left pleural space (Fig. 4.1B).
- Scout image shows right hydropneumothorax, drainage tube in pleural space and compression collapse of the right lung (Fig. 4.1C).
- CT chest shows air-fluid level in right pleural space. Section of drainage tube appears as a ring/circle in pleural space (Fig. 4.1D).
- CT chest shows hydropneumothorax, air-fluid level seen in right pleural space (Fig. 4.1E).

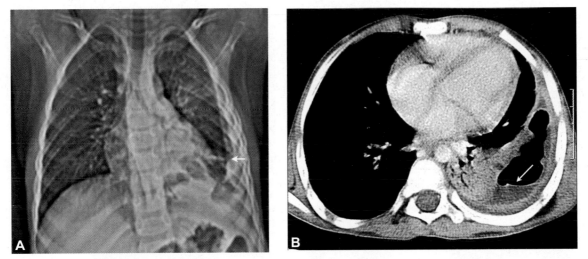

Figs 4.1A and B: CT thorax shows left loculated hydropneumothorax

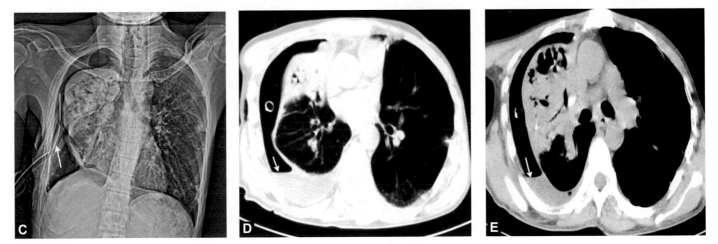

Figs 4.1C to E: Right hydropneumothorax

4.2 Hydropneumothorax 2

- Scanogram shows opaque right hemithorax with mediastinum shifted to the left. Oxygen hood, chest leads, central venous line and a drainage tube are seen *in situ* (Fig. 4.2A).
- CT image shows hydropneumothorax on right with air fluid level and drainage catheter *in situ*. Underlying collapse of the right lung is also depicted (Figs 4.2B to D).

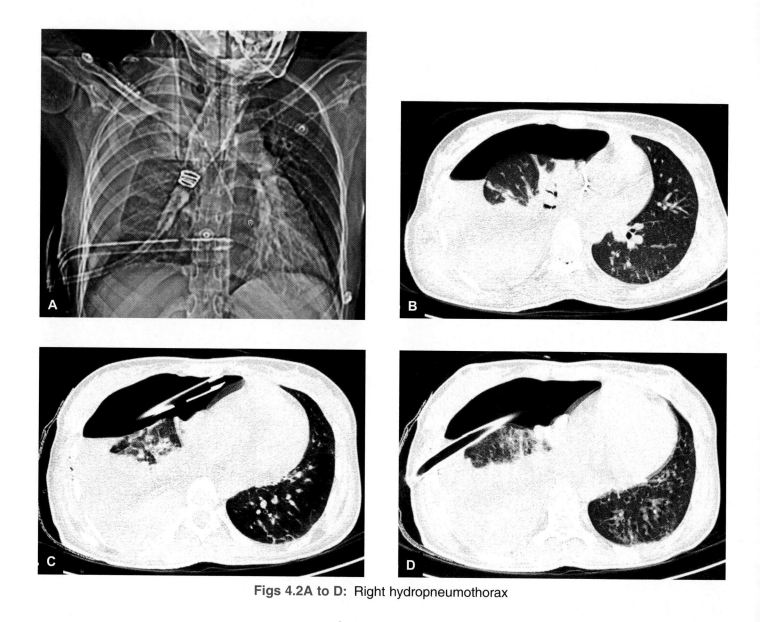

Figs 4.2A to D: Right hydropneumothorax

4.3 Pleural Calcification 1

Armor or sheet like bilateral pleural calcification (Figs 4.3A and B) with calcified pretracheal (Fig. 4.3C) and subcarinal (Fig. 4.3D) lymph nodes.

Pleural calcification is usually benign sequelae of pleural inflammation or asbestos exposure. It is suspected and diagnosed based on history and imaging studies.

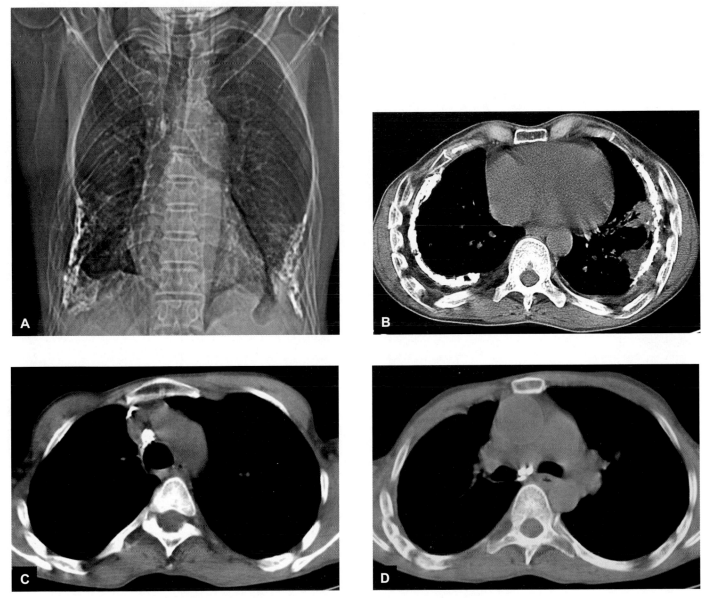

Figs 4.3A to D: CT chest shows bilateral pleural calcification

4.4 Pleural Calcification 2

Plain CT thorax shows thickened and calcified right pleura posteriorly (Fig. 4.4).

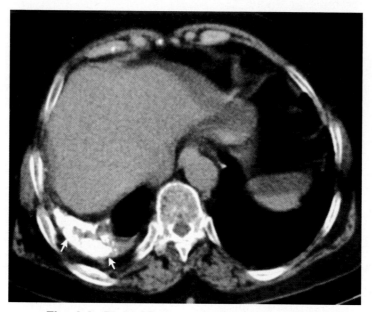

Fig. 4.4: Plain CT chest shows calcified pleura

5. TRAUMA

5.1 Pneumomediastinum

- Pneumomediastinum (vertical arrows) following tracheostomy (horizontal arrow) (Fig. 5.1A).
- Pneumomediastinum seen as air lucencies in mediastinum (Fig. 5.1B).

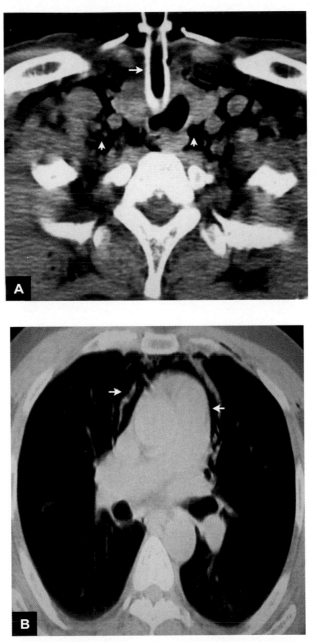

Figs 5.1A and B: CT chest shows pneumomediastinum

6. MISCELLANEOUS CHEST CONDITIONS

6.1 Bilateral Emphysematous Chest

X-ray and CT chest show bilateral emphysematous change (Figs 6.1A and B). In emphysematous chest there is increase beyond normal in the size of the air spaces distal to the terminal bronchioles, with dilatation and destruction of their walls which is depicted on imaging.

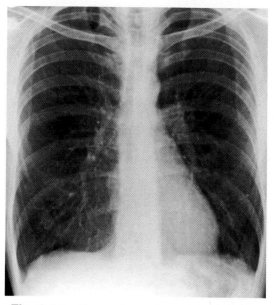

Fig. 6.1A: X-ray shows hyperlucent lungs

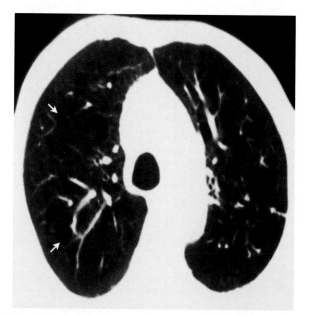

Fig. 6.1B: CT chest shows bilateral emphysematous changes

6.2 Eventration

- Shows elevated left hemidiaphragm (Fig. 6.2A).
- Axial CT Thorax shows stomach with oral contrast extending into chest (Fig. 6.2B).

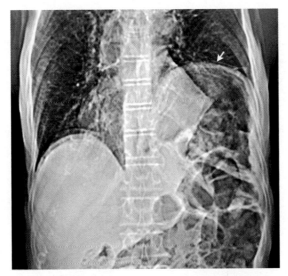

Fig. 6.2A: X-ray shows elevated left hemidiaphragm

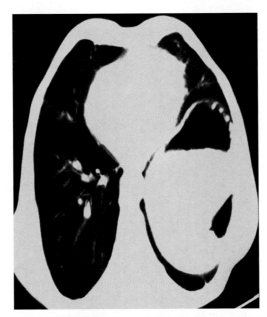

Fig. 6.2B: Axial CT chest shows infradiaphragmatic but thoracic position of stomach due to eventration

6.3 Giant Multiple Lung Bullae

Scout and HRCT chest images show giant multiple lung bullae in apices (Figs 6.3A to D).

   A giant bulla is a complication of emphysema. It is a large cavity of captured air. A giant bulla is a component of chronic obstructive pulmonary disease (COPD).

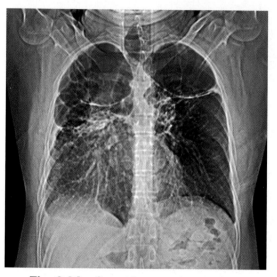

Fig. 6.3A: Scout image shows giant multiple lung bullae

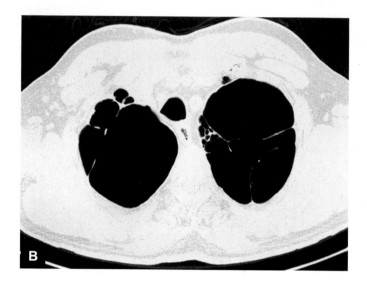

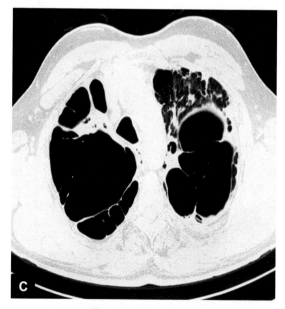

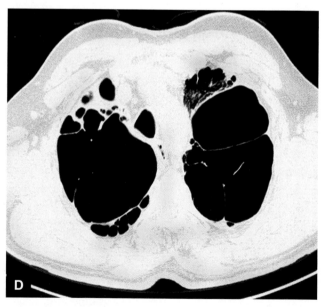

Figs 6.3B to D: HRCT chest images show giant multiple lung bullae

6.4 Bronchocele

- Chest topogram shows bronchocele seen as rounded parahilar opacity (Fig. 6.4A).
- CT chest shows bronchocele as sacccular dilatation radiating from the right hilum. A soft tissue mass is seen protruding into the right main bronchus (mediastinal window) (Fig. 6.4B).

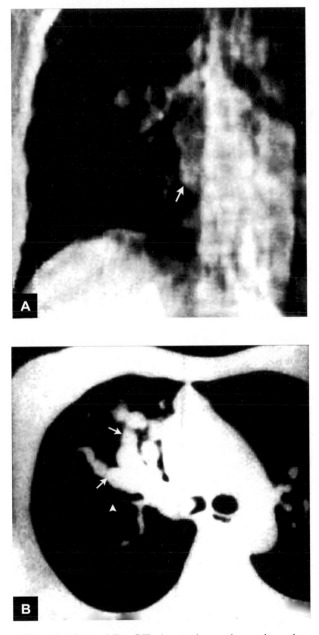

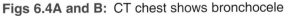

Figs 6.4A and B: CT chest shows bronchocele

6.5 Traction Bronchiectasis

HRCT Thorax shows traction bronchiectasis in both lungs (Figs 6.5A to D).

Traction bronchiectasis refers to bronchial dilation that occurs in patients with lung fibrosis or distorted lung architecture. Traction on the bronchial walls due to fibrous tissue results in irregular bronchial dilation (bronchiectasis). Usually segmental and subsegmental bronchi are involved, but small periperhal bronchi or bronchioles may also be affected. Commonly associated with honeycombing.

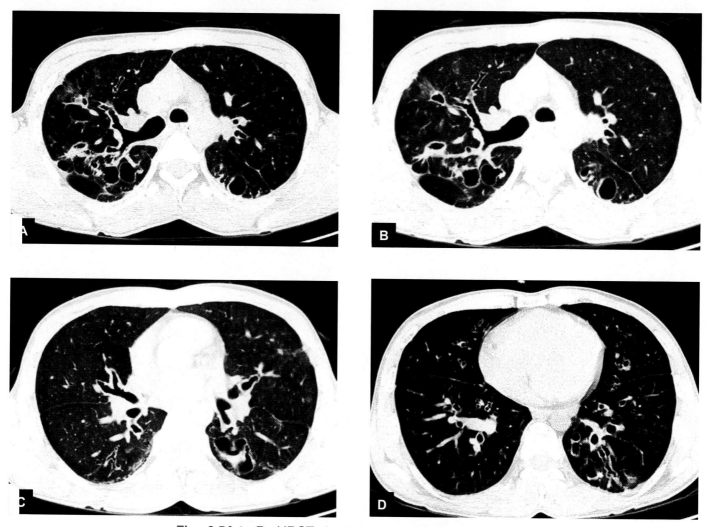

Figs 6.5A to D: HRCT chest shows traction bronchiectasis

6.6 Pre Tracheal Lymph Node

Pre tracheal lymph node 1 cm in diameter (Fig. 6.6).

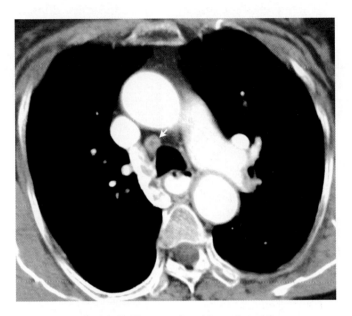

Fig. 6.6: Pre tracheal lymph node

6.7 Carcinoma Breast (Bilateral) with Metastases

Two large solid irregular marginated lesions seen in the left breast parenchyma infiltrating into the adjacent fat and pectoralis muscles with thickening of the skin. Multiple enlarged axillary nodes are present (Figs 6.7A to C). Right breast also shows two small nodular lesions (Fig. 6.7D) in the parenchyma infiltrating into the adjacent fat. Both sides nipples are retracted. Multiple nodular metastatic lesions are seen in lungs. Bilateral malignant pleural effusion is present. Sclerotic metastatic deposit is seen in the dorsal vertebral body(Figs 6.7E and F).

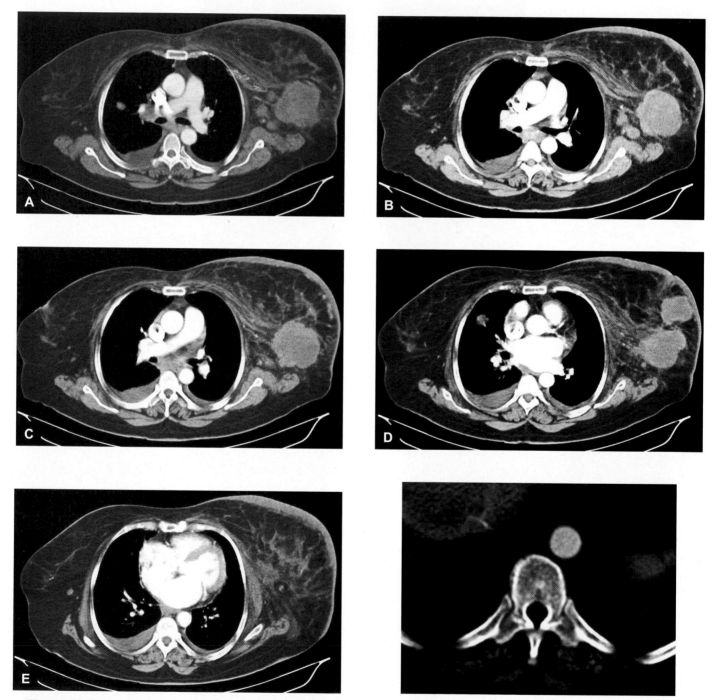

Figs 6.7A to E: CT chest shows nodular lesions in breasts and multiple enlarged axillary nodes

Fig. 6.7F: CT chest shows sclerotic metastatic vertebral body deposit

6.8 Idiopathic Interstitial Pulmonary Fibrosis 1

HRCT chest scout image (Fig. 6.8 A), mediastinal window images (Figs 6.8B and C), lung window images (Figs 6.8D and E).

There is reticulointerstitial prominence and subpleural areas of honeycombing in the posterior basal segments bilaterally suggestive of early phase of idiopathic interstitial pulmonary fibrosis (IIPF).

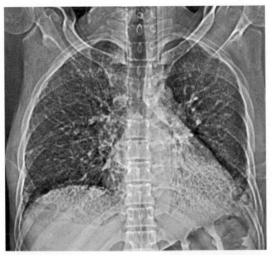

Fig. 6.8A: Scout image shows reticulointerstitial prominence

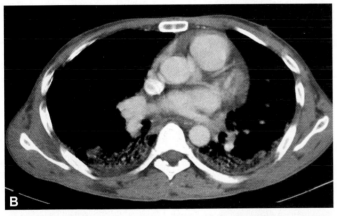
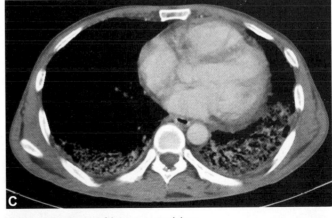

Figs 6.8B and C: CT images show subpleural areas of honeycombing

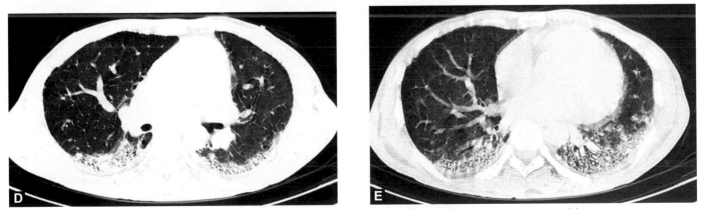

Figs 6.8D and E: Lung window images show subpleural areas of honeycombing

6.9 Idiopathic Interstitial Pulmonary Fibrosis 2

- HRCT chest scout image shows reticular prominence and cystic spaces. It is not possible to judge whether the cystic appearance is due to bronchiectasis or due to honeycombing (Fig. 6.9A).
- Show abundant areas of subpleural honeycombing. Interstitial thickening is also seen. These features are seen in IIPF. The patient presents with breathlessness and dry cough (Figs 6.9B and C).
- When patients of IIPF present with productive cough and increased breathlessness, superadded infection should be suspected as is seen here in form of alveolar opacities and increased ground glass opacification (Fig. 6.9D).

IIPF is a rare, chronic, progressive interstitial lung disease. It is a chronic fibrosing interstitial pneumonia characterized with abnormal and excessive deposition of fibrotic tissue in the pulmonary interstitium with minimal associated inflammation.

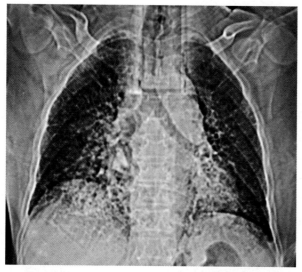

Fig. 6.9A: HRCT chest scout image shows reticular prominence and cystic spaces

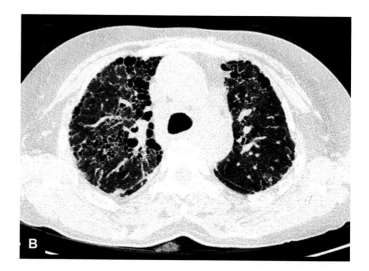

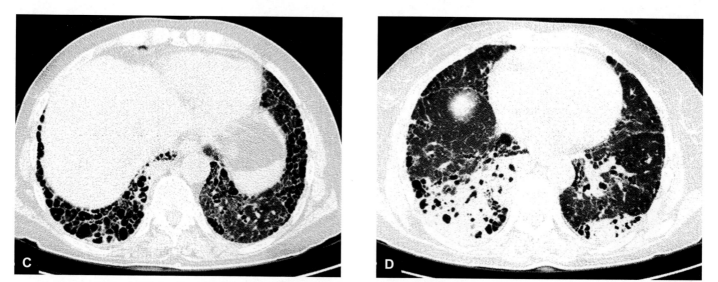

Figs 6.9B to D: HRCT chest shows subpleural honeycombing, interstitial thickening and ground glass opacification indicating superadded infection on IIPF

6.10 Idiopathic Interstitial Pulmonary Fibrosis 3

Subpleural honeycombing and septal thickening is seen (Figs 6.10A to D).

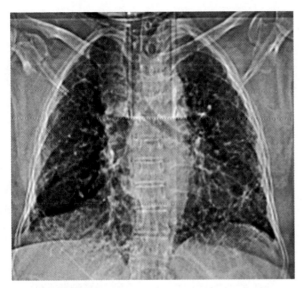

Fig. 6.10A: Scout image shows reticular prominence and cystic spaces

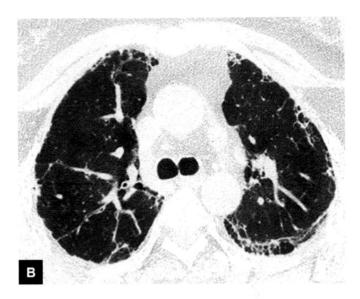

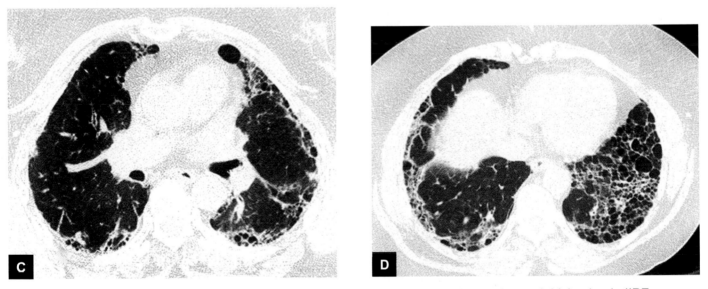

Figs 6.10B to D: HRCT chest images show subpleural honeycombing and septal thickening in IIPF

6.11 Pulmonary Embolism 1

- Soft tissue density filling defect with near complete occlusion of right pulmonary artery at its bifurcation extending into segmental branches (Fig. 6.11A to D).
- A wedge-shaped infarct is seen in the lateral segment right middle lobe (Fig. 6.11E).
- Lower lobe branch of left pulmonary artery also shows an embolus (Figs 6.11C and D).
  Patient had both lower limbs deep vein thrombosis, with left femoral vein thrombus extending into IVC.

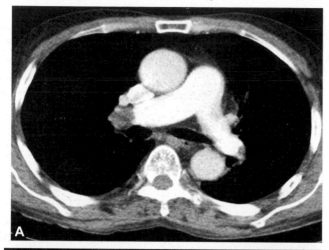

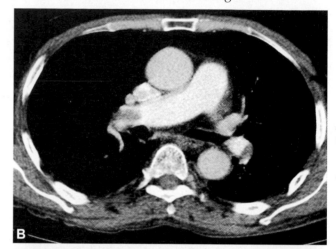

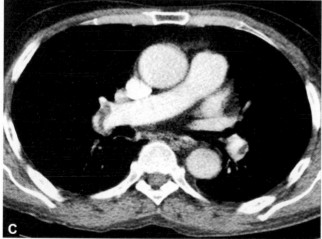

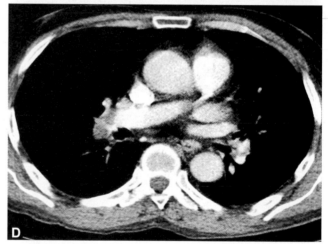

Figs 6.11A to D: Contrast CT shows embolus in right pulmonary artery and branch of left pulmonary artery

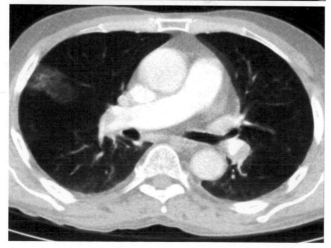

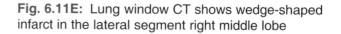

Fig. 6.11E: Lung window CT shows wedge-shaped infarct in the lateral segment right middle lobe

6.12 Pulmonary Embolism 2

- CT chest shows peripheral wedge-shaped patch of consolidation in right lung (Fig. 6.12A).
- CT pulmonary angiography image shows an embolus in right pulmonary artery as well as posterior branch of left pulmonary arteries (Fig. 6.12B).

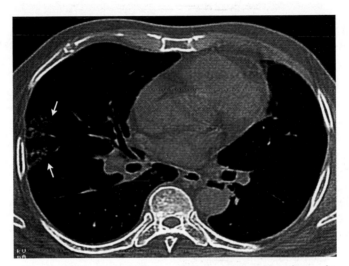

Fig. 6.12A: Lung window CT shows wedge-shaped consolidation in right lung

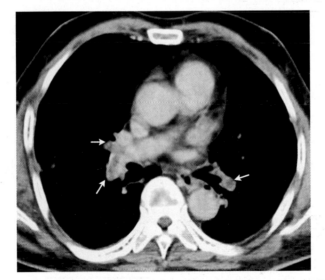

Fig. 6.12B: CT pulmonary angiography shows emboli in pulmonary artery branches

6.13 Pulmonary Embolism 3

Subpleural wedge-shaped consolidation right lung. Left pleural effusion is seen (Fig. 6.13A). Embolus is seen as a filling defect in right pulmonary artery supplying the consolidated portion of the lung (Figs 6.13B to D).

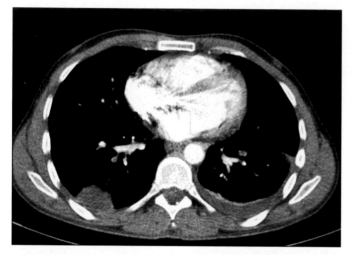

Fig. 6.13A: Lung window CT shows subpleural wedge-shaped consolidation right lung. Left pleural effusion is seen

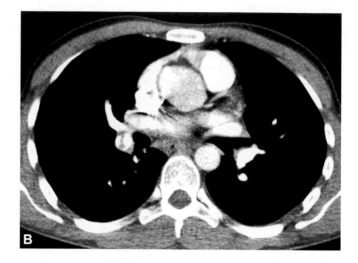

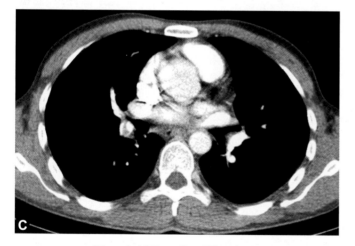

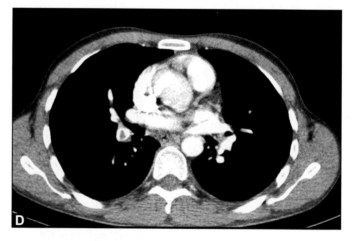

Figs 6.13B to D: CT pulmonary angiography shows an embolus in right pulmonary artery

6.14 Pulmonary Embolism 4

- Scout image (Fig. 6.14A).
- Pulmonary angiography image shows thrombosis in right and left main pulmonary artery branches (Fig. 6.14B).
- Pulmonary angiography image at same level as B, but with window settings adjusted to show distal atelectasis and consolidation secondary to embolus (Fig. 6.14C).
- Thrombosis is also seen in second order branches of right and left pulmonary arteries (Fig. 6.14D).

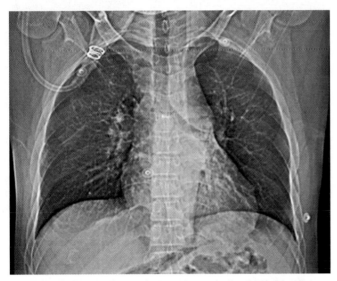

Fig. 6.14A: Scout image is apparently normal

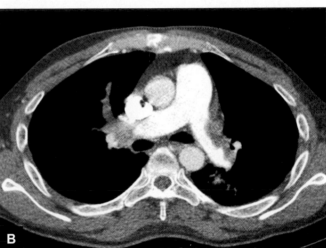

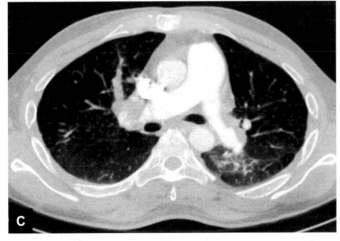

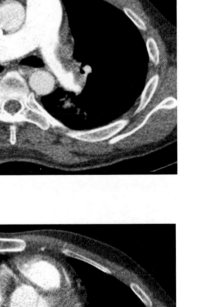

Figs 6.14B to D: CT pulmonary angiography shows emboli in both pulmonary artery branches

6.15 Pulmonary Embolism 5

CT Pulmonary angiography was done in a 70 years bed ridden patient who developed breathlessness suddenly.
- Nearly full lumen thrombosis is seen in the right as well as left main pulmonary arteries (arrow). Thrombosis is also seen in second order branches on right side (Figs 6.15A to C).
- Peripheral angiography done to find the cause of pulmonary embolism. It showed near full lumen thrombosis in left superficial femoral vein (arrow) seen as filling defect in the lumen. Only a peripheral rim of contrast is seen in the vessel lumen which was not completely blocked (Figs 6.15D and E).

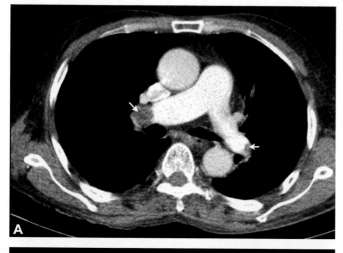

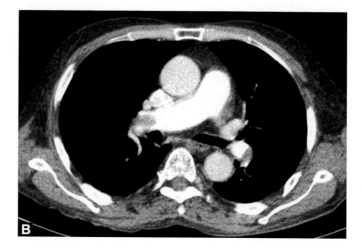

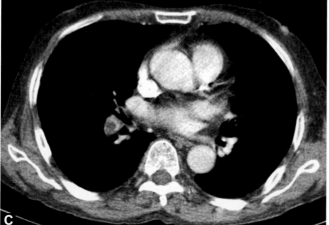

Figs 6.15A to C: CT pulmonary angiography shows emboli in both pulmonary artery branches

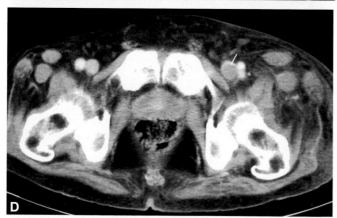

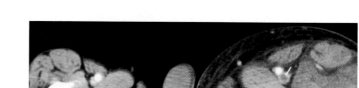

Figs 6.15D and E: CT lower limb venogram shows a thrombosis in left superficial femoral vein

6.16 Pneumoconiosis

Multiple small nodular dense opacities are seen in both lungs with bilateral effusion (Figs 6.16A and B) and hilar adenopathy (Fig. 6.16A) in a asbestos-cement factory worker (occupational lung disease).

In pneumoconiosis dust particles ingested by alveolar macrophages results in their breakdown with release of enzymes which produce fibrogenic response. It takes 10-20 years of exposure before appreciated on X-ray. Pneumoconiosis has a progressive course despite cessation to dust exposure. On imaging multiple diffuse small nodular rounded opacities 1-10 mm in size are seen, may have ground-glass appearance and may occasionally calcify. Lymph node enlargement is common.

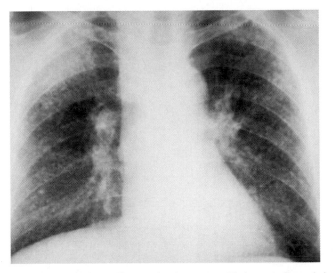

Fig. 6.16A: Plain radiograph shows multiple small nodular dense opacities in both lungs with hilar adenopathy

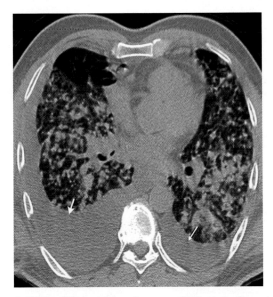

Fig. 6.16B: CT images show multiple small nodular dense opacities with bilateral pleural effusion

6.17 Pulmonary Arterial Hypertension

77 years male had breathlessness for 15 days. Plain X-ray chest showed enlarged cardiac silhouette and round upper paracardiac opacities. CT done to ascertain the nature of these opacities.

CT shows dilated pulmonary arteries which resulted in paracardiac opacities on X-ray chest as well as the scout image (Fig. 6.17A).

Main pulmonary artery (MPA) diameter measures 4.5 cm (Fig. 6.17B). Values for MPA greater than 3.37 cm is suggestive of pulmonary arterial hypertension, when viewed in an unenhanced axial 10 mm section on standard mediastinal window. Ratio of diameter of end-on segmental pulmonary artery and accompanying end-on bronchus (Figs 6.17E and F) is increased (>2). Normal ratio is 1:1. Segmental bronchi and pulmonary artery are arrowed in Figure 6.17F.

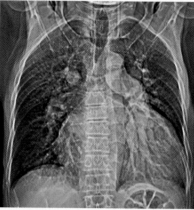

Fig. 6.17A: Scout image shows cardiomegaly and paracardiac opacities

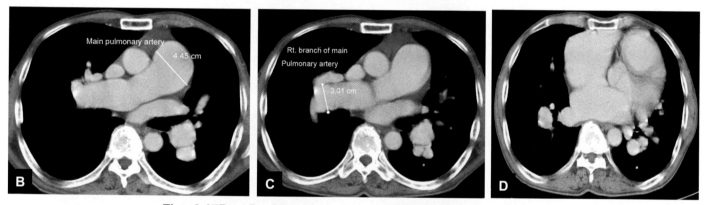

Figs 6.17B to D: CT shows markedly dilated pulmonary arteries

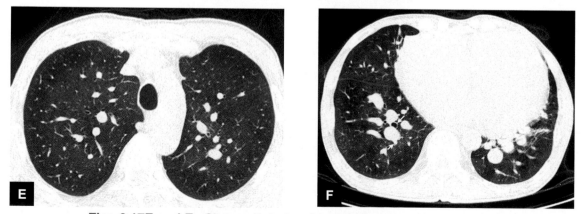

Figs 6.17E and F: Shows dilated end-on segmental pulmonary arteries

6.18 Jeune's Syndrome or Asphyxiating Thoracic Dystrophy

Jeune's syndrome is a rare genetic disorder, an autosomal recessive dysplasia also known as asphyxiating thoracic dystrophy. It is characterized by short limbs and a narrow rigid and abnormally small thoracic cage with reduced lung capacity. Ribs are short and have irregular and bulbous costochondral junctions. Chest diameter is significantly less (Figs 6.18A and B) as compared to abdominal diameter (Figs 6.18C and D) with reduced thoracic mobility and predominant abdominal breathing.

Jeune's syndrome often results in asphyxiation and associated kidney lesions may lead to renal failure. The most important area of medical care for an individual with Jeune's syndrome is preventing and treating respiratory infections.

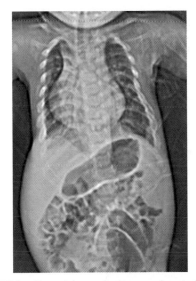

Fig. 6.18A: Scout image shows chest diameter significantly less than abdominal diameter

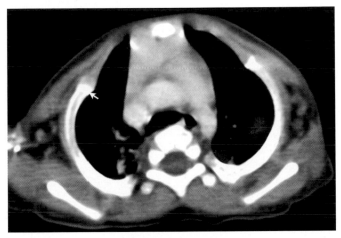

Fig. 6.18B: CT chest in Jeune's syndrome

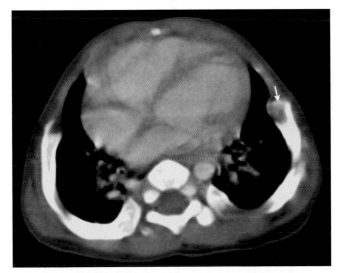

Fig. 6.18C: CT chest in Jeune's syndrome

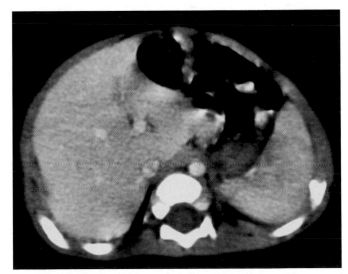

Fig. 6.18D: CT abdomen in Jeune's syndrome

Section 2

Cardiovascular System and Mediastinum

- Heart and Blood Vessels
- Mediastinum
- Thoracic Aorta
- Mediastinal Conditions

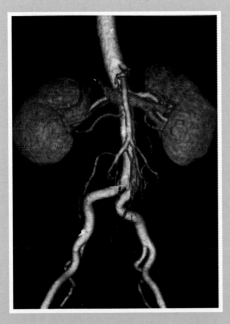
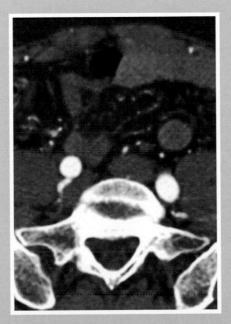
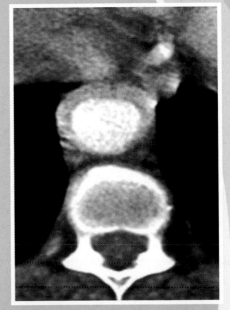

7. HEART AND BLOOD VESSELS

7.1 CT Coronary Angiography

Normal Anatomy

Heart imaging methods such as cardiac CT are allowing physicians to take a closer look at the heart and great vessels at little risk to the patient.

A traditional CT scan is an X-ray procedure which combines many X-ray images with the aid of a computer to generate cross-sectional views of the body. Cardiac CT uses advanced CT technology with or without intravenous iodine-based contrast to visualize cardiac anatomy, including the coronary arteries and great arteries and veins. With multi-detector scanning, it is possible to acquire high-resolution three-dimensional images of the heart and great vessels.

Cardiac CT is especially useful in evaluating the myocardium, coronary arteries, pulmonary veins, thoracic aorta, pericardium and cardiac masses such as thrombus of the left atrial appendage.

Coronary Arteries

The four main coronary arteries evaluated by CT are the right coronary artery (RCA), the left main coronary artery (LCA), the left anterior descending (LAD) artery and the left circumflex (LCx) artery (Figs 7.1A to I).

Whichever artery crosses the crux of the heart and gives off the posterior descending branches is considered to be the dominant coronary artery.

In approximately 85% of individuals, the RCA crosses the posterior interventricular groove and gives rise to the posterior descending branches (right dominance); in 7-8%, the LCx artery crosses the interventricular groove and gives rise to branches to the posterior right ventricular surface (left dominance); and in the remaining 7-8%, the inferior interventricular septum is perfused by branches from both the distal RCA and the distal LCx artery (co-dominance).

Right coronary artery: The RCA arises from the anterior right coronary sinus somewhat inferior to the origin of the LCA. The RCA passes to the right of and posterior to the pulmonary artery and then downward in the right atrioventricular groove toward the posterior interventricular septum.

In more than 50% of individuals, the first branch of the RCA is the conus artery, unless it (the RCA) has a separate origin directly from the right coronary sinus.

The second branches usually consist of the sinoatrial node/ nodal artery and several anterior branches that supply the free wall of the right ventricle.

The branch to the right ventricle at the junction of the middle and distal RCA is called the acute marginal branch.

The distal RCA divides into posterior descending artery (PDA) and posterior left ventricular branches (PLV) in a right dominant anatomy.

Left coronary artery: The LCA arises from the left posterior coronary sinus, is 5-10 mm long. The LCA passes to the left of and posterior to the pulmonary trunk and bifurcates into the LAD and LCx arteries. Occasionally, the LCA trifurcates into the LAD and LCx arteries and the ramus intermedius. The ramus intermedius has a course similar to that of the first diagonal branch of the LAD artery to the anterior left ventricle.

The LAD artery passes to the left of the pulmonary trunk and turns anteriorly to course in the anterior interventricular groove toward the apex. It provides the diagonal branches (D) to the anterior free wall of the left ventricle and the septal branches to the anterior interventricular septum.

The Left circumflex artery (LCx) courses in the left atrioventricular groove and gives off obtuse marginal branches (OM) to the lateral left ventricle.

In a left dominant or codominant anatomy, the LCx artery gives rise to the PDA or posterior left ventricular branches.

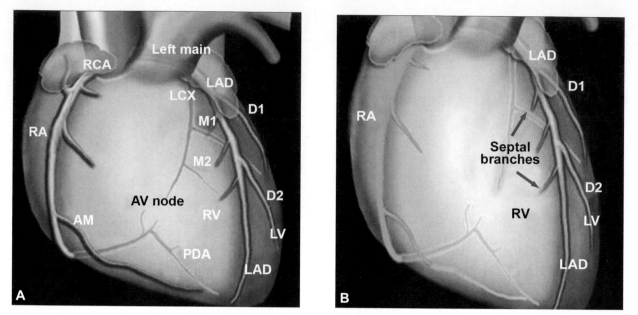

Figs 7.1A and B: Coronary arteries and their branches

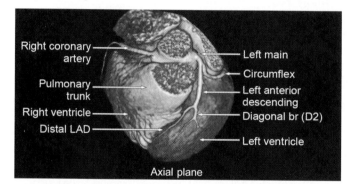

Fig. 7.1C: 3D Coronary CT in axial plane

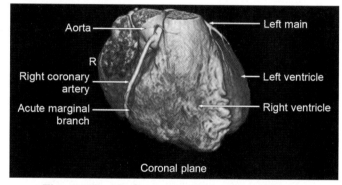

Fig. 7.1D: 3D Coronary CT in coronal plane

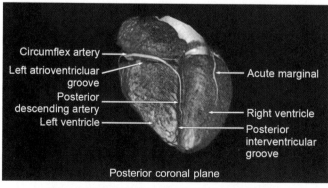

Fig. 7.1E: 3D Coronary CT in posterior coronal plane

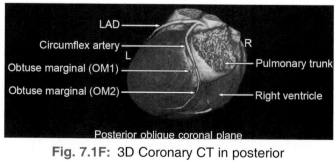

Fig. 7.1F: 3D Coronary CT in posterior oblique coronal plane

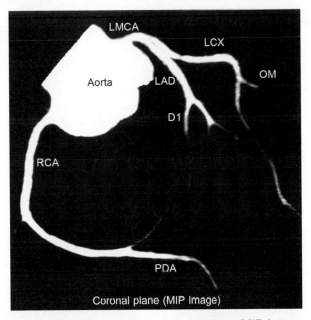

Fig. 7.1G: Coronary CT coronal plane MIP image

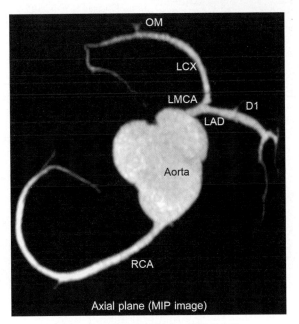

Fig. 7.1H: Coronary CT axial
plane MIP image

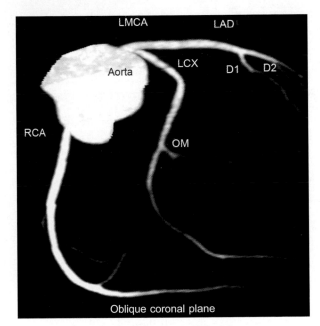

Fig. 7.1I: Coronary CT oblique
coronal plane MIP image

7.2 Normal Aortic Arch

Aortic Arch

- CT Aortic angiogram as seen from anterior aspect. In the most common branching pattern brachiocephalic trunk (BCT) is the first branch followed by left common carotid (CCA) and left subclavian artery (LSA) (Fig. 7.2A). Only 13% patients have a common origin as the first branch through which the brachiocephalic trunk and left CCA originate. Only 1-2% people have brachiocephalic trunks on both sides.
- CT Aortic angiogram as seen from left anterolateral aspect shows origin of brachiocephalic trunk, left CCA and left subclavian artery (Fig. 7.2B).

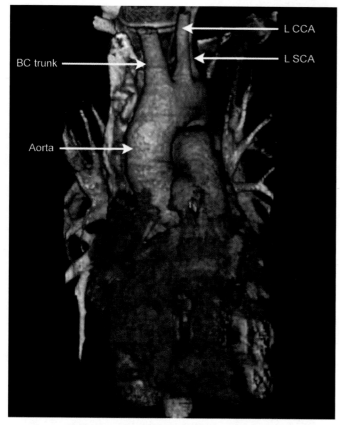

Fig. 7.2A: CT Aortic angiogram anterior aspect

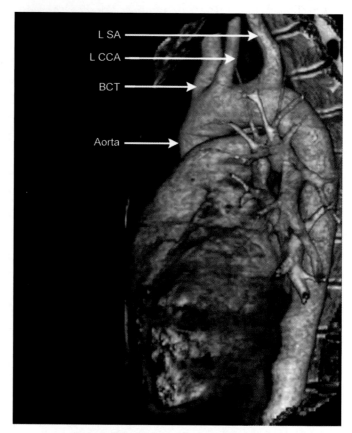

Fig. 7.2B: CT Aortic angiogram left anterolateral aspect

7.3 CT Arch Angiography (Fig. 7.3)

Branches of Aortic Arch

1. Brachiocephalic trunk
   i. Right subclavian artery
   ii. Right common carotid artery
   iii. Thyroidea ima artery
2. Left common carotid artery
   i. External carotid
   ii. Internal carotid
3. Left subclavian artery

Subclavian artery

On the *left*, the subclavian artery arises directly from the arch of aorta.

On the *right* the relatively short brachiocephalic artery (trunk) bifurcates into subclavian artery which gives out a branch, the vertebral artery and then the subclavian artery becomes the axillary artery at the lateral border of the first rib.

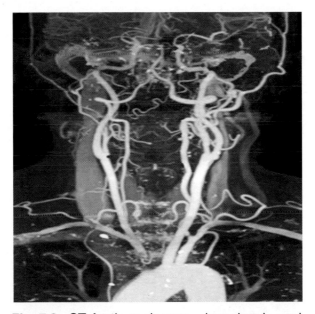

Fig. 7.3: CT Aortic angiogram – branches in neck

7.4 Normal CT Angiography Intracranial Vessels (Fig. 7.4)

Internal carotid artery and vertebrobasilar artery are the arteries that supply blood to the brain.

Branches from each portion of the internal carotid artery (C denotes the portion)

C1.   Branches from the cervical portion—none.

C2.   Branches from the petrous portion
   i.   Caroticotympanic arteries
   ii. Vidian artery

C3.   Branches from the lacerum portion—none

C4.   Branches from the cavernous portion
   i.   Branches of the meningohypophyseal trunk
   ii. Capsular branches—supplies wall of cavernous sinus
   iii. Branches of the inferolateral trunk.

C5.   Branches from the clinoid portion—none

C6.   Branches from the ophthalmic portion
   i.   Ophthalmic artery
   ii. Superior hypophyseal artery

C7.   Branches from the communicating portion
   i.   Posterior communicating artery
   ii. Anterior choroidal artery
   iii. Anterior cerebral artery
   iv. Middle cerebral artery

Basilar artery arises from the confluence of the two vertebral arteries and gives following branches.
   i.   Anterior inferior cerebellar arteries
   ii. Multiple pontine arteries
   iii. Posterior cerebral arteries
   iv. Superior cerebellar arteries

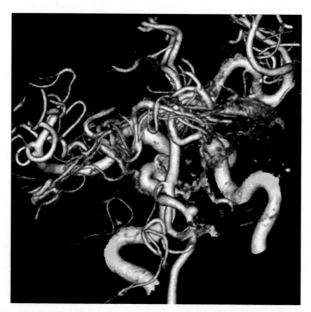

Fig. 7.4: Normal CT angiography intracranial vessels

7.5 Normal Abdominal Aorta

CT Angiography Abdominal Aorta (Figs 7.5A to D)

The branches of abdominal aorta (from above downwards) are divided into following groups (Figs 7.5E to G):

A. Anterior : Coeliac trunk (T12 Vertebral level)
Superior mesenteric trunk (L1 Vertebral level)
Inferior mesenteric (L3 Vertebral level)

B. Lateral : Inferior phrenic
Suprarenal
Renal
Gonadal
Spinal/Lumbar

C. Terminal : Right and left common iliacs
Median sacral
Aortic bifurcation into terminal branches occurs at L 4 vertebral level.

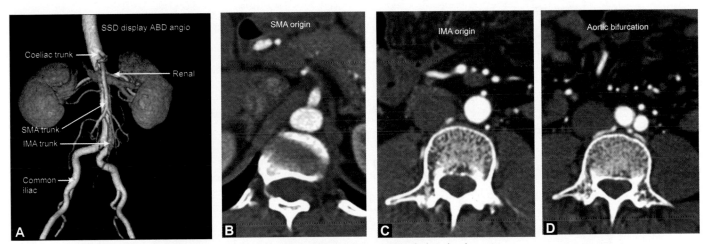

Figs 7.5A to D: CT angiography abdominal aorta

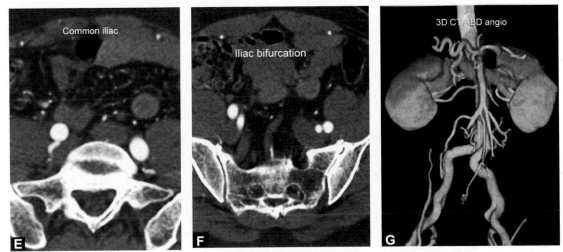

Figs 7.5E to G: CT angiography abdominal aorta with branches

7.6 Normal CT Angiography Abdominal Aorta (Figs 7.6A to J)

Abbreviations used in images :

- AA—Abdominal aorta
- CA—Coeliac artery
- Com.hep.a.—Common Hepatic artery
- SPL.a.—Splenic artery
- Rt.ren.a.—Right renal artery
- Lt.ren.a.—Left renal artery
- SMA—Superior mesenteric artery
- IMA—Inferior mesenteric artery
- Rt.com.iliac.a—Right common iliac artery
- Lt.com.iliac.a—Left common iliac artery

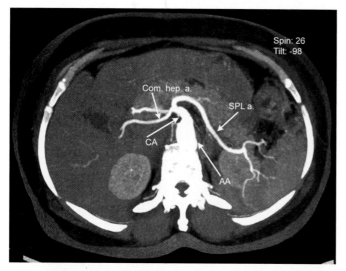

Fig. 7.6A: Axial CT angiogram showing coeliac artery

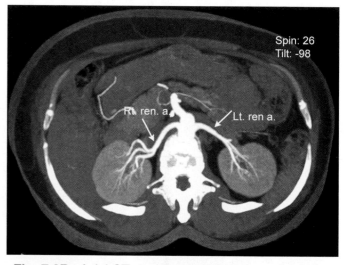

Fig. 7.6B: Axial CT angiogram showing renal arteries

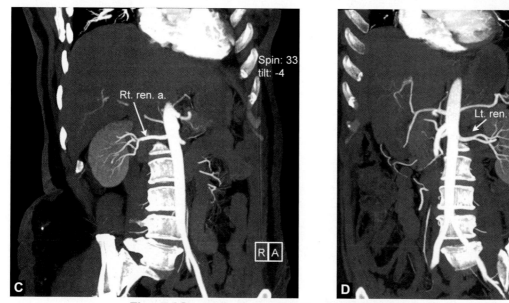

Figs 7.6C and D: Coronal CT angiogram showing renal arteries

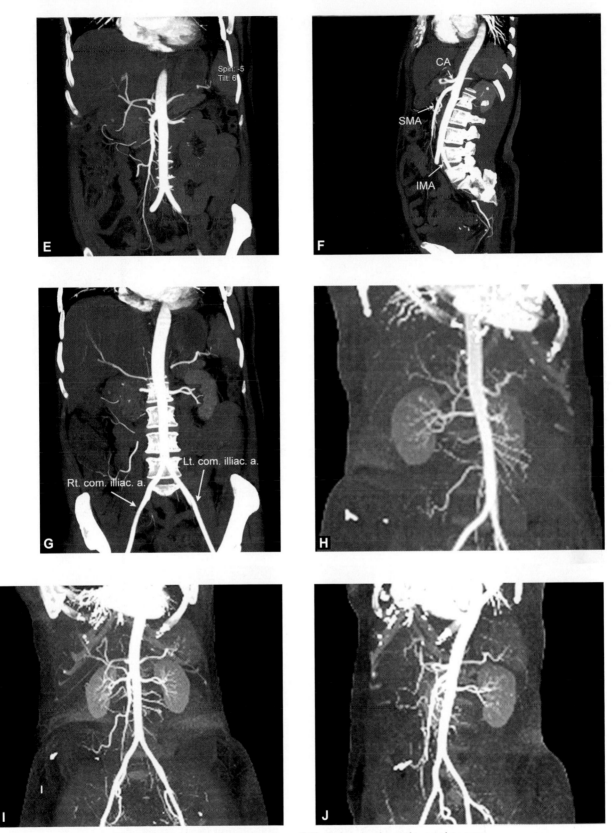

Figs 7.6E to J: Coronal recon CT abdominal aortic angiogram

7.7 Normal CT Angiography Lower Limb (Figs 7.7A to G)

Abbreviations used in images:

- Rt.prof.a—Right profunda femoris artery.
- Lt.prof.a—Left profunda femoris artery.
- Rt.SFA—Right superficial femoral artery.
- Lt.SFA—Left superficial femoral artery.
- Rt.pop.a—Right popliteal artery.
- Lt.pop.a—Left popliteal artery.
- Rt.ata—Right anterior tibial artery.
- Lt.ata—Left anterior tibial artery.
- Rt.per.a—Right peroneal artery.
- Lt.per.a—Left peroneal artery.
- Rt.PTA—Right posterior tibial artery.
- Lt.PTA—Left posterior tibial artery.

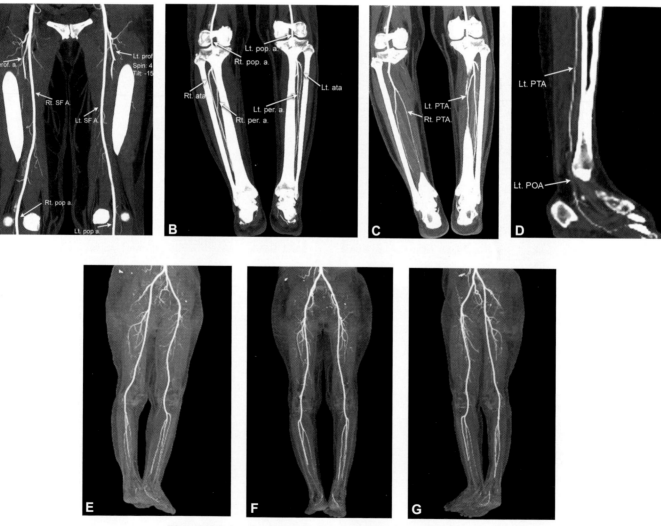

Figs 7.7A to G: Normal CT angiography lower limbs

8. MEDIASTINUM

8.1 Normal Anatomy (Figs 8.1A to I)

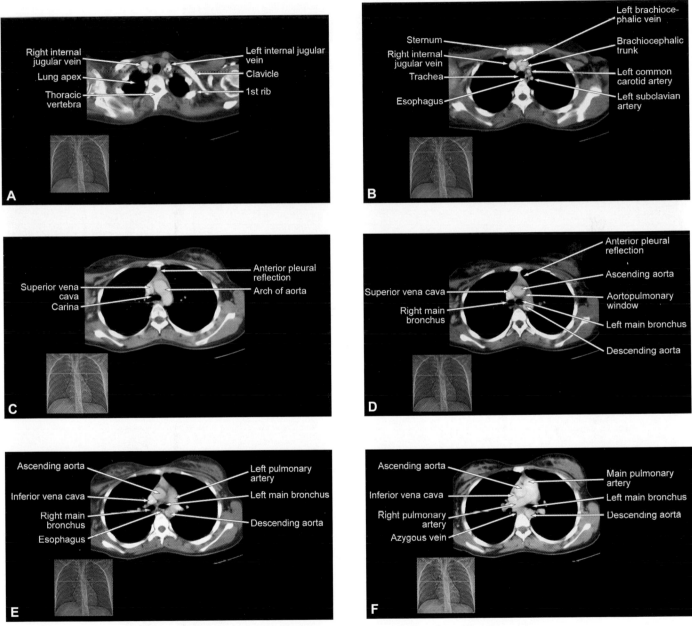

Figs 8.1A to F: Normal axial CT sections of mediastinum

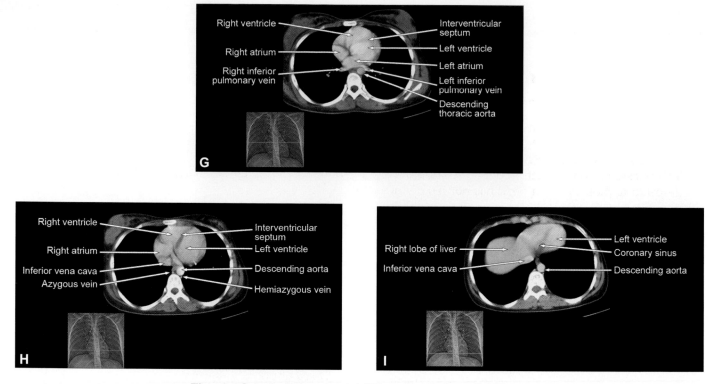

Figs 8.1G to I: Normal axial CT sections of mediastinum

9. THORACIC AORTA

9.1 Aortic Aneurysm

Case I : Aneurysm of Ascending Aorta

- Plain CT shows aneurysm of ascending aorta. Descending aorta has normal diameter (Fig. 9.1A).
- Contrast saggital reconstruction shows the extent of aneurysm of ascending aorta (AAA) up to the origin of brachiocephalic trunk (BCT) and left common carotid artery (CCA) (Fig. 9.1B).
- 3-Dimensional reconstruction demonstrating the aneurysm of ascending aorta (AAA) from posterior aspect. The descending thoracic aorta (DA) has normal diameter (Fig. 9.1C).

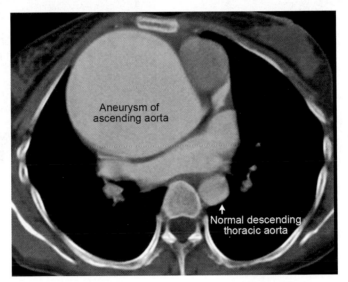

Fig. 9.1A: Axial CT shows aneurysm of ascending aorta

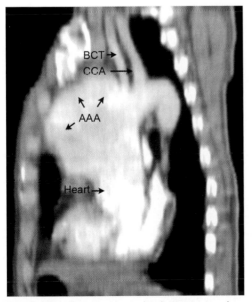

Fig. 9.1B: Contrast sagittal recon to show the extent of aneurysm

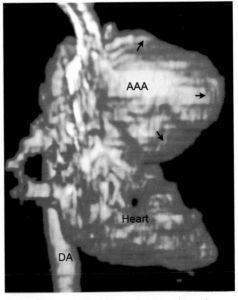

Fig. 9.1C: 3-Dimensional reconstruction demonstrating the aneurysm of ascending aorta from posterior aspect

Case II: Aneurysm of Descending Thoracic Aorta

- Plain CT scan shows aneurysm of descending thoracic aorta. Calcification is seen in the wall (Fig. 9.1D).
- Contrast CT of the same patient shows that the lumen of aneurysmal segment is entirely filled with contrast except at periphery, which has hypodense non-enhancing thrombus *in situ* (Fig. 9.1E)

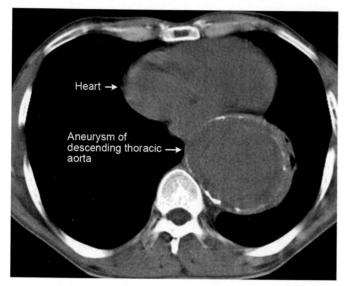

Fig. 9.1D: Plain CT scan shows aneurysm of descending thoracic aorta

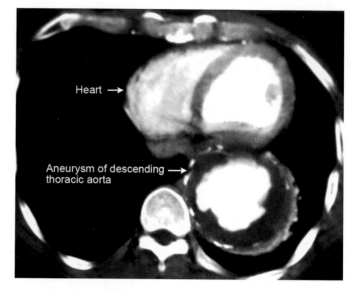

Fig. 9.1E: Contrast CT scan shows aneurysm with thrombus component of descending thoracic aorta

Aortic Aneurysm

Aneurysmal enlargement of aorta is generally defined as a permanent dilatation to at least 150% of normal size. True aneurysms comprise of all the layers of the aortic wall, while false aneurysms comprise just adventitia with surrounding fibrosis and organised hematoma. They may be a) *Saccular aneurysms*: These are localized aneurysms of aorta b) *Fusiform aneurysms*: These are diffuse dilatation of aorta.

CT signs of aneurysms of the aorta include:

a. Saccular or fusiform dilatation of a variable segment of aorta.
b. Calcification in the aortic wall.
c. Intraluminal thrombus.
d. Displacement of adjacent mediastinal structures.

The signs of impending perforation on CT are rapid increase in aortic diameter, high attenuation crescent in aortic thrombus and intramural hematoma.

Aneurysms with a wide mouth have lower risk of rupture. False aneurysms have a narrow mouth and a higher risk of rupture.

False aneurysms are treated surgically. True aneurysms are often managed medically.

9.2 Atherosclerosis Aorta

- Plain CT abdomen. No clear demarcation is seen between the wall and lumen of aorta (Fig. 9.2A).
- Contrast CT abdomen clearly demarcates the aortic wall thickening and patent lumen (Fig. 9.2B).

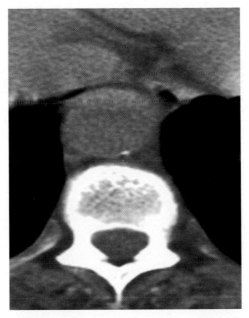

Fig. 9.2A: Contrast CT shows aorta but no information about wall thickening

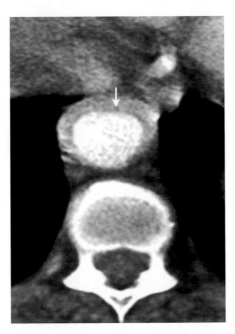

Fig. 9.2B: Contrast CT showing aortic wall thickening and patent lumen

9.3 Coarctation of Aorta

CT Aortic angiography in a case of post-ductal coarctation of aorta.
- Aortic arch shows reduction in diameter of descending aorta as compared to ascending-aorta (Fig. 9.3A).
- The diameter of ascending aorta (upright arrow) is maintained but that of descending aorta (down pointing arrow) has abruptly reduced (Figs 9.3B and C).
- Return of normal caliber of descending aorta (Fig. 9.3D).
- Sagittal and coronal reformatted image shows the actual site and extent of coarctation (Figs 9.3E and F).
- Color coded CT angiogram shows exact location of narrowing (Fig. 9.3G).

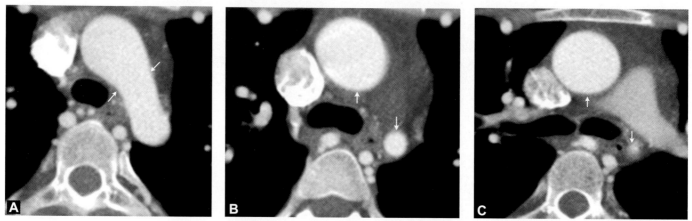

Figs 9.3A to C: CT Aortic angiography of post-ductal coarctation of aorta

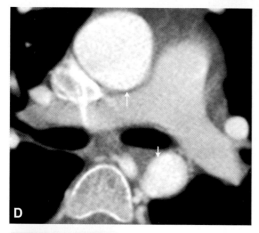

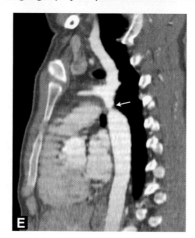

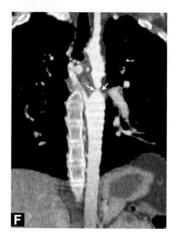

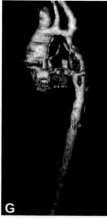

Figs 9.3D to G: CT Aortic angiography showing post-ductal coarctation of aorta

9.4 Redundant and Tortuous Aorta

Scout CT image of chest shows prominent descending aorta raising a suspicion of aneurysm (Fig. 9.4A). Aortic reconstruction following contrast CT abdomen shows no aneurysm but only tortuous dilatation of thoracic aorta (Fig. 9.4B).

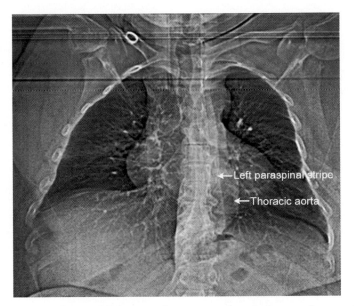

Fig. 9.4A: Scout CT image shows prominent descending aorta

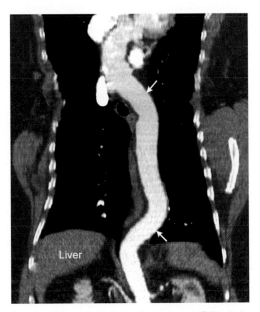

Fig. 9.4B: Aortic reconstruction of contrast CT abdomen shows tortuous dilatation of thoracic aorta

9.5 Sternal Sutures (Figs 9.5A to C)

Polydioxanone suture (PDS) in sternal closure protect against development of aseptic sternal complications like sternal dehiscence and wound instability.

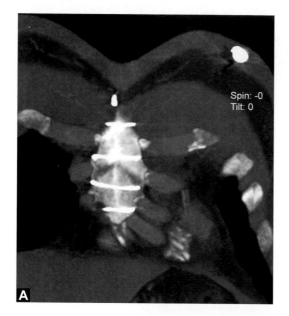

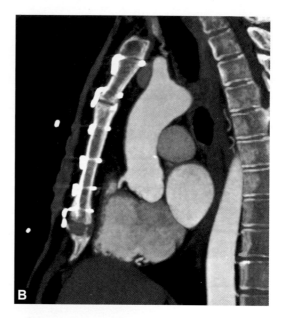

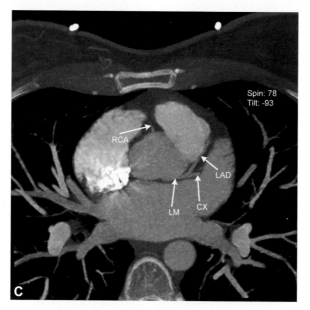

Figs 9.5A to C: Sternal sutures

10. MEDIASTINAL CONDITIONS

10.1 Hodgkin's Lymphoma

Contrast CT in a proven case of Hodgkin's lymphoma (Figs 10.1A and B).
Intrathoracic group of nodes are involved in patients with lymphoma, the most common are a) Prevascular and paratracheal group b) Hilar group c) Subcarinal nodes.

Lymph node enlargement is more common in Hodgkin's than in non-Hodgkin's lymphoma. Any intrathoracic lymph nodal group may be involved, but the anterior mediastinal and middle mediastinal nodes (paratracheal groups) of nodes are most frequently involved. In most cases the involvement is bilateral and asymmetrical. The posterior mediastinal nodes are infrequently involved.

On CT, individual mediastinal lymph nodes are easily identified as discrete, round or oval soft tissue attenuation structures within the mediastinal fat.

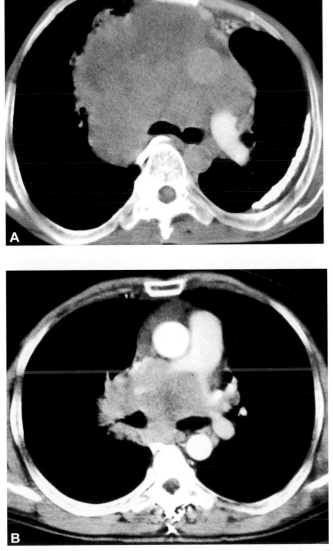

Figs 10.1A and B: Contrast CT in case of Hodgkin's lymphoma

10.2 Non-Hodgkin's Lymphoma

Figures 10.2A, B and C show anterior mediastinal lymph nodal mass encasing the major vessels of the mediastinum in a case of non-Hodgkin's lymphoma.

In Hodgkin's disease the anterior mediastinal and paratracheal group of lymph nodes are involved. In non-Hodgkin's lymphoma involvement of other lymph nodal groups like posterior lymph nodal groups and hilar lymph nodes is more common.

Non-Hodgkin's disease affects single lymph node group more commonly and presents as a focal mass, unlike the diffuse multi-nodular mass seen frequently in Hodgkin's disease.

Tracheal and carinal compression is more common in patients with non-Hodgkin's lymphoma due to close proximity of enlarged mediastinal nodes with these vital mediastinal structures.

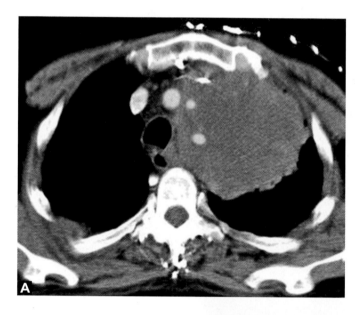
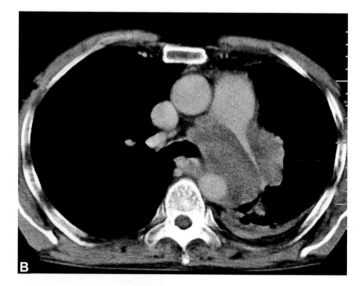
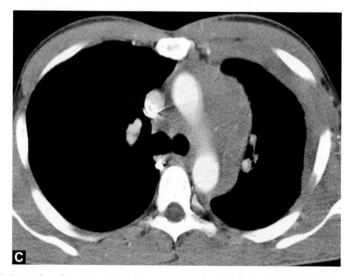

Figs 10.2A to C: Contrast CT shows anterior mediastinal lymph nodal mass encasing the major vessels of the mediastinum

10.3 Hydatid Cyst

- Hydatid cyst in anterior mediastinum with daughter cysts having calcified walls (Fig. 10.3A).
- Hydatid cyst in right lower lobe with daughter cysts (Fig. 10.3B).

Hydatid cyst is caused by the parasite echinococcus granulosus. Though commonly found in liver, the lung and mediastinum are also involved. Calcification may be seen.

Other features which aid in diagnosis are
a. *Meniscus sign*: Radiolucent crescent in the uppermost part of the cyst.
b. *Air-fluid level*: Rupture of cyst walls with air entering in the endocyst.
c. *Water-lily sign*: Completely collapsed cyst membrane floating on the cyst fluid.
d. *Combo sign*: Air-fluid level in the endocyst with air between the pericyst and endocyst with an "onion-peel" appearance.

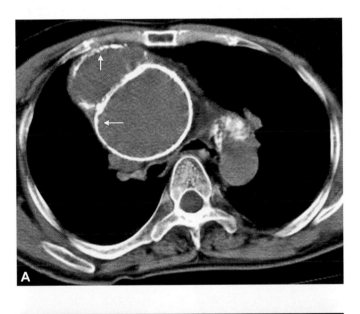

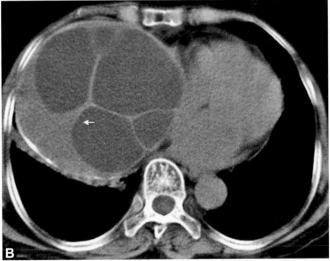

Figs 10.3A and B: Hydatid cyst with daughter cysts

10.4 Nerve Sheath Tumor

- CT scan shows a peripheral nerve sheath tumor—Neurofibroma (Fig. 10.4A).
- CT scan shows a posterior mediastinal mass, proved as schwannoma on FNAC (Fig. 10.4B).

Nerve sheath tumors are the commonest posterior mediastinal masses and neuroblastomas are the most common amongst them. They are classified according to their origin:

a. Peripheral nerves (neurofibroma, schwannoma and their malignant counterparts).
b. Sympathetic ganglia (ganglioneuroma, ganglioneuroblastoma, neuroblastoma).
c. Paraganglia (chemodectoma, pheochromocytoma).

On CT, the attenuation depends on their histologic characteristics. They frequently have low attenuation secondary to cystic degeneration, xanthomatous features or confluent areas of hypocellularity or myxoid stroma. They show soft tissue attenuation value on plain CT with central areas of cystic degeneration or fat within.
Neurofibromas have low attenuation on CT scans and enhance heterogeneously on postcontrast scans. Schwannomas have attenuation similar to that of muscles on CT scans and enhance mildly with contrast. Approximately, 10% of nerve sheath tumors grow through the intervertebral foramen into the spinal canal producing a "dumbbell" configuration.

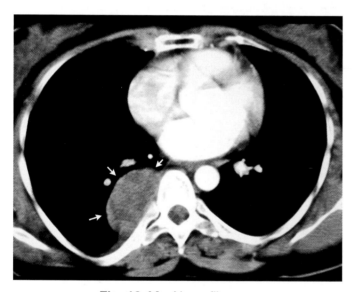

Fig. 10.4A: Neurofibroma

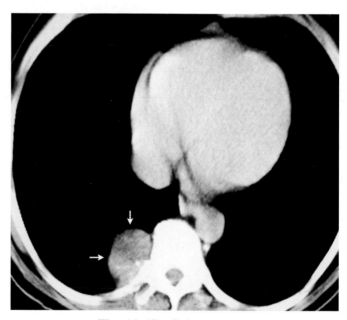

Fig. 10.4B: Schwannoma

10.5 Pericardial Cyst

Pericardial cyst is a fluid-filled cyst of the parietal pericardium consisting of a single layer of mesothelial cells generally asymptomatic and is an incidental finding (Fig. 10.5). On imaging it is sharply marginated, round or oval measuring from 3 to 8 cm in size. On CT, the attenuation value is 20-30 HU.

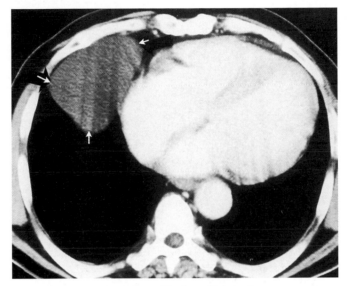

Fig. 10.5: Pericardial cyst

10.6 Teratoma

CT shows a rounded, mixed attenuation enhancing mass lesion measuring 12 x 10 cm in anterior mediastinum. This mass has few fat components having attenuation value (–)80 to (–)110 HU, calcific foci of attenuation value 150 to 190 HU and soft tissue component with attenuation value of 30 to 45 HU. Confirmed as mature teratoma on histopathology (Fig. 10.6).

Teratomas comprise of ectodermal, mesodermal and endodermal components.

Germ cell tumors/teratomas arise from primordial germ cells that undergo aberrant midline migration during embryologic development. They are divided into seminomatous and nonseminomatous tumors and both these groups have benign and malignant varieties.

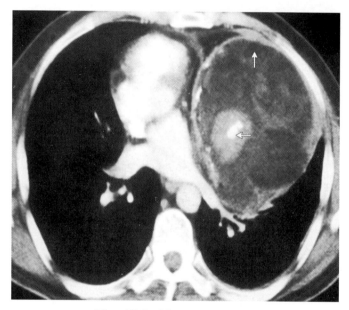

Fig. 10.6: Mature teratoma

10.7 Thymoma

• Contrast CT images of two different patients with invasive thymoma (Figs 10.7A and B).

Thymoma is a lymphoepithelial neoplasm. 15-30% are malignant. Approximately 35% of patients with thymomas have myasthenia gravis and approximately 15% of myasthenia gravis patients have thymoma. They usually arise in the upper anterior mediastinum, but may project into the adjacent middle mediastinum.

CT Scan shows a homogenous density with uniform enhancement, may occasionally be cystic. Invasion of the adjacent pleura may be identified with malignant thymomas. Calcifications can occasionally be seen.

Benign thymomas are smooth or have lobulated border and show homogenous enhancement with areas of decreased attenuation caused by cysts, necrosis or fibrosis.

Calcifications can be seen in both benign and malignant varieties.

Thymic hyperplasia usually enlarges the gland but maintains its normal pyramidal shape.

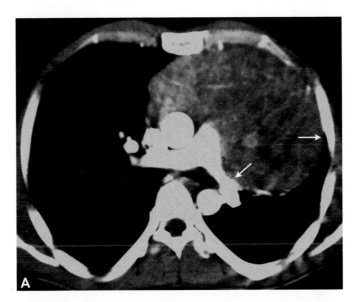

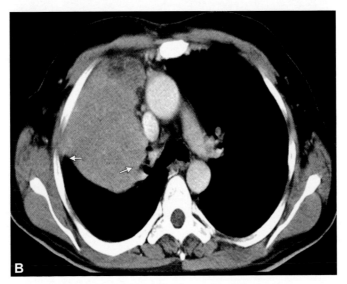

Figs 10.7A and B: Invasive thymoma

10.8 CT Guided FNAC

- FNAC from an anterior mediastinal mass (Fig. 10.8A)
- FNAC from posterior mediastinal mass (Fig. 10.8B)

FNAC

Percutaneous FNAC of the mediastinum is a diagnostically helpful, minimally invasive procedure that can be performed in patients of all ages as part of the evaluation of a mediastinal mass lesion.

Pneumothorax develops as a minor complication but generally resolves spontaneously.

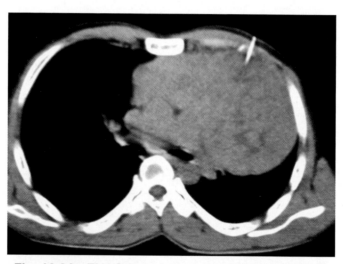

Fig. 10.8A: FNAC from an anterior mediastinal mass

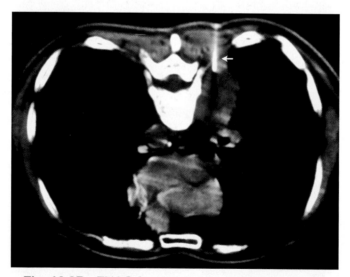

Fig. 10.8B: FNAC from posterior mediastinal mass

Section 3

Abdomen and Gastrointestinal System

- Normal Anatomy
- Esophagus
- Stomach
- Intestine
- Liver
- Biliary System
- Pancreas
- Spleen
- Adrenals
- Miscellaneous

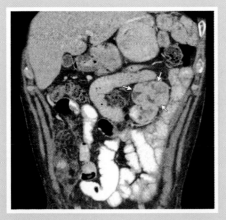
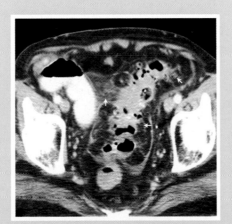
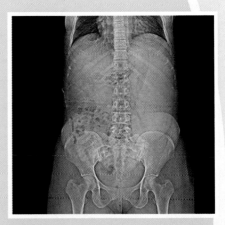

11. NORMAL ANATOMY

Axial CT Section of Abdomen (Figs 11.1 to 11.14)

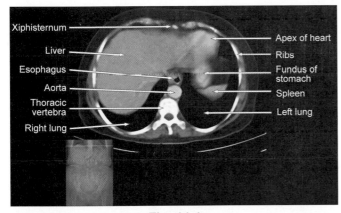

Fig. 11.1

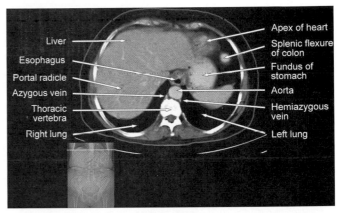

Fig. 11.2

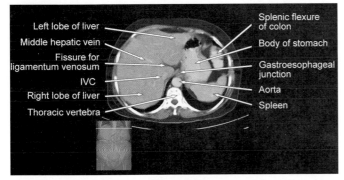

Fig. 11.3

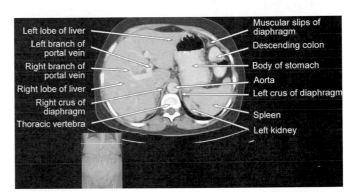

Fig. 11.4

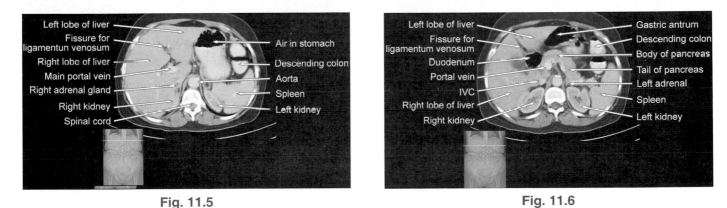

Fig. 11.5

Fig. 11.6

Figs 11.1 to 11.6: Axial CT sections of abdomen

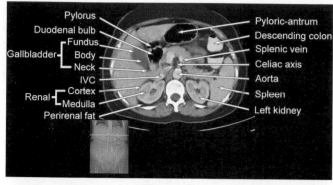

Pylorus
Duodenal bulb
Gallbladder — Fundus
Body
Neck
IVC
Renal — Cortex
Medulla
Perirenal fat

Pyloric-antrum
Descending colon
Splenic vein
Celiac axis
Aorta
Spleen
Left kidney

Fig. 11.7

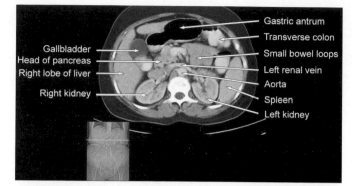

Gallbladder
Head of pancreas
Right lobe of liver
Right kidney

Gastric antrum
Transverse colon
Small bowel loops
Left renal vein
Aorta
Spleen
Left kidney

Fig. 11.8

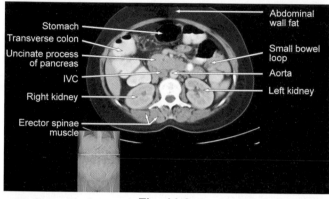

Stomach
Transverse colon
Uncinate process of pancreas
IVC
Right kidney
Erector spinae muscle

Abdominal wall fat
Small bowel loop
Aorta
Left kidney

Fig. 11.9

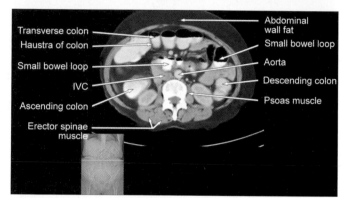

Transverse colon
Haustra of colon
Small bowel loop
IVC
Ascending colon
Erector spinae muscle

Abdominal wall fat
Small bowel loop
Aorta
Descending colon
Psoas muscle

Fig. 11.10

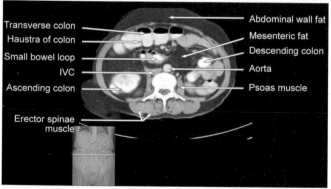

Transverse colon
Haustra of colon
Small bowel loop
IVC
Ascending colon
Erector spinae muscle

Abdominal wall fat
Mesenteric fat
Descending colon
Aorta
Psoas muscle

Fig. 11.11

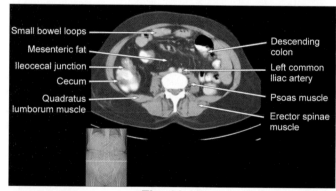

Small bowel loops
Mesenteric fat
Ileocecal junction
Cecum
Quadratus lumborum muscle

Descending colon
Left common Iliac artery
Psoas muscle
Erector spinae muscle

Fig. 11.12

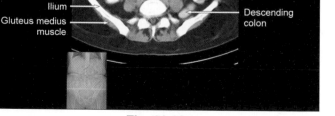

Small bowel loop
Mesenteric fat
Small bowel loop
Ilium
Gluteus medius muscle

Rectus abdominis muscle
Small bowel loop
Descending colon

Fig. 11.13

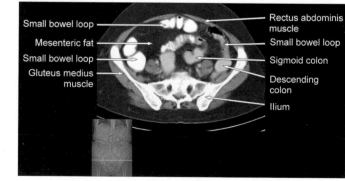

Small bowel loop
Mesenteric fat
Small bowel loop
Gluteus medius muscle

Rectus abdominis muscle
Small bowel loop
Sigmoid colon
Descending colon
Ilium

Fig. 11.14

Figs 11.7 to 11.14: Axial CT sections of abdomen

Axial CT Section Showing Appendix (Figs 11.15A and B)

Normal appendix is a narrow, worm-shaped tube which originates from the apex of the cecum (Figs 11.15A and B) and may extend to any of the several directions: upward behind the cecum; to the left behind the ileum and mesentery or downward into the lesser pelvis. It varies from 2 to 20 cm in length, average being about 8.3 cm. It is retained in position by a fold of peritoneum (mesenteriole) derived from the mesentery. Histologically, the appendix has the same basic structure as the large intestine.

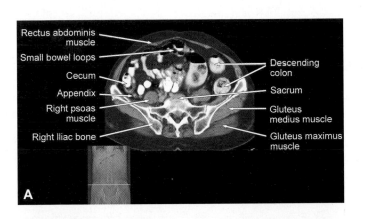

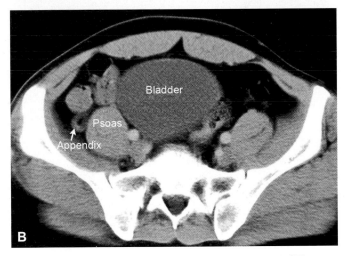

Figs 11.15A and B: Normal appendix on CT

12. ESOPHAGUS

12.1   Hiatus Hernia

Herniation of the stomach through the esophageal hiatus is known as hiatus hernia.

It is commonly caused by laxity and stretching of phrenoesophageal ligament and widening of the esophageal hiatus. It can be of sliding or paraesophageal variety.

CT scan (Fig. 12.1) revealed presence of portion of proximal stomach into the lower posterior mediastinum with an abnormally wide esophageal hiatus and a diagnosis of sliding hiatus hernia was made.

In paraesophageal hernias, the stomach and other abdominal structures herniated, lie alongside the gastroesophageal junction, which itself lies below the diaphragm. Paraesophageal hernias can undergo serious complications.

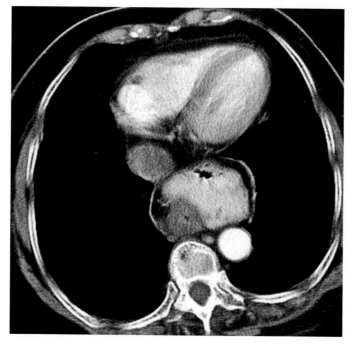

Fig. 12.1: Hiatus hernia

12.2 Carcinoma Esophagus 1

- CT shows prestenotic dilatation of esophagus with air fluid (contrast) level (arrow) (Fig. 12.2A).
- CECT chest shows circumferential wall thickening of mid esophagus with loss of fat planes with bronchus, pulmonary artery and aorta. The esophageal lumen is narrowed (arrow) (Fig. 12.2B).

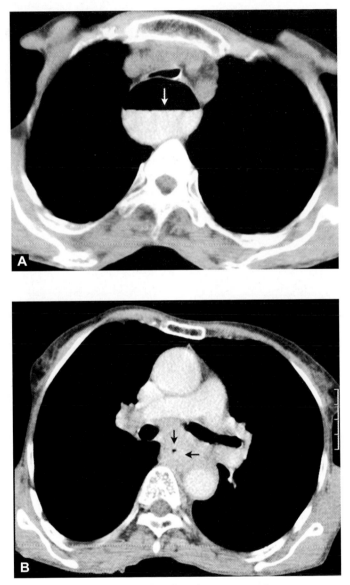

Figs 12.2A and B: Carcinoma esophagus

12.3 Carcinoma Esophagus 2

Well defined asymmetric circumferential wall thickening of the esophagus is seen in midthoracic region causing marked luminal narrowing (Figs 12.3A to D).

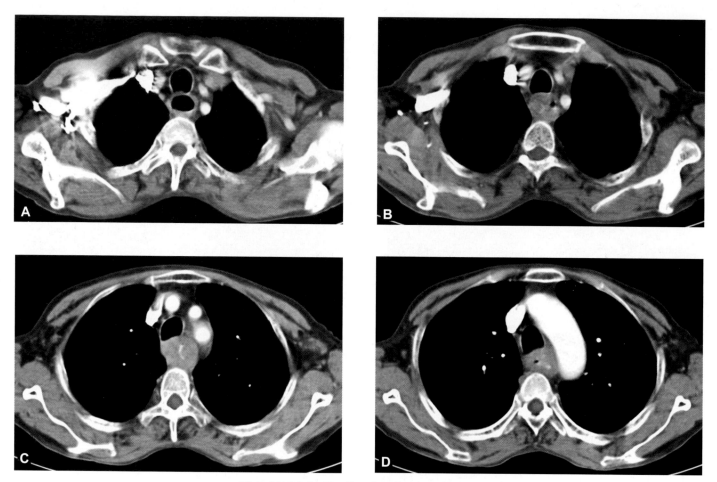

Figs 12.3A to D: Carcinoma esophagus

13. STOMACH

13.1 Carcinoma

- Homogenously enhancing circumferential thickening of almost entire stomach wall is seen. Few enlarged lymph nodes are also present. Vertebral bodies show degenerative change (Figs 13.1A to F).
- Images are in right oblique decubitus position (Figs 13.1E and F).

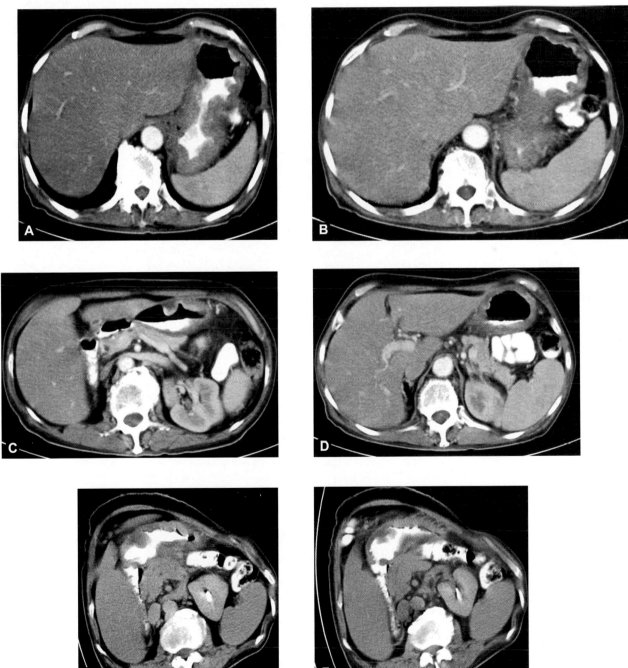

Figs 13.1A to F: Carcinoma stomach

13.2 Carcinoma Pylorus (Figs 13.2A and B)

CT images in right lateral recumbent position show circumferential thickening of pylorus with the growth extending into antrum and duodenum. Prepyloric lymph node is seen (arrow).

Carcinoma of the pylorus may simulate benign duodenal obstruction. Complete reliance should not be placed on history of duodenal ulcer. Persistent obstruction despite intensive medical treatment is suggestive of pyloric carcinoma and imaging examinations are confirmatory.

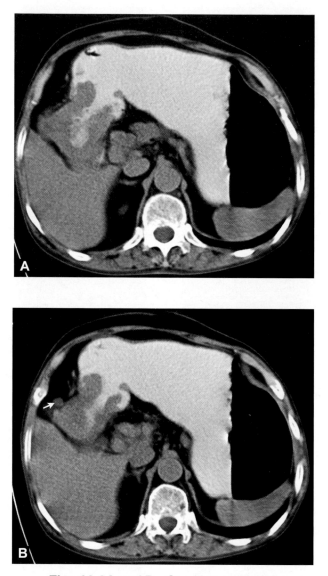

Figs 13.2A and B: Carcinoma pylorus

13.3 Lymphoma

- Contrast CT shows diffuse thickening of walls of stomach with narrowing of lumen (Fig. 13.3A).
- Contrast CT also shows splenomegaly with splenic infarcts (arrow) in this case of gastric lymphoma (Fig. 13.3B).

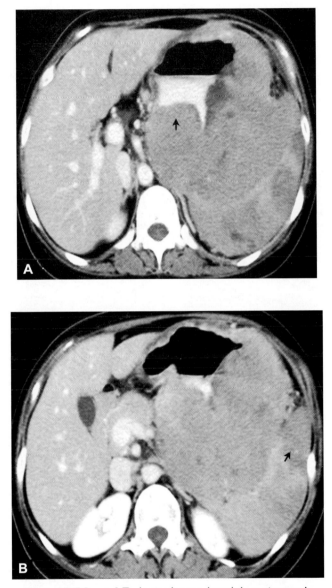

Figs 13.3A and B: Lymphoma involving stomach

13.4 Krukenberg Tumor

36 years old female with partial gastrectomy and under treatment for carcinoma of stomach. Follow up scan shows: Bilateral pleural effusion (Fig. 13.4A). Recurrence of carcinoma stomach and massive malignant ascites (Fig. 13.4B). Ascites and bilateral ovarian deposits (Krukenberg tumor) (Figs 13.4C and D).

Krukenberg tumor classically refers to a metastatic ovarian malignancy whose primary site is gastrointestinal tract or breast. Krukenberg tumors are often found in both ovaries. Microscopically they are characterized by appearance of mucin secreting signet ring cells.

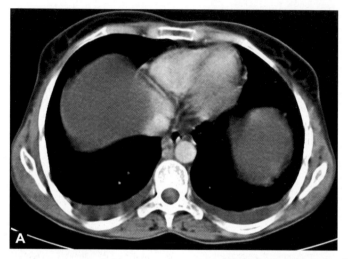 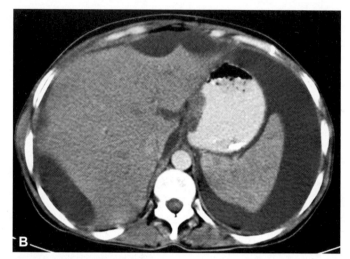

Figs 13.4A and B: Bilateral pleural effusion

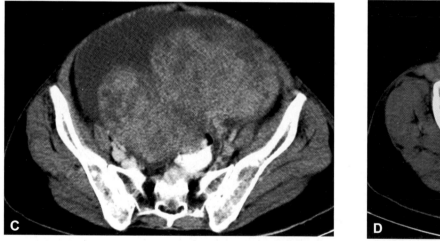 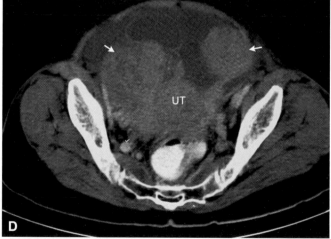

Figs 13.4C and D: Ascites and bilateral ovarian deposits (Krukenberg tumor)

14. INTESTINE

14.1 Infective-Inflammatory

1. Abdominal Koch's 1

A 29 years male presented with abdominal discomfort and distension. He had loss of appetite.

Matting of bowel loops and shaggy appearance of mesentery is seen. There is massive ascites and bilateral pleural effusion (Figs 14.1A to F).

CT has the ability to demonstrate changes in the peritonium, mesentery, lymph nodes, bowel and solid organs hence it is being increasingly used for primary evaluation of abdominal tuberculosis.

Peritoneal involvement is the most common feature with ascites (wet peritonitis). Other features are mesenteric or omental thickening or mass formation, lymphadenopathy mainly of diffuse nature, bowel wall thickening and solid organ involvement.

These features in appropriate clinical setting, should help optimize the correct diagnosis.

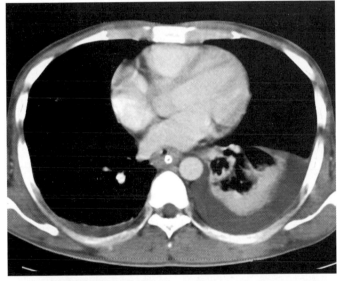

Fig. 14.1A: Bilateral pleural effusion

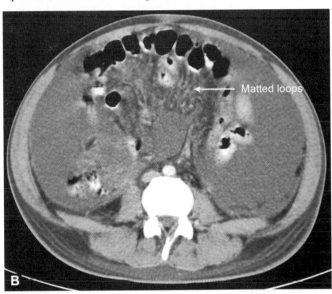

Matted loops

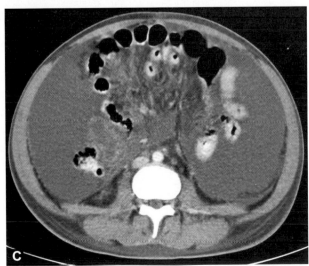

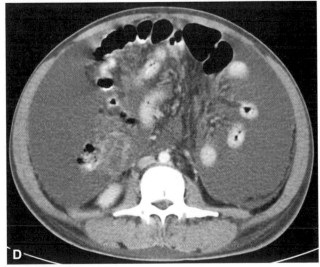

Figs 14.1B to D: Abdominal Koch's 1

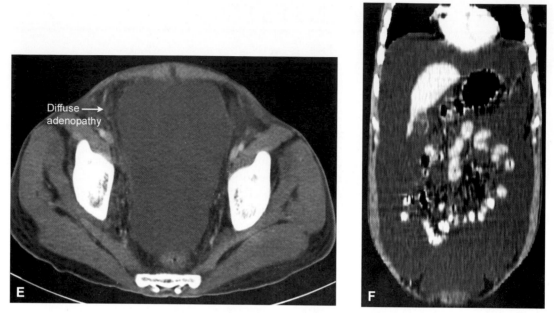

Figs 14.1E and F: Abdominal Koch's 1

2. Abdominal Koch's 2

41 years male with decreased appetite and sensation of abdominal discomfort.

Contrast CT shows mesenteric fat stranding in addition to mesenteric and retroperitoneal lymphadenopathy (Figs 14.1G and H).

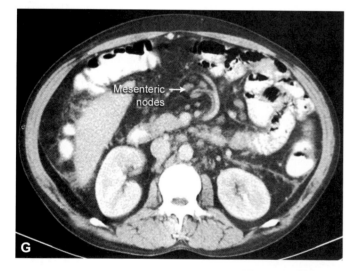
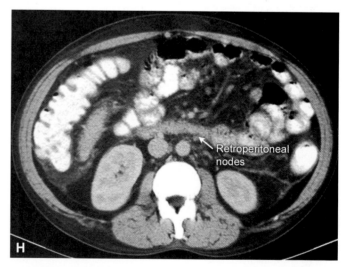

Figs 14.1G and H: Abdominal Koch's 2

3. Abdominal Koch's 3

40 years old female had recurrent episodes of diarrhea and abdominal discomfort. CT shows bilateral pleural effusion, ascites and thickening of colonic wall. Areas of narrowing and dilatation of bowel loops is seen (Figs 14.1I to L).

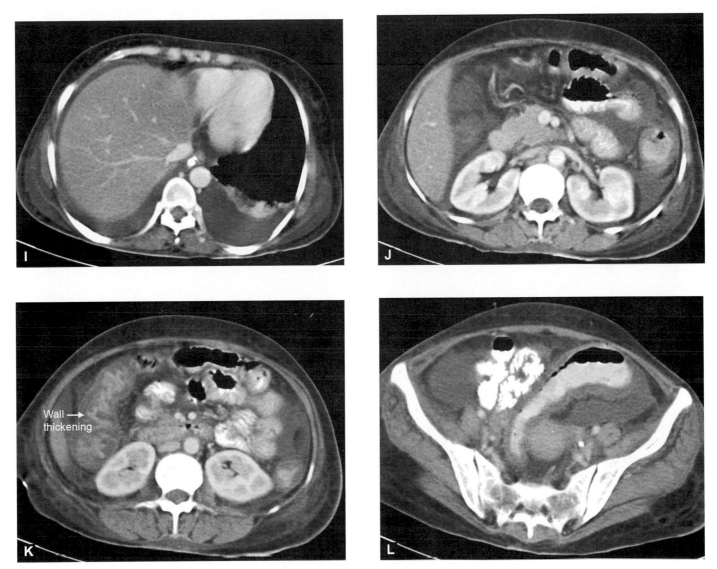

Wall → thickening

Figs 14.1I to L: Abdominal Koch's 3

4. Abdominal Koch's 4

CT shows bilateral pleural effusion (Fig. 14.1M). Figures 14.1N to R show ascites, colonic wall thickening, mesenteric fat stranding (arrow) and lymphadenopathy which are indicators of Koch's abdomen.

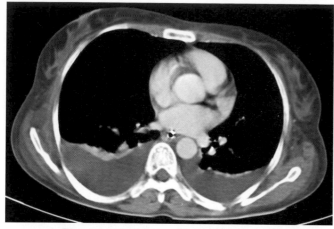

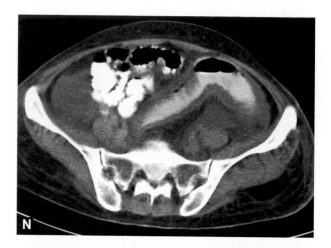

Fig. 14.1M: Bilateral pleural effusion

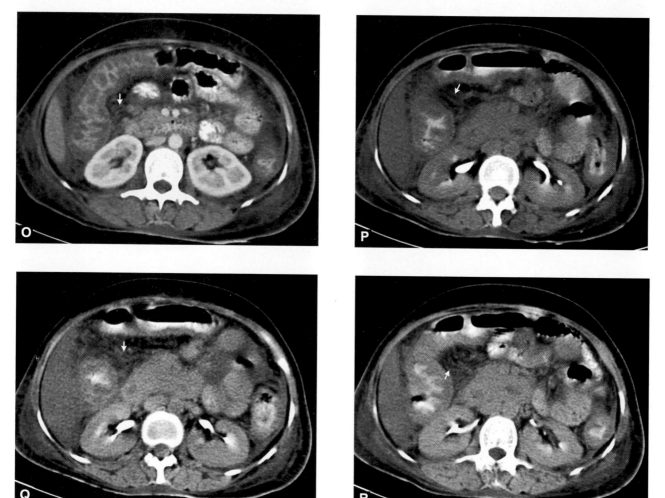

Figs 14.1N to R: Abdominal Koch's 4

5. Sigmoid Diverticulitis

- CT pelvis shows inflammed diverticuli of sigmoid colon (horizontal arrows) and pericolic abscess (vertical arrow) (Figs 14.1S and T).
- Loculated pelvic abscess (Fig. 14.1U).

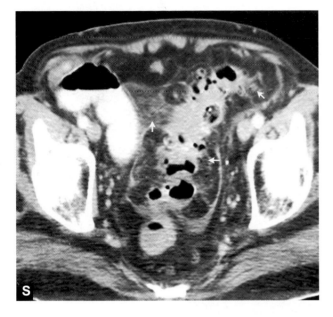
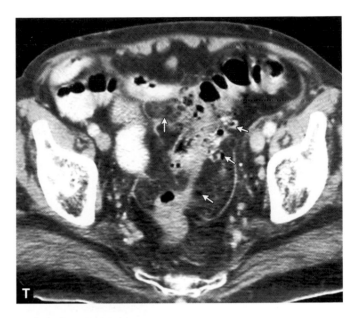
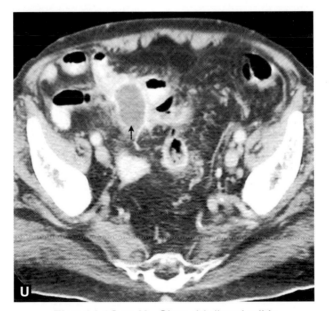

Figs 14.1S to U: Sigmoid diverticulitis

6. Appendix

- Plain CT scan with oral contrast shows contrast filled normal non-inflamed appendix (Fig. 14.1V).
- Contrast CT abdomen shows enlarged inflamed appendix and adjacent fat stranding (Fig. 14.1W).
- Contrast CT abdomen shows enlarged inflamed appendix with gas in lumen and early stage of appendicular lump formation (Fig. 14.1X).

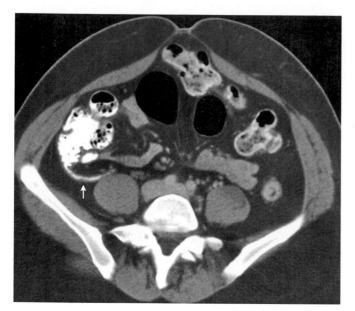

Fig. 14.1V: Normal barium filled appendix

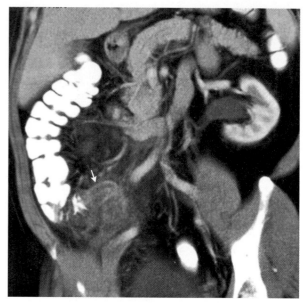

Fig. 14.1W: Inflamed appendix with adjacent fat stranding

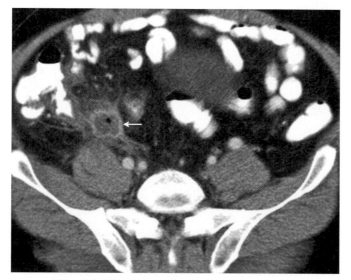

Fig. 14.1X: Appendicular lump formation

7. Nontoxic Megacolon

CT images in a 10 years female who had no bladder or bowel complaints. A lower abdominal lump was incidentally found on palpation. Ultrasound was inconclusive. CT demonstrated massive distension of rectosigmoid and descending colon loaded with faeces. Anal canal was normal and sudden dilatation of rectosigmoid was noted. The walls and surrounding fat of dilated bowel segment did not show any signs of inflammation (Figs 14.1Y to AC) and diagnosed as asymptomatic megacolon (Nontoxic megacolon).

Nontoxic megacolon is defined as severe dilatation of a segment or the entire colon unaccompanied by signs or symptoms of colon toxicity.

Mechanical factors (volvulus, anastomosis, diverticulosis, carcinoma) are responsible for the nontoxic megacolon or may have pseudo obstruction as in this case. Colonoscopy for decompression should be considered as the initial treatment for nontoxic megacolon prior to surgical intervention.

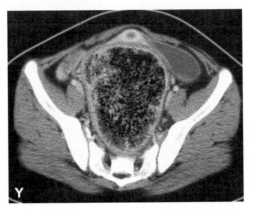

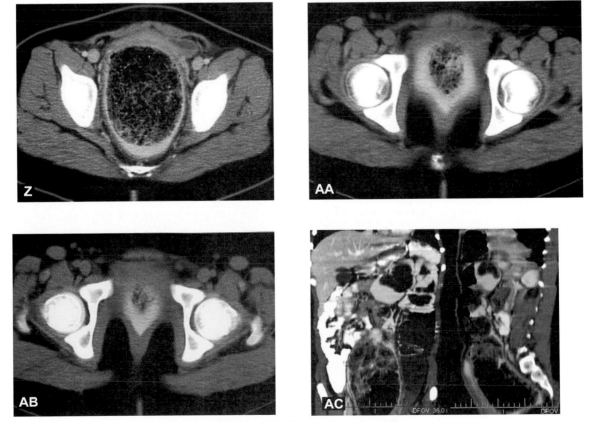

Figs 14.1Y to AC: Nontoxic megacolon

14.2 Neoplastic

1. Carcinoma Duodenum

CT images show hepatic metastases (Figs 14.2A to C) in a patient with duodenal carcinoma (Figs 14.2B to D). Post-cholecystectomy status (Figs 14.2E and F).

Adenocarcinoma of the duodenum gives rise to nonspecific gastrointestinal tract symptoms and diagnosis is often delayed. It is generally considered to have a low resectability rate. The Whipple procedure may still be curative for patients with positive lymph nodes. There is an increased risk in patients with familial adenomatous polyposis and adenomas in the duodenum.

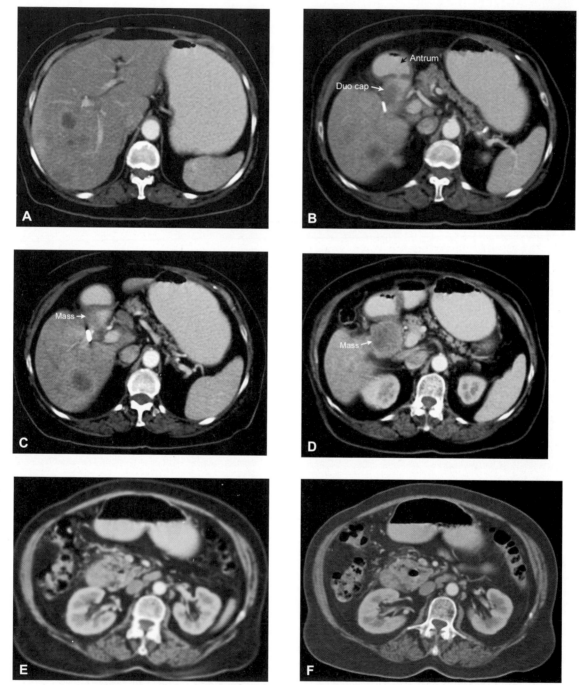

Figs 14.2A to F: Duodenal carcinoma with hepatic metastases

2. Jejunal Angiodysplasia

It is an arterio-venous malformation or venous ectasia. It is seen at antimesenteric border.

Elderly patients have chronic intermittent bleed in stools. Hence they sometimes present with severe anemia.

Coronal (Fig. 14.2G) and sagittal (Fig. 14.2H) reconstructions in a patient of jejunal angiodysplasia. Intense enhancement of the tumor is seen. Early opacification and engorgement of draining vein is seen in such case.

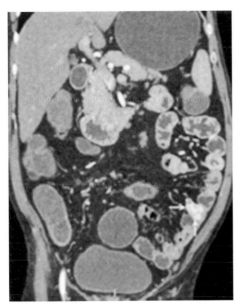

Fig. 14.2G: Coronal reconstruction in a patient of jejunal angiodysplasia

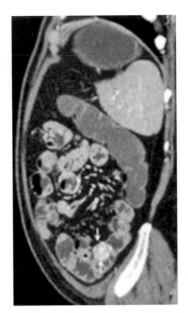

Fig. 14.2H: Sagittal reconstruction in a patient of jejunal angiodysplasia

3. Gastrointestinal Stromal Tumor (GIST)

GIST is a benign neoplasm of intestinal mucosa. There is bowel wall thickening of focal segment. No spread is seen to the mesentery. Nodes are not involved.

Post contrast axial CT (Fig. 14.2I) and coronally reconstructed CT (Fig. 14.2J) shows GIST.

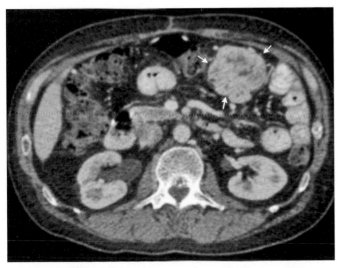

Fig. 14.2I: Post contrast axial CT shows GIST

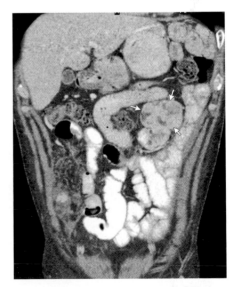

Fig. 14.2J: Coronally reconstructed CT shows GIST

4. Adenocarcinoma of Ileum

Axial (Fig. 14.2K) and coronal reconstruction (Fig. 14.2L) CT images show an enhancing mass in terminal ileum. Proved as adenocarcinoma on histopathology.

Mesentery and lymph nodes are involved.

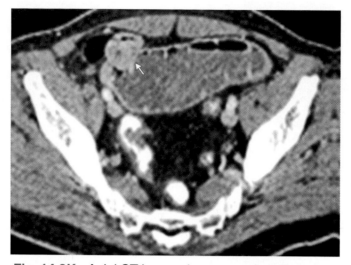

Fig. 14.2K: Axial CT image shows an enhancing mass in terminal ileum proved as adenocarcinoma

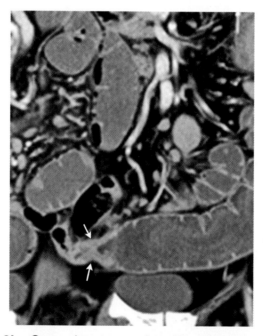

Fig. 14.2L: Coronal reconstruction of ileal adenocarcinoma

5. Abdominal Sarcoma

50 years male presented with massive distension of abdomen. Figures 14.2M to P, CT images show a large heterogeneous abdomino-pelvic soft tissue mass lesion. It involves the anterior abdominal walls and extends behind to encase the ureter.

Biopsy proved it to be a sarcoma.

A sarcoma is a malignant tumor of the connective tissue (bone, cartilage, fat) resulting in mesodermal proliferation. This is in contrast to carcinomas, which are of epithelial origin (breast, colon, pancreas). The term soft tissue sarcoma is used to describe tumors of soft tissue, which includes elements that are in connective tissue but not derived from it (such as muscles and blood vessels).

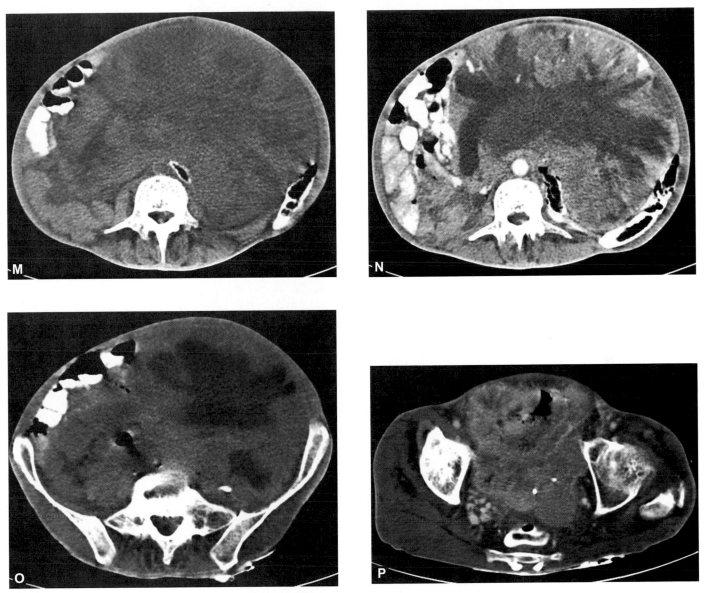

Figs 14.2M to P: Abdominal sarcoma

6. Mesenteric and Peritoneal Non-Hodgkin's Lymphoma

- CT abdomen shows peritoneal and omental thickening (Fig. 14.2Q).
- Peritoneal and mesenteric thickening and mass like appearance with bowel narrowing in a proved case of Non-Hodgkin's lymphoma (Fig. 14.2R).

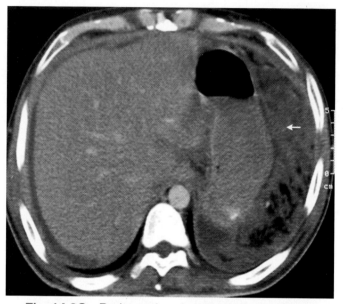

Fig. 14.2Q: Peritoneal and mesenteric thickening

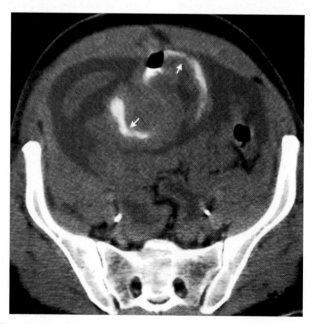

Fig. 14.2R: Mass like appearance with bowel narrowing in Non-Hodgkin's lymphoma

7. Carcinoma Sigmold Colon

CT images show circumferential irregular intraluminal growth in the distal sigmoid colon that turned out to be carcinoma. No adjacent lymphadenopathy or pericolic fat stranding seen (Figs 14.2S to X).

The disease has its highest incidence between the ages of 60 and 70 years. Women are more prone.

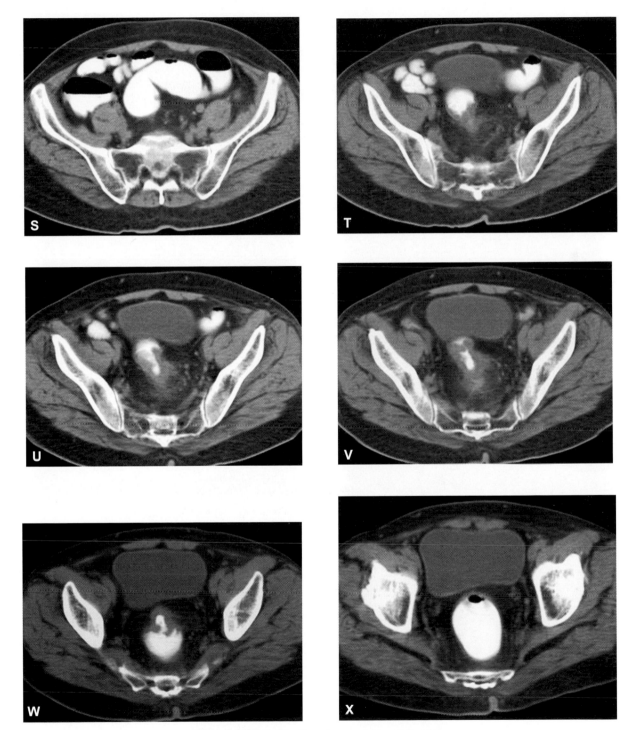

Figs 14.2S to X: Carcinoma sigmoid colon

8. Carcinoma Rectum with Metastases

Figures 14.2Y and Z show a rectal mass causing intraluminal filling defect in the contrast column. Biopsy proved this to be a rectal carcinoma. Metastatic inguinal lymphadenopathy is also seen. Figures 14.2AA and AB show hepatic metastases.

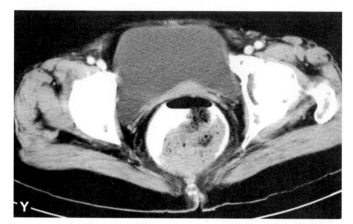
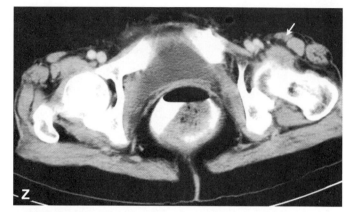

Figs 14.2Y and Z: Rectal mass

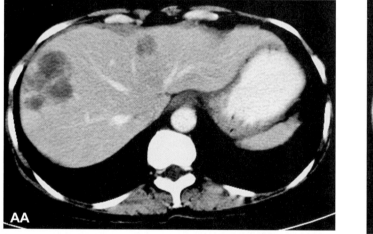
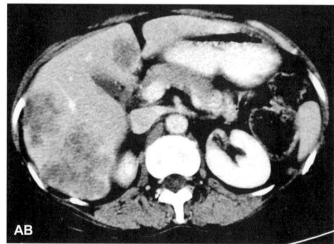

Figs 14.2AA and AB: Hepatic metastases in carcinoma rectum

9. Carcinoma Rectum

CT pelvis, the delayed post contrast images (Figs 14.2AC and AD) show thickening of wall of rectum with the growth projecting into the lumen. There is perirectal fat stranding, lymph node involvement and extension of growth into the posterior bladder wall (arrow).

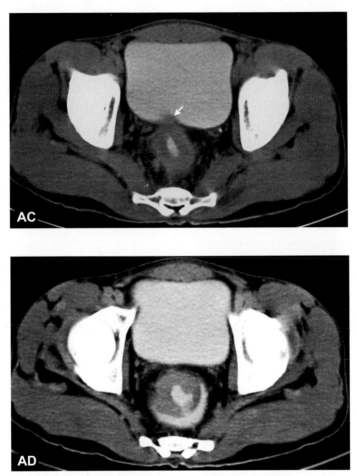

Figs 14.2AC and AD: Carcinoma rectum

14.3 Miscellaneous

1. Direct Inguinal Hernia (Figs 14.3A to E)

On CT scan inguinal hernia is usually an incidental finding. CT shows the course, contents and status of vascularity in complicated unreducible hernia where ultrasound may not be effective due to reverberation artifacts of bowel gas.

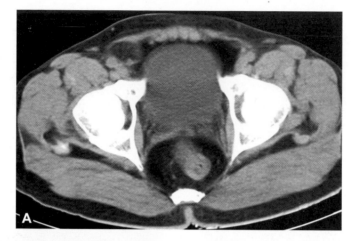

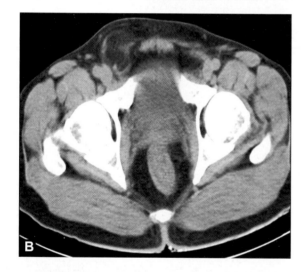

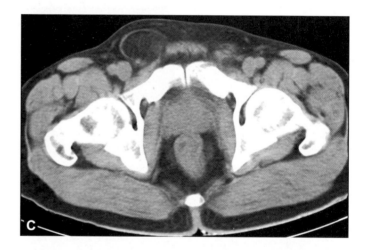

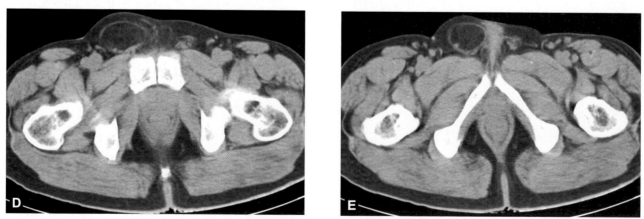

Figs 14.3A to E: Direct inguinal hernia

2. Superior Mesenteric Artery (SMA) Syndrome

Normal distance between aorta and SMA is more than 13.5 mm (Fig. 14.3F).

Normal angle between aorta and SMA is > 28° (Fig. 14.3G).

When either the distance is less than 10 mm (Fig. 14.3H) or the angle becomes less than 20° (Fig. 14.3I), third portion of duodenum undergoes extrinsic vascular compression so that the patient presents with abdominal cramps and repeated vomiting.

This compression is characteristically relieved in prone or elbow-knee position.

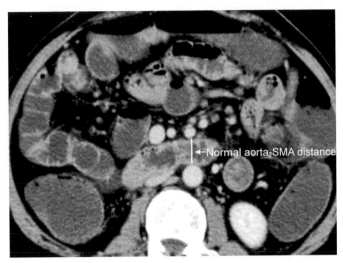

Fig. 14.3F: Axial CT showing normal distance between aorta and SMA

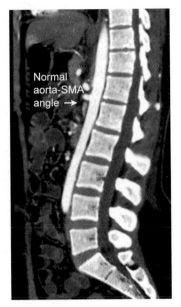

Fig. 14.3G: Coronal CT showing normal angle between aorta and SMA

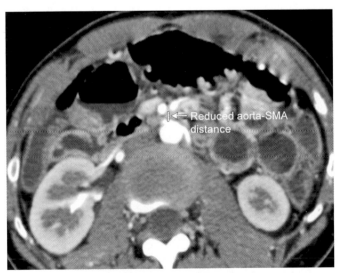

Fig. 14.3H: Axial CT in superior mesenteric artery syndrome

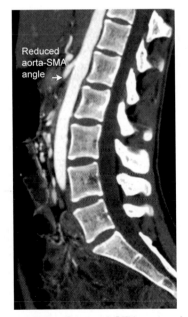

Fig. 14.3I: Coronal CT in superior mesenteric artery syndrome

3. Small Bowel Strangulation

Radially distributed dilated bowel loops are seen in the scout image (Fig. 14.3JA) and coronal recon CT image (Fig. 14.3JB) in a patient who presented with abdominal pain.

Exploratory surgery confirmed strangulated small bowel obstruction.

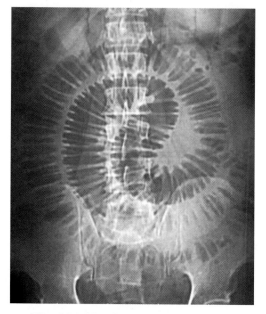

Fig. 14.3JA: Scout image showing small bowel strangulation

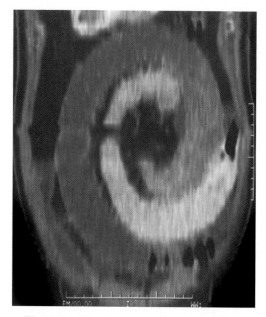

Fig. 14.3JB: Coronal recon CT image showing small bowel strangulation

4. Thrombosis of Superior Mesenteric Vessels

Contrast CT images showing
- Thrombus only in proximal part of superior mesenteric artery (SMA). Distal SMA is patent (Fig. 14.3K).
- Partial thrombosis in superior mesenteric artery. Lumen is patent (Fig. 14.3L).
- Complete thrombosis of SMA (Fig. 14.3M).
- Thrombosed superior mesenteric vein (SMV) (Fig. 14.3N).

Thrombosis of intra-abdominal vessels leads to bowel ischemia and edema of bowel loops. Commonest presentation is in the form of abdominal pain.

Most definitive finding is the presence of thrombus in artery or vein seen as a non-enhancing filling defect in the vessel lumen.

Other associated findings are:
- Mesenteric fat stranding due to mesenteric ischemia.
- Intense mucosal enhancement of bowel wall.
- Bowel wall thickening.
- Bowel distension and intraluminal fluid accumulation.

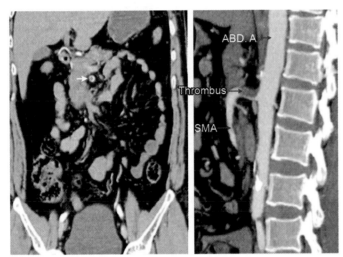

Fig. 14.3K: Thrombus only in proximal part of SMA. Distal SMA is patent

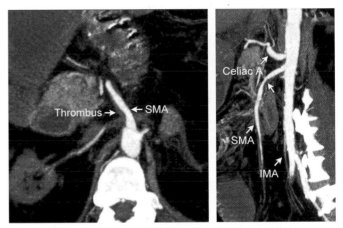

Fig. 14.3L: Partial thrombosis in superior mesenteric artery. Lumen is patent

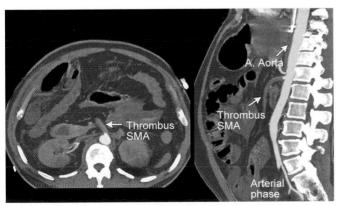

Fig. 14.3M: Complete thrombosis of SMA

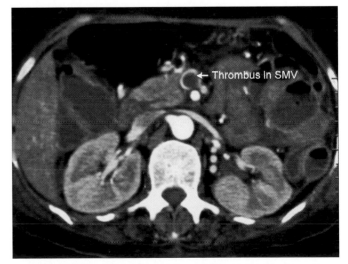

Fig. 14.3N: Thrombosed superior mesenteric vein

15. LIVER

15.1. Normal

Normal Liver Segments

Segmental Anatomy of Liver (Figs 15.1A to H)

The Couinaud classification of liver anatomy divides the liver into eight functionally indepedent segments. Each segment has its own vascular inflow, outflow and biliary drainage. In the center of each segment there is a branch of the portal vein, hepatic artery and bile duct. The numbering of the segments is in a clockwise manner.

Segment 1 (caudate lobe) is located posteriorly and extends between fissure of the ligamentum venosum anteriorly and the inferior vena cava posteriorly.

The longitudinal plane of the right hepatic vein divides segment 8 from segment 7 in the superior portion of the liver and in the inferior portion of the liver segment 5 from segment 6.

The longitudinal plane of the middle hepatic vein through the gallbladder fossa separates segment 4a from segment 8 in the superior liver and segment 4b from segment 5 in the inferior liver.

The longitudinal plane of the left hepatic vein and fissure of the ligamentum teres separates segment 4a from segment 2 in the superior liver and segment 4b from segment 3 in the inferior liver.

The axial plane of the left portal vein separates segment 4a superiorly from segment 4b inferiorly and segment 2 superiorly from segment 3 inferiorly in the left lobe.

The axial plane of the right portal vein separates segment 8 and segment 7 superiorly from segment 5 and segment 6 inferiorly in the right lobe.

The segment 1 caudate lobe is anatomically divided into 3 parts: Spiegel's lobe (segment 1a), paracaval portion (segment 1b), and caudate process (segment 1c).

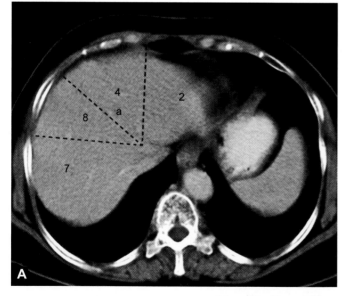 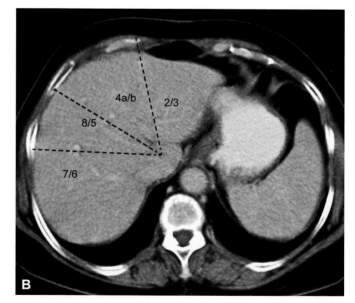

Figs 15.1A and B: Segmental anatomy of liver

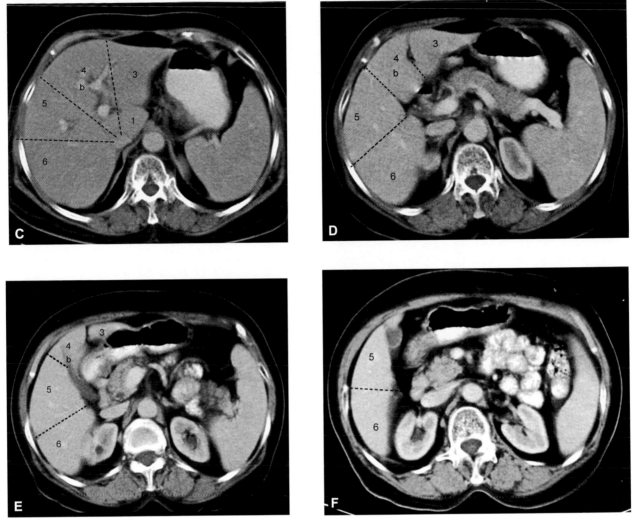

Figs 15.1C to F: Segmental anatomy of liver

Liver Segments

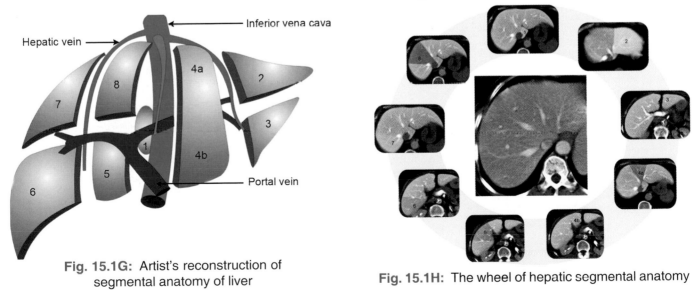

Fig. 15.1G: Artist's reconstruction of segmental anatomy of liver

Fig. 15.1H: The wheel of hepatic segmental anatomy

15.2. Infective-Inflammatory

1. Calcified Focus in Liver (Fig. 15.2A)

Calcification in old granuloma, simple cysts and hemangiomas can have this type of appearance.

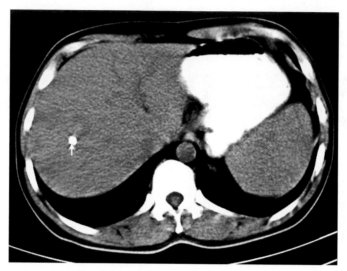

Fig. 15.2A: Calcified focus in liver

2. Amoebic Liver Abscesses

Plain (Fig. 15.2B) and contrast (Figs 15.2C to E) CT abdomen shows multiple, irregular, hypodense lesions with minimally enhancing thin walls and mild perilesional edema in the enlarged liver. Reactionary bilateral pleural effusion and ascites are also seen. Aspirate had anchovy sauce appearance.

Amoebic abscess should be included in the differential diagnosis when CT shows one or more cystic or complex masses within the liver, especially when there is evidence of extrahepatic extension. The presence of pleural effusion and/or perihepatic fluid in association with a cystic or complex hepatic mass is certainly not specific for amoebic abscess and can be seen with many inflammatory and neoplastic hepatic lesions.

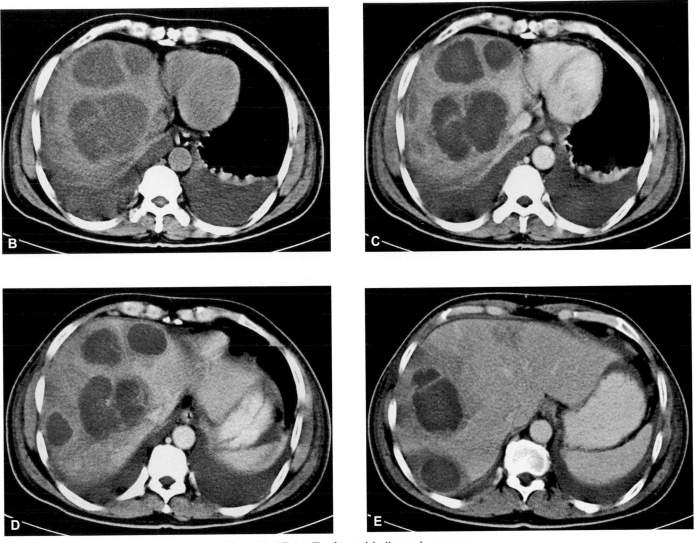

Figs 15.2B to E: Amoebic liver abscesses

3. Hepatic Abscess (Figs 15.2F to I)

Abscess is seen as a hypodense non-enhancing thin walled lesion in liver. Sympathetic right pleural effusion is seen. The etiology can be bacterial/fungal/parasitic and evaluation of the aspirate alone can give confirmation.

At an early stage, the lesion is usually confined. As a lesion develops, tissues in the abscess are liquidized and merge to form a pus cavity and plain CT scans show low attenuation with CT values less than 20 HU and enhanced CT scans show clearer and smoother edges and the wall of the pus cavity can enhance. The lesion develops further forming a typical liver abscess. At this stage, the wall of the pus cavity has a 3 layer structure, fresh granulation tissue, old fibrous-granulation tissue and an outer inflammatory edema layer. Typically, the wall of an abscess displays iso-attenuation in plain CT scans and single or double-ring signs in enhanced CT scans. Larger lesions are prone to have septa, which are uneven in thickness and diversified in shape.

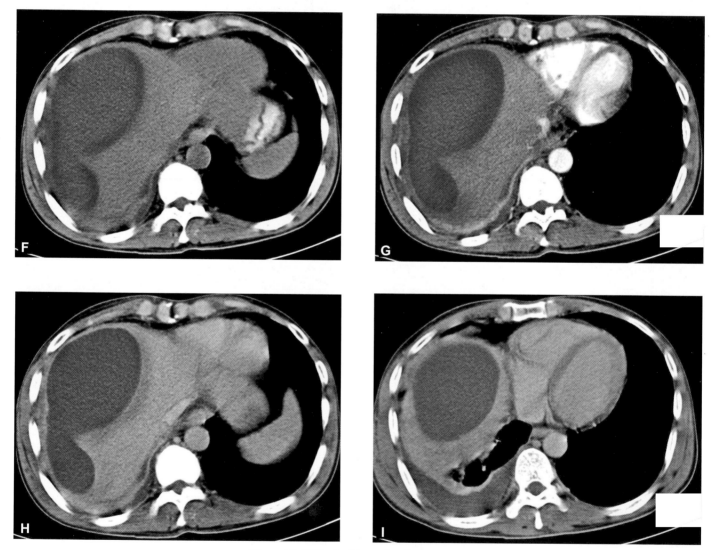

Figs 15.2F to I: Hepatic abscesses

4. Hydatid Cyst Liver (Figs 15.2J and K)

CT images show heterogeneous well-defined space occupying lesion in anterosuperior segment of right hepatic lobe with internal and capsular calcification and retraction of hepatic capsule in a case of burnt out hydatid cyst.

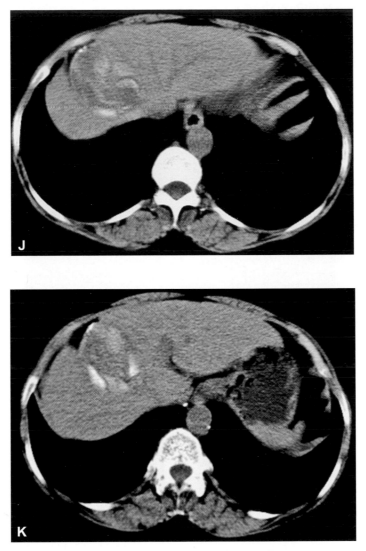

Figs 15.2J and K: Hydatid cyst liver

15.3 Trauma

1. Hepatic Laceration

Images show laceration of right hepatic lobe with subcapsular collection secondary to fracture of overlying rib (Fig. 15.3A). There is associated contusion in small bowel mesentery (Fig. 15.3B) and subcutaneous fat (Fig. 15.3C) in lower abdomen in a case of blunt trauma abdomen.

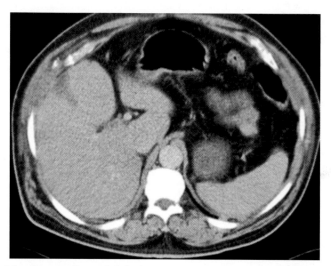

Fig. 15.3A: Laceration of right hepatic lobe with subcapsular collection

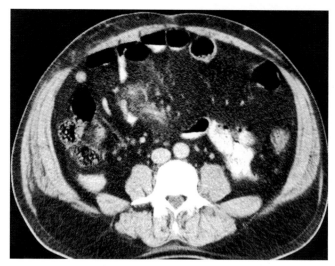

Fig. 15.3B: Contusion in small bowel mesentery

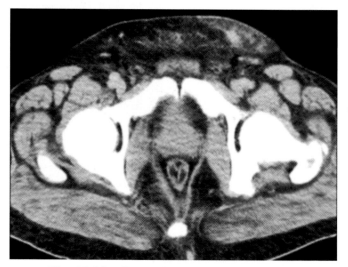

Fig. 15.3C: Contusion in subcutaneous fat

2. Hepatic Trauma

Liver is the second most frequently injured abdominal organ.
Posterior segment of right lobe is the most frequent site (near spine and ribs).
Lacerations extending to bare area may only have retroperitoneal finding.

- Contrast CT abdomen shows small contusions in liver (Fig. 15.3D).
- Contrast CT abdomen shows lacerated liver (Fig. 15.3E).
- CT images in a patient with diaphragmatic rupture with herniation of liver into the thorax (Fig. 15.3F).

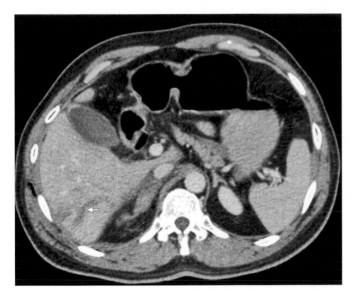

Fig. 15.3D: Hepatic contusion

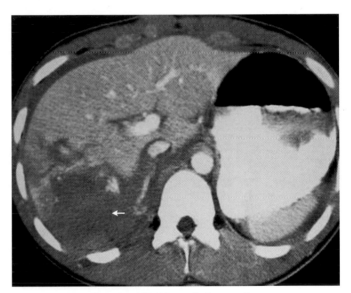

Fig. 15.3E: Hepatic laceration

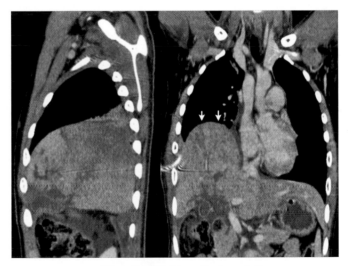

Fig. 15.3F: Hepatic herniation

15.4 Neoplastic

1. Hemangioma Liver 1

Well-defined hyperdense lesion is seen in liver that shows peripheral enhancement in arterial phase and progressive centripetal fill in, in delayed phases.

Plain CT image (Fig. 15.4A), CT image in arterial phase (Fig. 15.4B), CT image in portal phase (Fig. 15.4C), CT image in venous phase (Fig. 15.4D), CT image at 3 minutes phase after contrast (Fig. 15.4E), CT image at 5 minutes phase after contrast (Fig. 15.4F).

Hemangioma is the most common benign tumor of the liver. The classic findings of hemangioma on CT shows hypoattenuation similar to that of vessels; on dynamic contrast-enhanced CT peripheral globular enhancement and a centripetal fill in pattern with the attenuation of enhancing areas identical to that of the aorta.

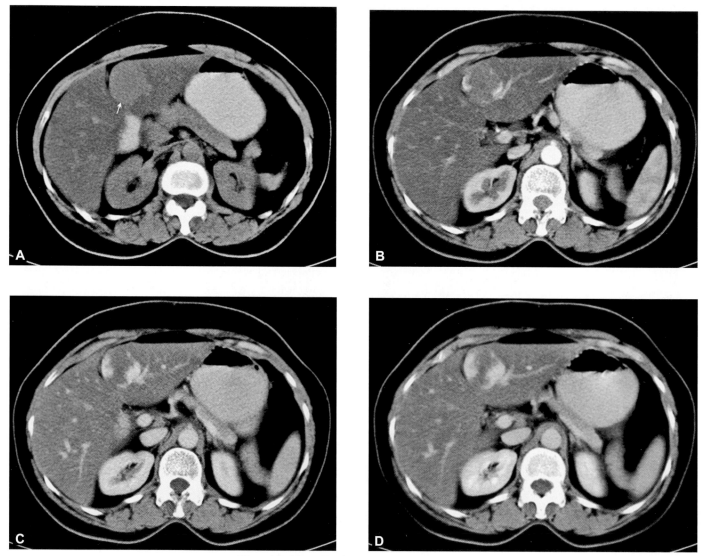

Figs 15.4A to D: Hepatic hemangioma

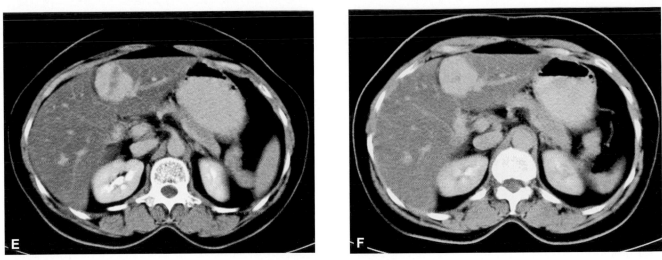

Figs 15.4E and F: Hepatic hemangioma

2. Hemangioma Liver 2 (Figs 15.4G to I)

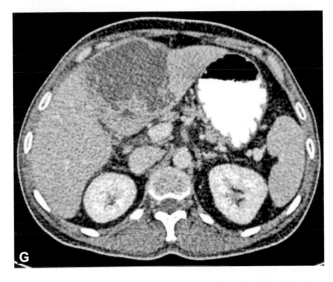
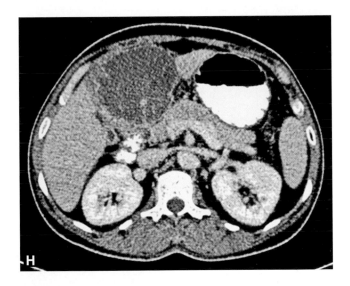

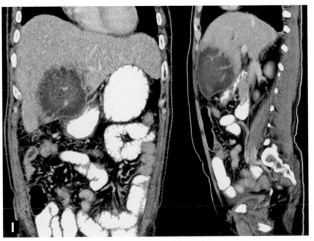

Figs 15.4G to I: Hepatic hemangioma

3. Hemangioma Liver 3 (Figs 15.4J to L)

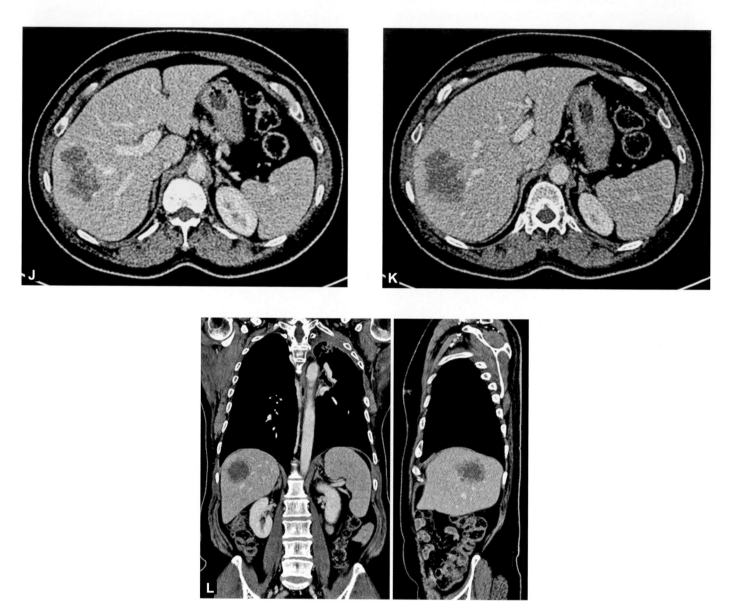

Figs 15.4J to L: Liver hemangioma

4. Focal Nodular Hyperplasia (FNH)

- Plain CT – shows isodense solid mass in liver with hypodense central scar (Fig. 15.4M).
- Arterial phase – shows mild enhancement (Fig. 15.4N).
- Venous phase – hypodense central scar shows vascularity (Fig. 15.4O).
- Portal phase – central scar shows increased vascularity (Fig. 15.4P).
- Angiogram – central scar shows vascular malformation (Fig. 15.4Q).
- Angiogram – central scar shows vascular malformation (Fig. 15.4R).

Focal nodular hyperplasia is benign lesion and does not require treatment unless causing mass effect or pain. It is common under the liver surface. On USG, the lesion appears hypoechoic. On unenhanced CT, lesion is hypodense to liver and shows significant enhancement on arterial phase and becomes isodense to liver on portal venous phase and delayed phase. The central scar may enhance on delayed images. Small lesions may not demonstrate the central scar and may be difficult to differentiate from malignant lesions.

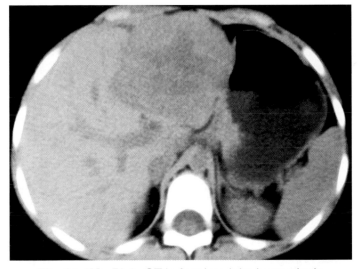

Fig. 15.4M: Plain CT in focal nodular hyperplasia

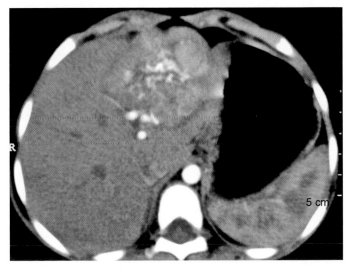

Fig. 15.4N: Arterial phase CT in focal nodular hyperplasia

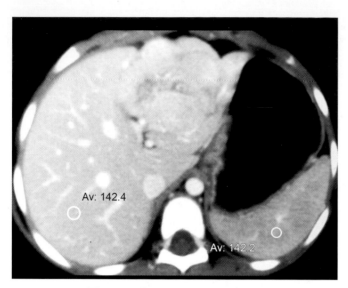

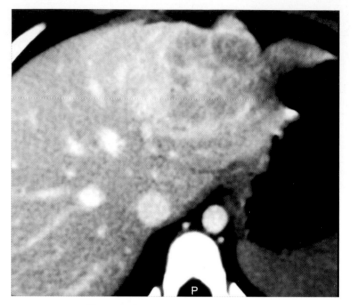

Fig. 15.4O: Venous phase CT in focal nodular hyperplasia

Fig. 15.4P: Portal phase CT in focal nodular hyperplasia

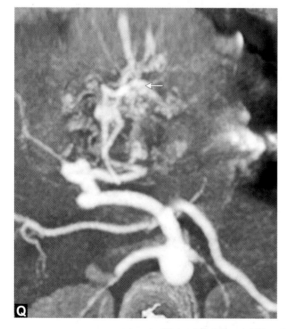

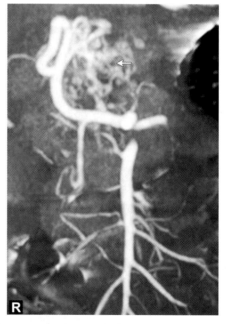

Figs 15.4Q and R: Angiogram shows central scar due to vascular malformation

5. Hepatic Adenoma

They are usually solitary and benign in nature. The capsule is hypervascular.

Internal hemorrhage is common. It is known to be associated with glycogen storage disorder. It is common in females, especially those on oral contraceptives.

Resection is indicated due to possibility of rupture.

On post contrast CT it shows mixed density. Central and peripheral filling can be seen without persistence of contrast enhancement.

Plain (Fig. 15.4S) and post-contrast (portal phase) (Fig. 15.4T) images of an hepatic adenoma.

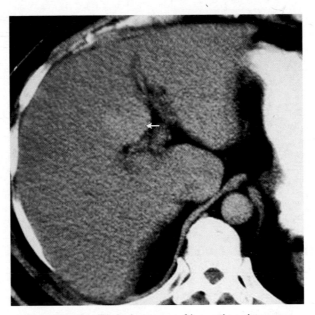

Fig. 15.4S: Plain images of hepatic adenoma

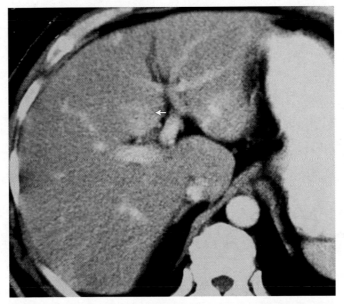

Fig. 15.4T: Post-contrast (portal phase) image of hepatic adenoma

6. Hepatocellular Carcinoma

Elderly female had right upper quadrant pain.

- Plain CT abdomen shows mass in liver (Fig. 15.4U).
- Arterial phase CT shows enhancement in the mass. A hypodense scar is also seen (arrow) (Fig. 15.4V).
- Venous phase CT shows enhancement in the mass as well as the scar (arrow) (Fig. 15.4W).
- In delayed phase CT there is persistence of contrast in the scar. This differentiates it from fibronodular hyperplasia (Fig. 15.4X).

Excised mass was found to be a hepatocellular carcinoma.

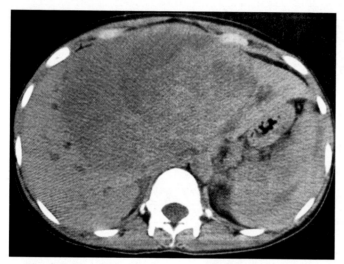

Fig. 15.4U: Plain CT in a hepatocellular carcinoma

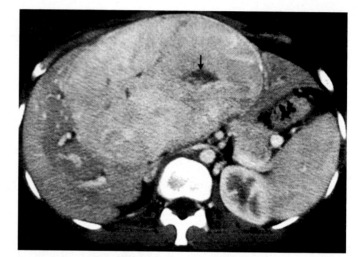

Fig. 15.4V: Arterial phase CT in a hepatocellular carcinoma

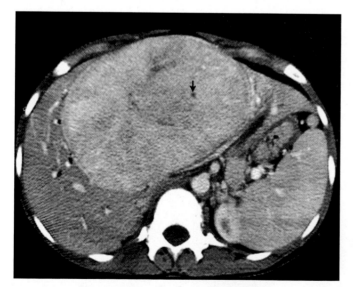

Fig. 15.4W: Venous phase CT in a hepatocellular carcinoma

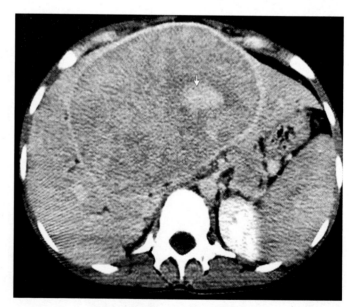

Fig. 15.4X: Delayed CT in a hepatocellular carcinoma

7. Hepatic Metastasis 1

Liver metastases are malignant tumors that originated at sites remote from the liver and generally spread to the liver via the bloodstream.

Common primary tumors that may spread to the liver are from gastrointestinal tract (colon and stomach), pancreas, breast, lung, eye and melanoma and are generally multiple. Gastrointestinal tract primary tumors often spread to the liver because blood flows directly from these organs to the liver and malignant cells have a direct path. Liver metastases may be present before primary malignancy is diagnosed or at the time the primary malignancy is diagnosed or they may occur months or years after the primary tumor is removed. The cells in a metastatic tumor resemble those in the primary tumor and hence suggest the site of primary malignancy. CT is the study of choice for evaluating liver metastases (Figs 15.4Y to AB).

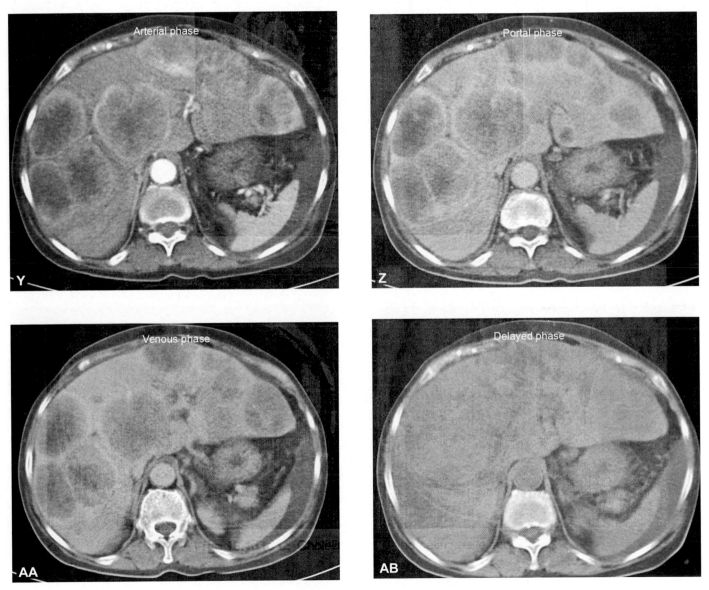

Figs 15.4Y to AB: Liver metastases

8. Hepatic Metastasis 2

Hepatic Metastasis from Mucinous Carcinoma of Transverse Colon

- Plain CT abdomen shows amorphous calcification in left lobe of liver (Fig. 15.4AC).
- Contrast CT abdomen shows differential enhancement in the left lobe and an ill-defined low density mass (Fig. 15.4AD).
- Contrast CT abdomen shows lesion in transverse colon which was diagnosed as mucinous carcinoma (Fig. 15.4AE).
- Necrotic preaortic (horizontal arrow) and aortocaval (vertical arrow) lymph nodes are also seen (Fig. 15.4AF).

    Mucinous carcinoma is an uncommon type of carcinoma of colon. However it has typical mottled calcification in the primary as well as the distant metastasis. Low density mass and nodes are also typically seen in them as more than half of the lesion is made up of extracellular mucin.

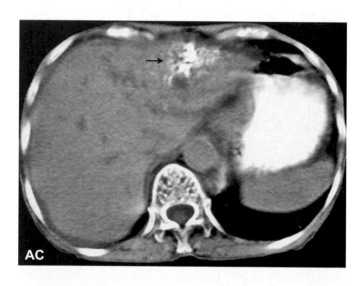
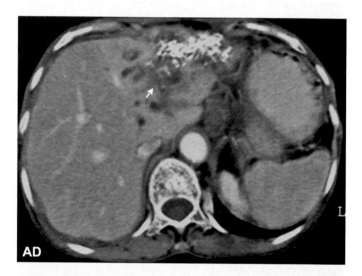
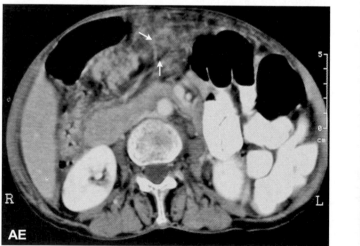
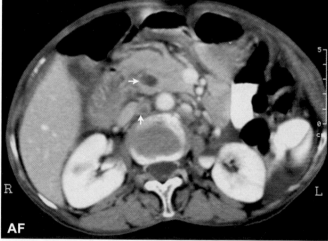

Figs 15.4AC to AF: Hepatic metastasis from mucinous carcinoma of transverse colon

9. Hepatic Metastases 3

Multiple hypodense lesions are seen scattered in the liver. Plain (Fig. 15.4AG), arterial phase (Fig. 15.4AH), portal phase (Fig. 15.4AI) and delayed venous phase (Fig. 15.4AJ).

Multidetector helical CT scanning remains the dominant modality in the evaluation of suspected hepatic metastases and for preoperative planning, treatment monitoring and post treatment follow-up.

The liver is the most common site of metastases that arise from malignancies of gastrointestinal tract, breast, lung, pancreas and melanoma. On CT scans, the appearance of metastatic disease of the liver depends on the vascularity of the tumor compared to the normal liver parenchyma. Larger tumors may have central low attenuation from necrosis or cystic degeneration as well as calcifications. Hypovascular lesions such as metastases from colorectal adenocarcinoma are best detected during the portal venous phase of liver enhancement.

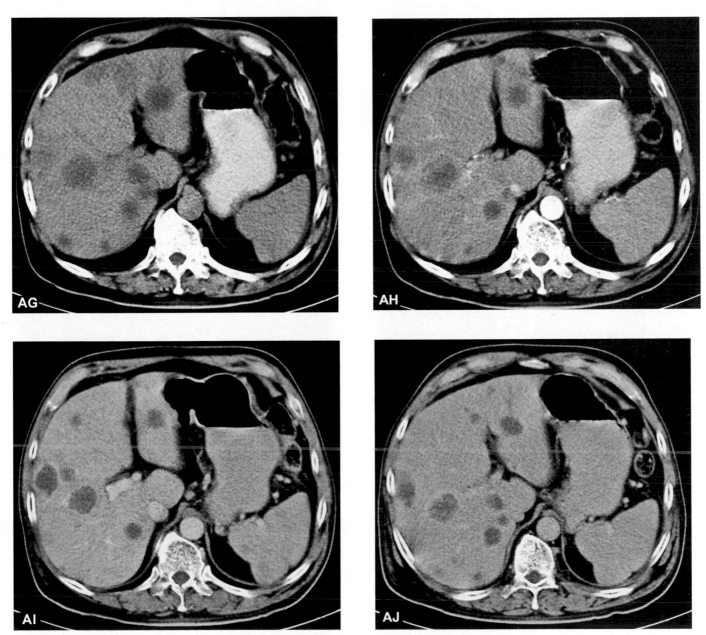

Figs 15.4AG to AJ: Hepatic metastases

10. Hepatic Metastasis 4

Abdominal CT images in various phases of contrast study. Plain scan (Fig. 15.4AK), arterial phase (Fig. 15.4AL), portal phase (Fig. 15.4AM), venous phase (Fig. 15.4AN), delayed phase (Fig. 15.4AO).

Enlarged liver shows multiple round hypodense non enhancing metastatic lesions in both the lobes. Those of which are more hypodense in center indicate onset of necrosis. The primary remained unknown.

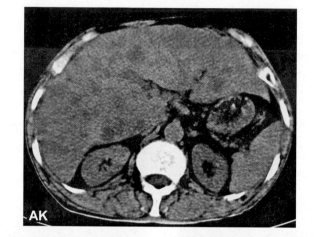

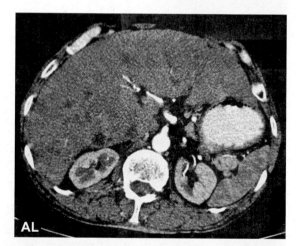

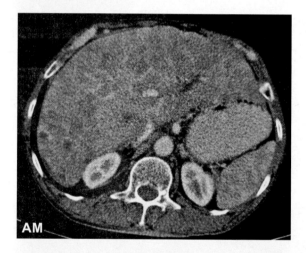

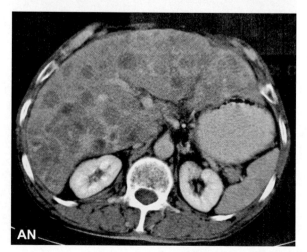

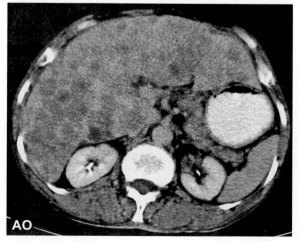

Figs 15.4AK to AO: Hepatic metastases

11. Regenerating Hepatic Nodule (Figs 15.4AP to AR)

Regenerating nodule (arrows) is seen in left lobe of cirrhotic liver. Dilated main portal vein and splenomegaly is present.

Most benign regenerating nodules show hyperattenuation on CT and this could be a tool for differentiating regenerating nodules from tumors.

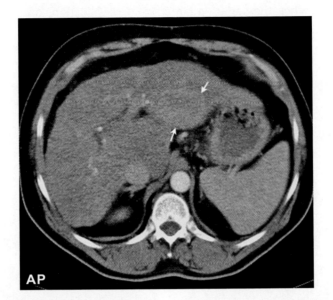

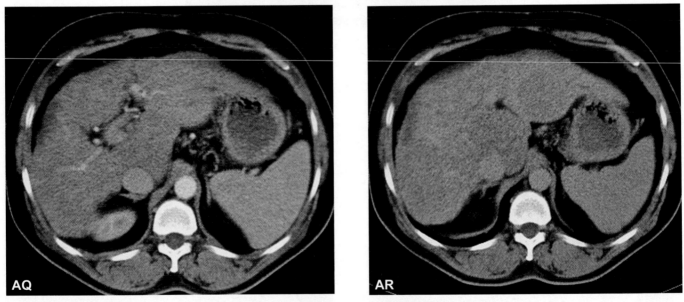

Figs 15.4AP to AR: Regenerating hepatic nodule

12. Simple Hepatic Cyst

Plain and contrast CT abdomen shows a large thin walled hypodense (12 HU) cystic lesion in the liver with smooth margins. No septae or calcifications are seen (Figs 15.4AS and AT).

CT abdomen of another case shows two different simple cysts. Ascitis is present (Fig. 15.4AU).

Liver cysts are benign congenital malformations resulting from isolated aberrant biliary ducts. The cyst contents are usually clear serous fluid. They do not invade biliary or vascular elements but may cause obstruction or compression atrophy of the liver parenchyma when they attain a large size. Complications are hemorrhage, rupture, torsion and infection.

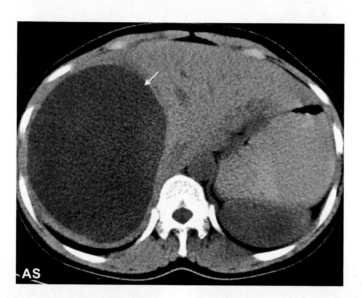

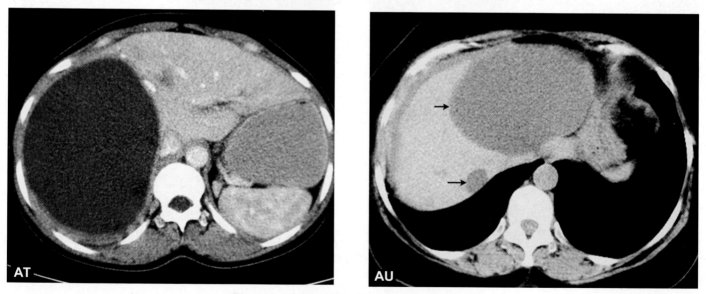

Figs 15.4AS to AU: Simple hepatic cyst

13. Pneumobilia

Pneumobilia i.e. air is seen as hypodensities (arrow) along the course of biliary radicals (Fig. 15.4AV). Stent (arrow) is seen in the CBD having distal end in duodenum (Figs 15.4AW and AX).

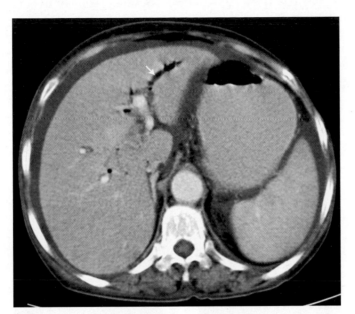

Fig. 15.4AV: Pneumobilia

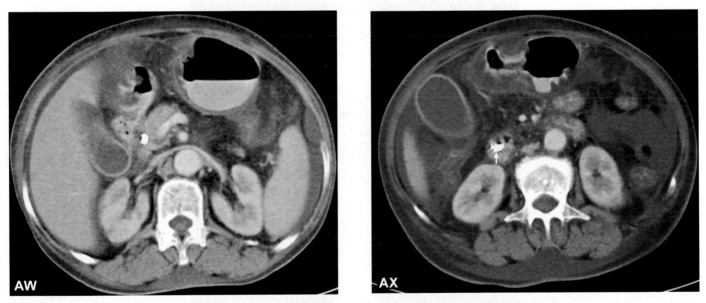

Figs 15.4AW and AX: Stent in the CBD having distal end in duodenum

15.5. Miscellaneous

1. Diffuse Fatty Infiltration of Liver

Plain and contrast enhanced images show diffusely low hepatic parenchymal attenuation value relative to spleen suggesting diffuse fatty infiltration of liver (Figs 15.5A and B). The attenuation of liver is lower than the blood in inferior vena cava on both plain and contrast images.

Fatty infiltration of liver, also known as fatty liver disease or fatty degeneration (FD) is a reversible condition where large vacuoles of triglyceride fat accumulate in liver cells and occurs worldwide in those with excessive alcohol intake and obesity. Morphologically it is difficult to distinguish alcoholic FD from non alcoholic FD and both show microvesicular and macrovesicular fatty changes at different stages.

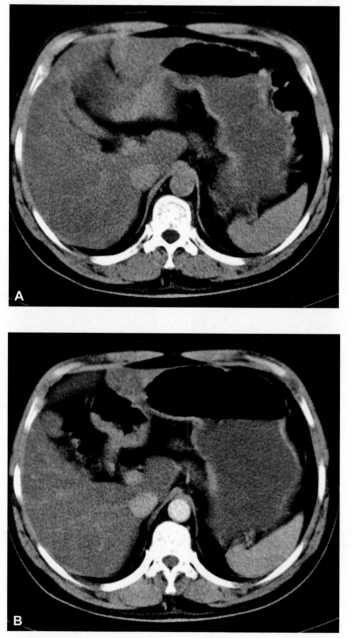

Figs 15.5A and B: Diffuse fatty infiltration of liver

2. Focal Fatty Infiltration Liver

Fat deposition can occur in liver. It can either be focal or diffuse.
- Plain CT shows hypodensity involving entire left lobe (Fig. 15.5C).
- Arterial phase CT shows normal arterial branches traversing lesion (Fig. 15.5D).
- Portal venous phase CT shows enhancement lesser than adjacent liver. Left portal vein is seen coursing through the lesion (Fig. 15.5E).
- Hepatic venous phase CT shows left hepatic vein coursing through the lesion (Fig. 15.5F).

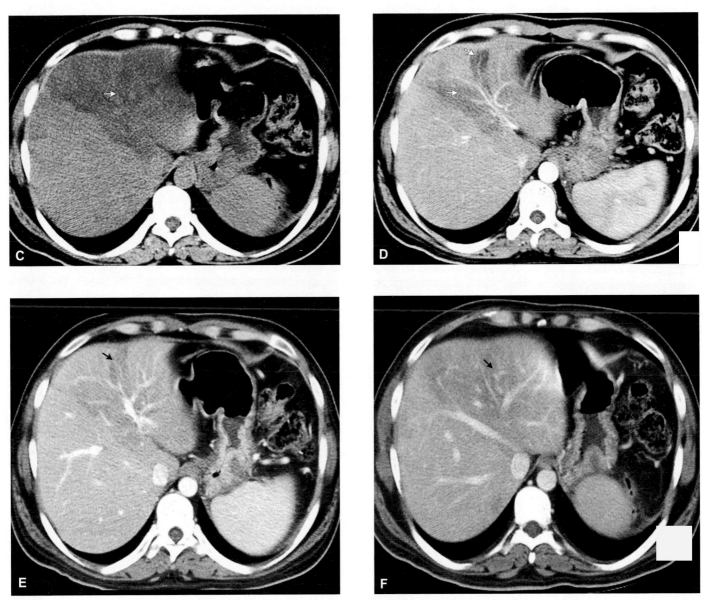

Figs 15.5C to F: Focal fatty infiltration of liver

3. Transient Hepatic Attenuation Difference (THAD)

THAD is an attenuation difference of the liver appearing during bolus-enhanced dynamic CT usually not corresponding to any mass. It is generally seen as an area of high attenuation on the hepatic arterial phase image (Figs 15.5G and H) that returns to normal attenuation on the portal venous phase (Figs 15.5I and J) images.

THADs that are associated with hepatic tumors are generally characteristic of malignant tumors.

However, benign focal lesions, such as hemangiomas, focal nodular hyperplasia, pyogenic abscesses and focal eosinophillic necrosis may accompany THADs.

THAD is not associated with following focal lesions:
1. Portal hypoperfusion due to portal branch compression or thrombosis.
2. Flow diversion caused by arterioportal shunt.
3. Anomalous blood supply.
4. Inflammation of the biliary vessels or adjacent organs.

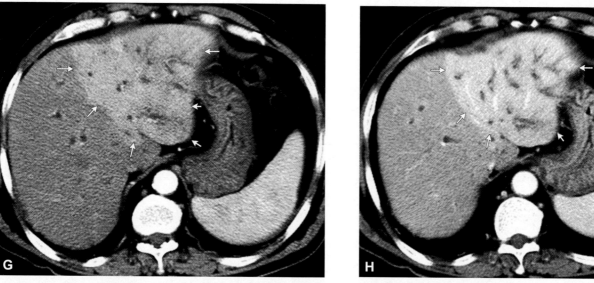

Figs 15.5G and H: Transient hepatic attenuation difference in arterial phase image

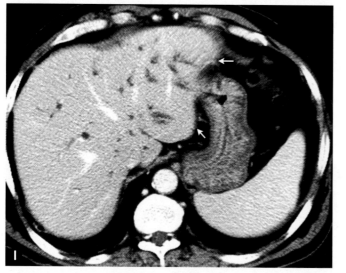

Figs 15.5I and J: Transient hepatic attenuation difference in portal venous phase

4. Liver Cirrhosis

Shrunken liver with nodular contour, esophageal and spleno-portal collaterals (arrow) are seen along with massive ascites indicating portal hypertension (Figs 15.5K and L).

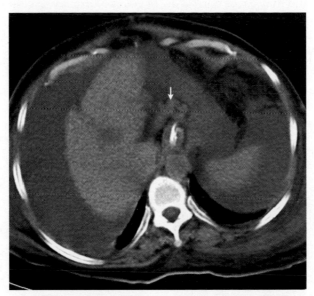

Fig. 15.5K: Liver cirrhosis and collaterals

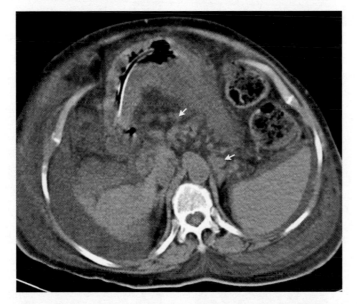

Fig. 15.5L: Ascites and collaterals in cirrhosis of liver

5. Gaucher's Disease

Gaucher's Infiltration in Liver

Deposition of foamy cells in the liver and spleen occurs commonly in Gaucher's disease. Focal deposition of these cells may sometimes be seen in perivenular location. These deposits are seen as hypodense minimally enhancing areas predominantly at liver periphery and may cause narrowing of veins. Normal vessels are usually seen traversing through these areas.

- Contrast CT in arterial phase showing hypodense area of Gaucher cell infiltration (Fig. 15.5M).
- CT image shows narrowing of veins in the region of cell deposition (Fig. 15.5N).
- CT images show vessels traversing the lesion (Figs 15.5O and P).

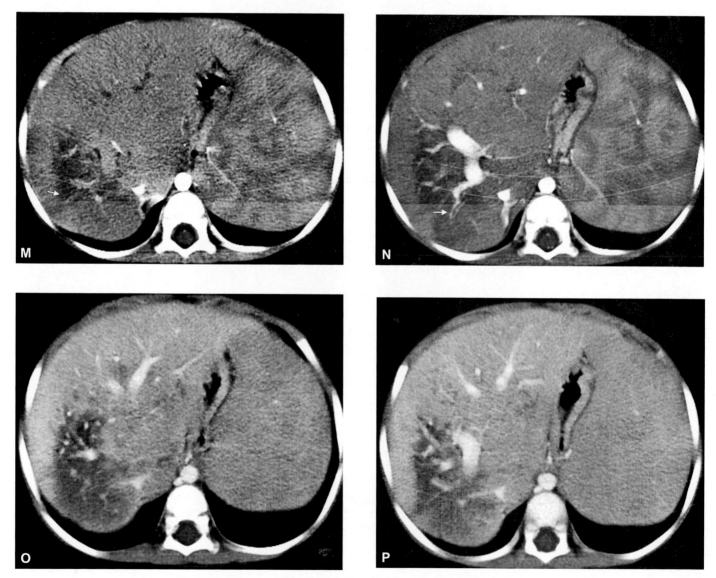

Figs 15.5M to P: CT shows Gaucher's disease infiltrating liver

6. Portal Vein Thrombosis

No fill up of contrast is seen in left branch of portal vein indicating thrombosis (Fig. 15.5Q).

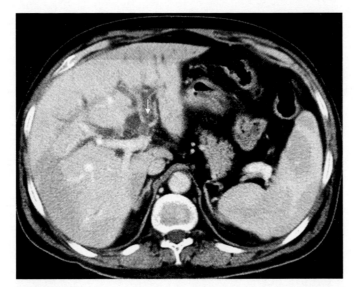

Fig. 15.5Q: CT shows thrombosed left branch of portal vein

16. BILIARY SYSTEM

16.1 Infective-Inflammatory

1. Gallstones

- Plain CT scan shows a large stone as a hyperdense (superior arrow) structure in the lumen of gallbladder. Common bile duct is distended (inferior arrow) (Fig. 16.1A).
- Plain CT showing two gallstones as hyperdensities in the lumen. Ascites is also present (Fig. 16.1B).

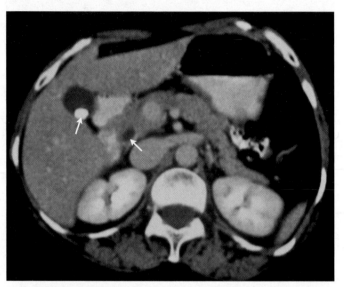

Fig. 16.1A: Plain CT shows a gallstone and distended common bile duct

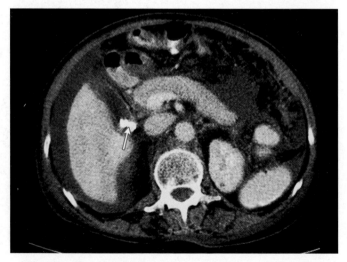

Fig. 16.1B: Plain CT shows gallstones and ascites

2. Acute Calculus Cholecystitis

CT images shows optimally distended gallbladder with multiple hyperdense calculi and thickened wall especially in the region of fundus associated with soft tissue stranding in the adjacent greater omental fat in a case of cholelithiasis with acute cholecystitis (Figs 16.1C to E).

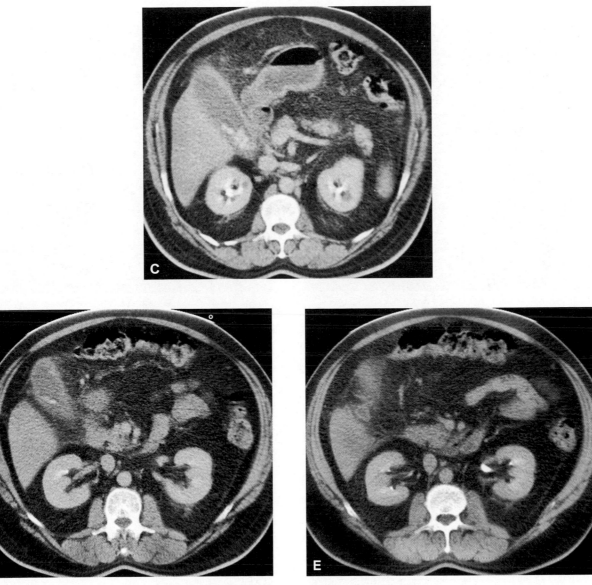

Figs 16.1C to E: Acute calculus cholecystitis

3. Acute Acalculus Cholecystitis

Six mm thickened edematous gallbladder wall reveals nodular enhancement with soft tissue strands into adjacent fat (Figs 16.1F to I).

Acute cholecystitis in the appropriate clinical setting on CT scan present with gallbladder distention, gallbladder wall thickening > 3 mm and pericholecystic abnormality (either fluid or abnormal fat strands).

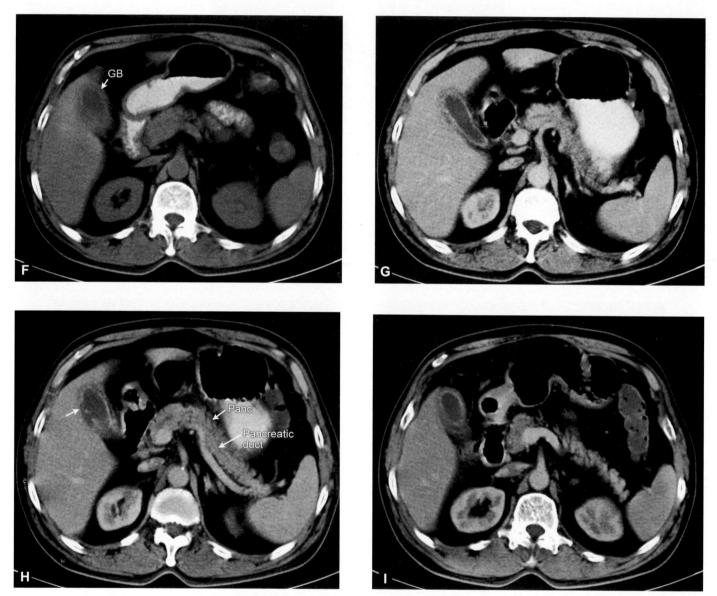

Figs 16.1F to I: Acute acalculus cholecystitis

4. Cholelithiasis in a Porcelain Gallbladder

- Plain CT abdomen shows hyperdense appearance in the dependent part of gallbladder due to multiple small calculi (Fig. 16.1J). There is calcification of the wall of the gallbladder (Porcelain gallbladder).
- In right lateral decubitus position the calculi have shifted to the now dependent position (Fig. 16.1K).
- Contrast CT shows no enhancement of walls of gallbladder. This rules out cholecystitis (Fig. 16.1L).
  CT scan is less valuable in visualizing gallstones, as bile and stones are isodense on CT scan and difficult to distinguish.
It is estimated that only 60% of gallstones are detected by CT scan.

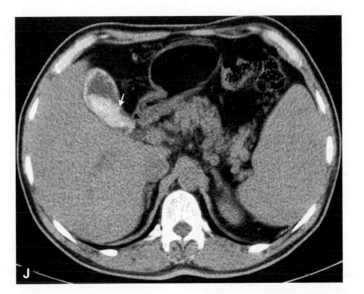

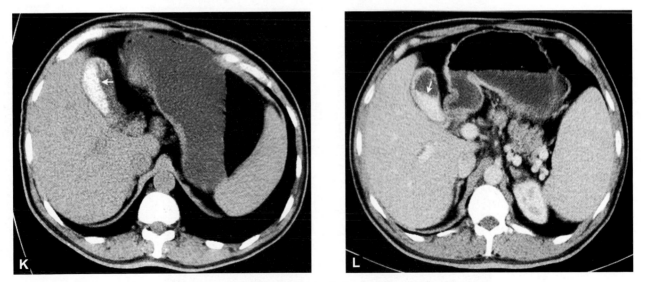

Figs 16.1J to L: Cholelithiasis in a porcelain gallbladder

5. Cholecystitis

CT scan of different patients show
- Calculus cholecystitis (Fig. 16.1M)
- Acalculus cholecystitis (Fig. 16.1N)
- Emphysematous cholecystitis (Fig. 16.1O)
- Cholecystitis due to worm infestation (Fig. 16.1P)
- Obstructive biliopathy due to worm infestation (Fig. 16.1Q).

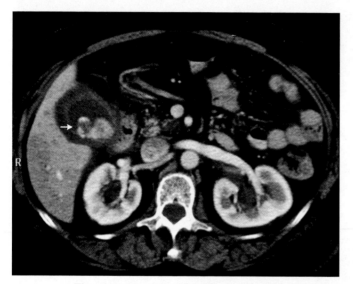

Fig. 16.1M: Calculus cholecystitis

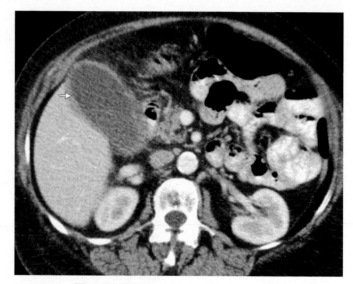

Fig. 16.1N: Acalculus cholecystitis

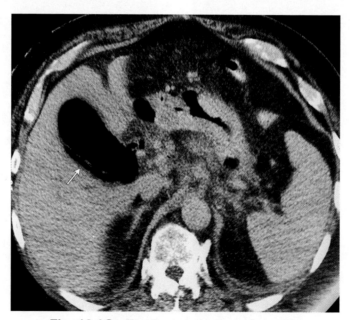

Fig. 16.1O: Emphysematous cholecystitis

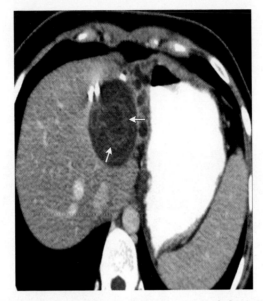

Fig. 16.1P: Cholecystitis due to worm infestation

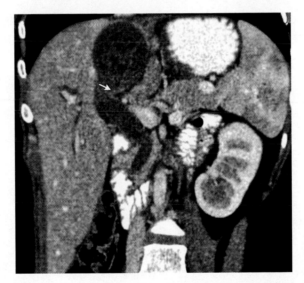

Fig. 16.1Q: Obstructive biliopathy due to worm infestation

16.2 Miscellaneous

1. Common Bile Duct Calculus (Figs 16.2A and B)

Obstructive biliopathy due to a stone impacted in extrahepatic common bile duct causing dilatation of proximal CBD and intrahepatic biliary radicals.

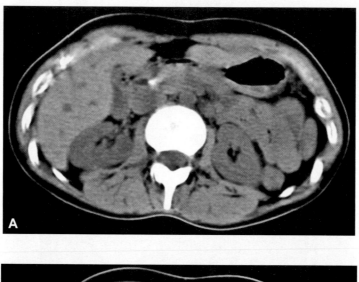

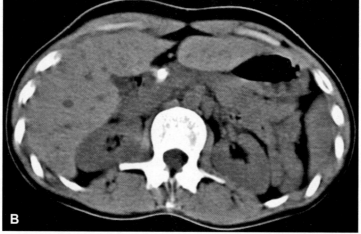

Figs 16.2A and B: Common bile duct calculus

2. Obstructive Calculus Biliopathy

Figures 16.2C to F are plain CT images and Figures 16.2G to H are post-contrast images.

Massive dilatation of intrahepatic biliary radicals and CBD is seen secondary to an intraluminal calculus in distal CBD.

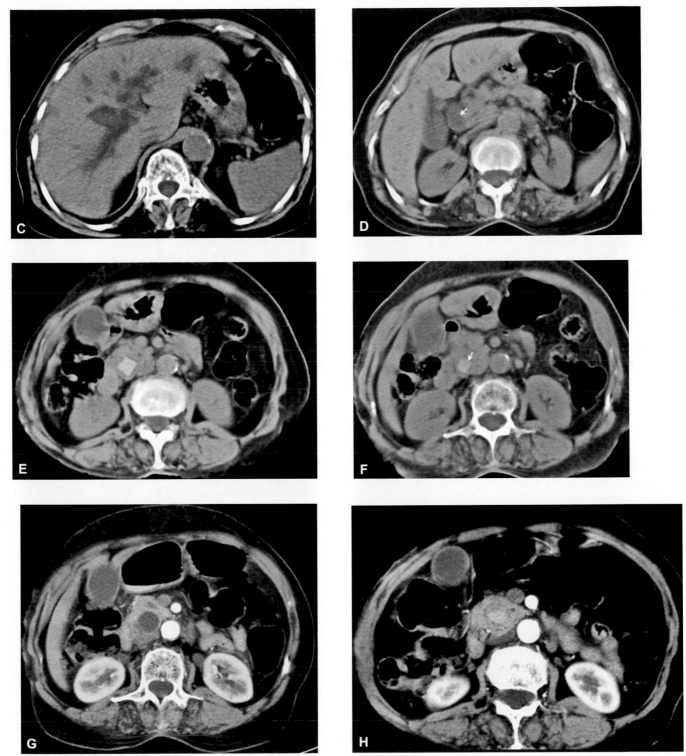

Figs 16.2C to H: Distal CBD calculus causing obstructive biliopathy

16.3 Neoplastic

1. Biliary Cystadenoma

CT images of biliary cystadenoma (phase wise) plain (Fig. 16.3A), arterial (Fig. 16.3B), venous (Fig. 16.3C) and parenchymal (Fig. 16.3D); show ill-defined nonenhancing hypodense lesion with thick enhancing septae without any solid component or calcification.

It is a rare biliary ductal neoplasm, common in young women. Low density intrahepatic multilocular mass is seen on plain CT scan. Solid enhancing mural nodule, papillary projections and presence of calcification favor diagnosis of cystadenocarcinoma.

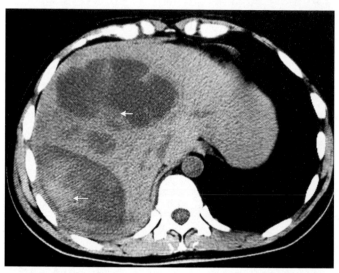

Fig. 16.3A: Plain CT image in biliary cystadenoma

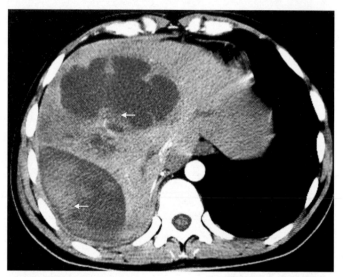

Fig. 16.3B: Arterial phase image of biliary cystadenoma

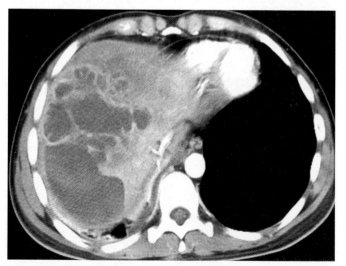

Fig. 16.3C: Venous phase image of biliary cystadenoma

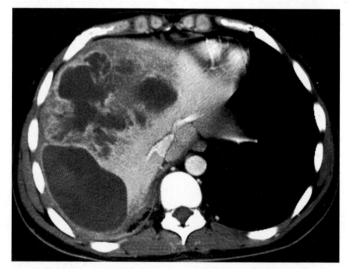

Fig. 16.3D: Parenchymal phase image of biliary cystadenoma

2. Cholangiocarcinoma

The intra and extrahepatic biliary tract and the gallbladder are distended. An enhancing solid mass is seen in the distal end of common bile duct. The biopsy confirmed it as cholangiocarcinoma. Figures 16.3E to G show cholangiocarcinoma causing obstructive biliopathy.

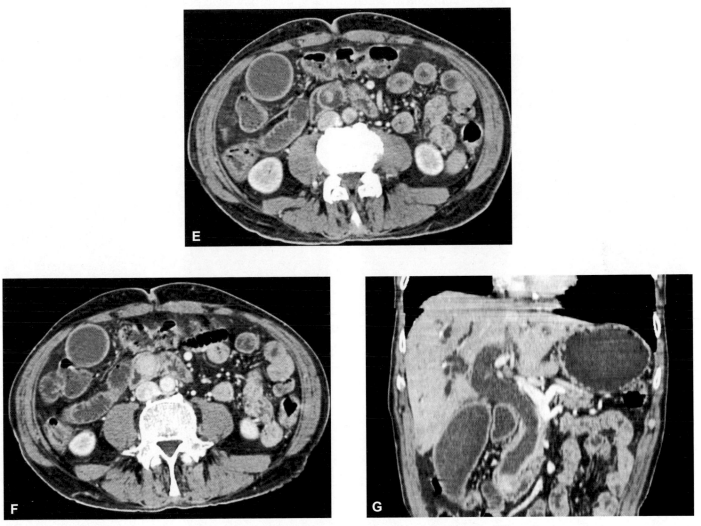

Figs 16.3E to G: Cholangiocarcinoma causing obstructive biliopathy

3. Operable Hilar Cholangiocarcinoma

- Venous phase CT shows patent left portal vein and dilated intrahepatic biliary radicals (Fig. 16.3H). No mass is seen.
- Delayed phase CT shows a vague minimally enhancing mass that was subsequently proven to be a cholangiocarcinoma (Fig. 16.3I).
- Contrast CT in another patient shows dilated intrahepatic biliary radicals in left lobe (Fig. 16.3J). No obvious mass is seen.
- Delayed CT in same patient shows subtle enhancement in mass and thrombosed portal vein (Fig. 16.3K).

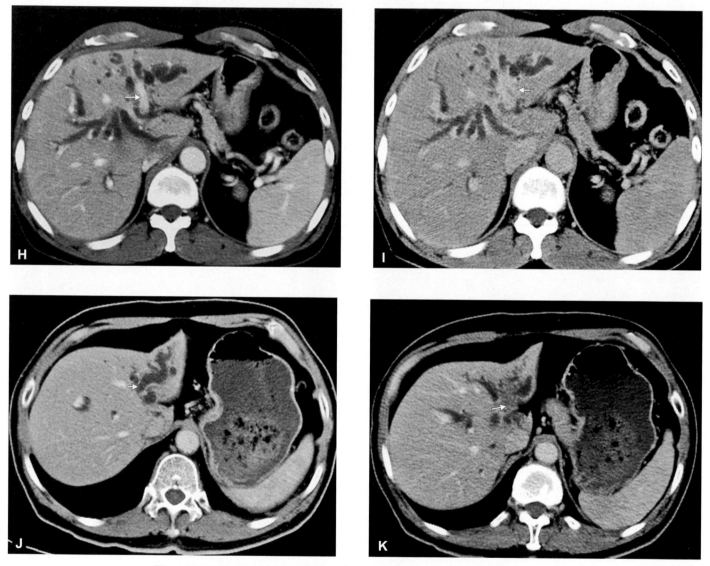

Figs 16.3H to K: Cholangiocarcinoma causing obstructive biliopathy

4. Intrahepatic Cholangiocarcinoma

50 years old female had progressive jaundice since 2 months.

CT scan shows a hypodense peripherally enhancing lesion in arterial phase (Fig. 16.3L) with gradual centripetal filling in on delayed scans (Fig. 16.3L to 16.3O).

It is thus a large, irregular, hypo attenuating mass with thin or thick band like contrast enhancement around the tumor at the early phase and progressive and concentric filling of contrast material in the later phase.

This is explained by slow diffusion into the interstitial spaces of the tumor.

Fibrotic component within this type of cholangiocarcinoma also contributes to the delayed tumoral contrast enhancement.

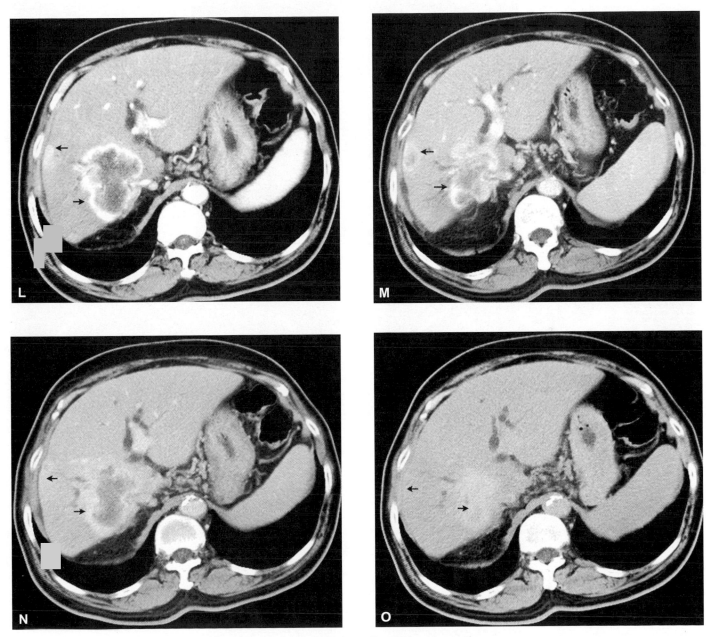

Figs 16.3L to O: Intrahepatic cholangiocarcinoma

17. PANCREAS

17.1 Normal Pancreas

- Plain and contrast CT shows normal pancreas. Uncinate process is shown by horizontal arrow (Figs 17.1A and B).
- CT shows thinned out pancreas in an elderly patient. Splenic vein is shown by horizontal arrow (Fig. 17.1C).

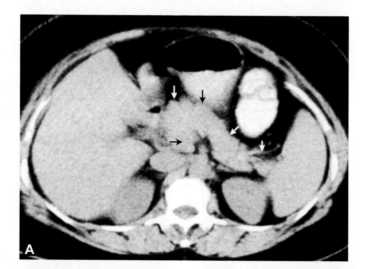

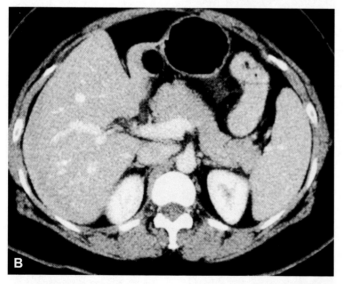
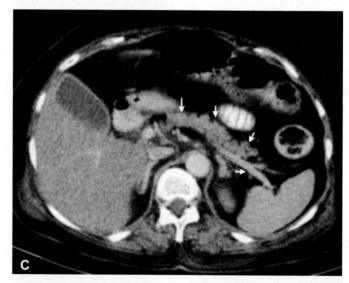

Figs 17.1A to C: Normal pancreas

17.2 Infective Inflammatory

1. Atrophic Pancreatitis

Plain CT show reduced parenchymal bulk of pancreas with diffuse punctate calcifications (white flecks) within it (Fig. 17.2A). No overt signs of acute inflammation are present. Findings are consistent with chronic atrophic calcific pancreatitis.

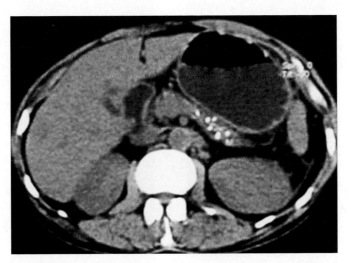

Fig. 17.2A: Chronic atrophic calcific pancreatitis

2. Acute Pancreatitis

Contrast CT shows bilateral pleural effusion and loculated peripancreatic and intra-abdominal fluid collections (Fig. 17.2B). Pancreas itself is irregular, heterogeneous, swollen and associated with fat stranding (Fig. 17.2C).

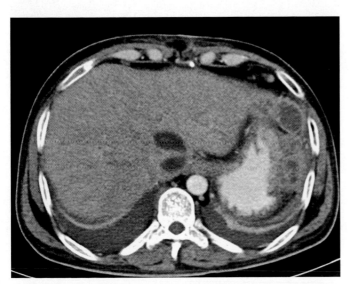

Fig. 17.2B: Bilateral pleural effusion and loculated intra-abdominal fluid collections

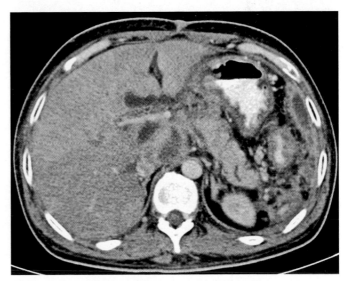

Fig. 17.2C: Acute pancreatitis

3. Acute Edematous Pancreatitis

- Bilateral mild pleural effusion (Fig. 17.2D).
- Thin walled fluid collections in region of stomach bed, anterior to pancreas and extending inferior to tail of pancreas and anterior to Gerota's fascia. The pancreas is bulky and edematous (Figs 17.2E to G).

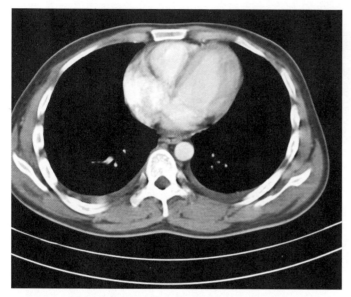

Fig. 17.2D: Bilateral pleural effusion

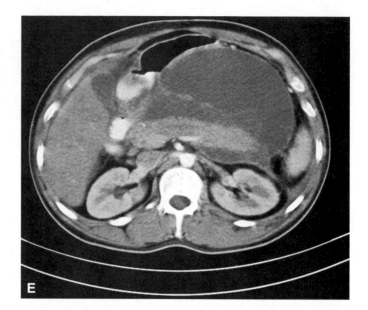

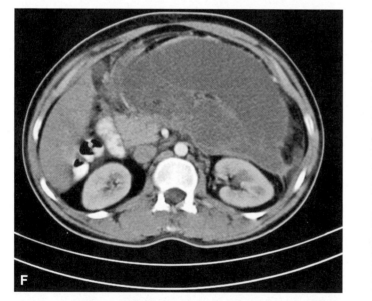

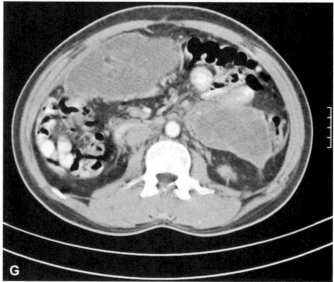

Figs 17.2E to G: The pancreas is bulky and edematous. Adjacent fluid collections are also seen

4. Pseudocyst of Pancreas

- Contrast CT abdomen shows a hypodense cyst with thick enhancing walls in the lesser sac anterior to body and tail of pancreas which are barely perceptible (Fig. 17.2H).
- Contrast CT abdomen of another patient shows a large pseudocyst lying anterior to the thinned out body and tail of pancreas and pushing the bulky pancreatic head posterolaterally (Fig. 17.2I).

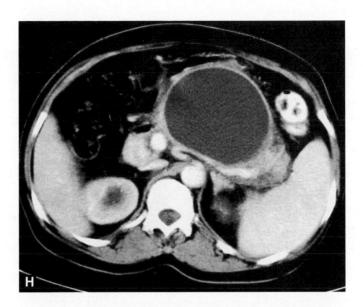

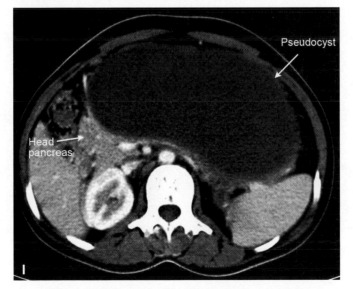

Figs 17.2H and I: Pseudocyst of pancreas

5. Pancreatic Inflammation with Pseudocyst and Psoas Abscess

- Pancreas shows few hypodense non enhancing areas suggestive of infective foci (Fig. 17.2J).
- Hypodense collection with thick walls and minimal enhancement towards the tail of pancreas. This is an infected pancreatic pseudocyst (Fig. 17.2K).
- Images show another retroperitoneal hypodense collection having intraluminal air and enhancing walls. It is located in the anterior part of left psoas muscle and is placed lateral to ureter. Minimal adjacent fat stranding is present (Figs 17.2L and M).

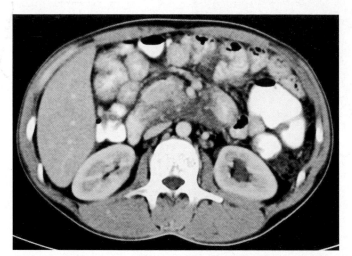

Fig. 17.2J: Pancreatic inflammation

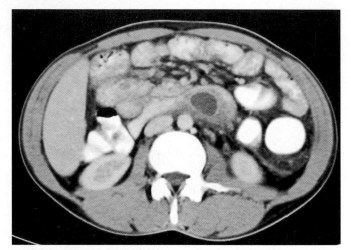

Fig. 17.2K: Pseudocyst of pancreas

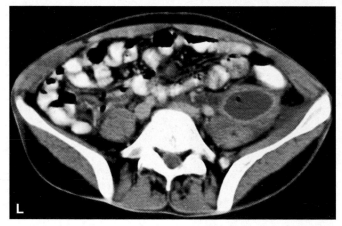

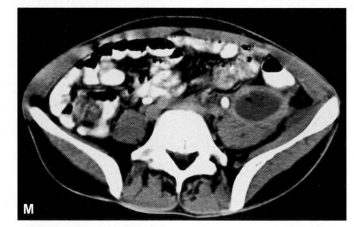

Figs 17.2L and M: Psoas abscess in the same patient

17.3 Trauma

Transection of Pancreas

Image shows complete transection of the neck of pancreas in a patient of blunt trauma abdomen (Fig. 17.3).

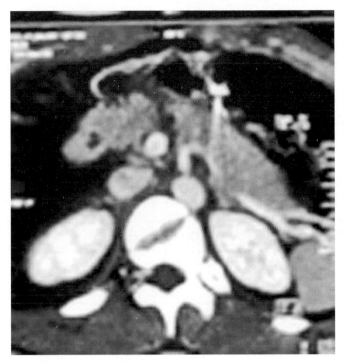

Fig. 17.3: Transection of the neck of pancreas

17.4 Carcinoma Pancreas (Figs 17.4A to D)

Large mixed attenuation lesion in the region of head and body of pancreas. An enhancing solid mass is seen within a large cystic component. The mass displaces the stomach and liver laterally and extends to the anterior abdominal wall.

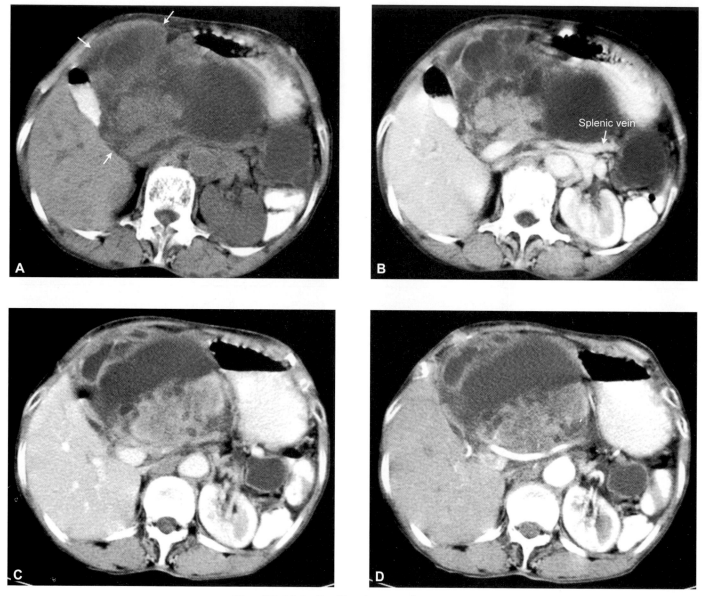

Figs 17.4A to D: Carcinoma of pancreas

17.5 Miscellaneous

1. Focal Fatty Infiltration Pancreas

Pre and post contrast images show presence of focal fatty infiltration in the head of pancreas with no mass effect (Figs 17.5A and B).

Focal fatty infiltration of the pancreas is most prominent in the head of the pancreas and seen as a region of decreased attenuation on computed tomography. CT helps to differentiate between focal fatty infiltration and actual pancreatic tumors.

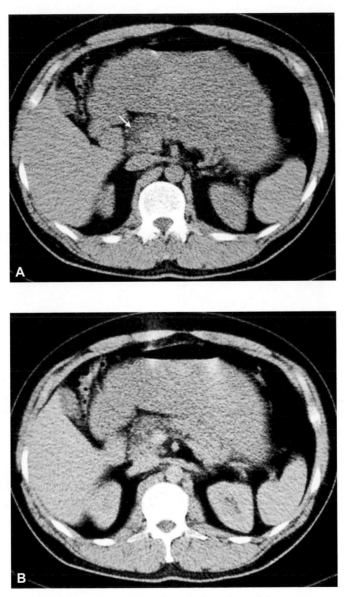

Figs 17.5A and B: Focal fatty infiltration of the pancreas

2. Pancreatic Duct Calcification and Dilatation

- CT showing necklace of pancreatic duct calcification involving the body and tail (Fig. 17.5C).
- CT shows dilated pancreatic duct in another patient having terminal obstruction due obstructive biliopathy (Fig. 17.5D).

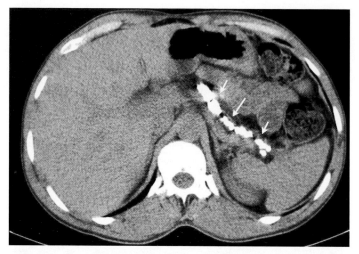

Fig. 17.5C: Pancreatic duct calcification

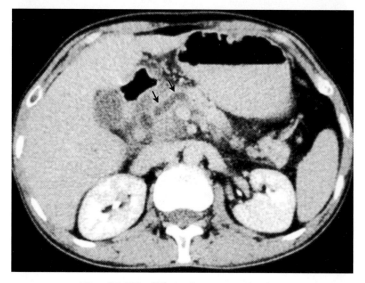

Fig. 17.5D: Dilated pancreatic duct

18. SPLEEN

18.1 Splenunculus

Figures 18.1A and B plain and contrast CT images show a small round structure medial to spleen, the splenunculus. It has same density as spleen in plain and contrast images.

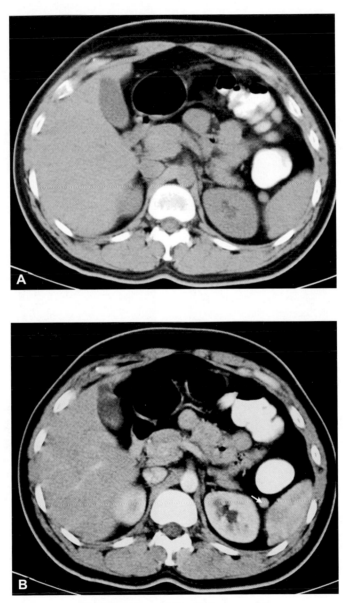

Figs 18.1A and B: Splenunculus

18.2 Splenic Trauma

Spleen is the most frequently injured abdominal organ.
Mirvis et al. Radiology 1989;171:34 gave the following CT-based criteria and severity grading of blunt splenic injury.

CT grade   I: Capsular avulsion, laceration(s), or sub-capsular hematoma < 1 cm diameter (Fig. 18.2A)

CT grade   II: Laceration(s) 1–3 cm deep, central/sub-capsular hematoma 1–3 cm diameter (Fig. 18.2B)

CT grade   III: Laceration(s) 3–10 cm deep, central/sub-capsular hematoma >3 cm diameter (Fig. 18.2C)

CT grade   IV: Laceration(s) >10 cm deep, central/sub-capsular hematoma >10 cm diameter, massive lobar maceration or devascularization (Fig. 18.2D)

CT grade   V: Bilobar tissue maceration or revitalization (Fig. 18.2E)

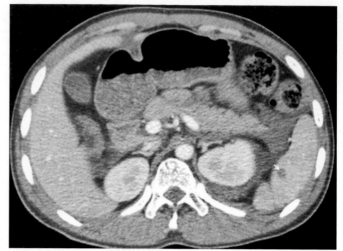

Fig. 18.2A: CT grade I splenic injury

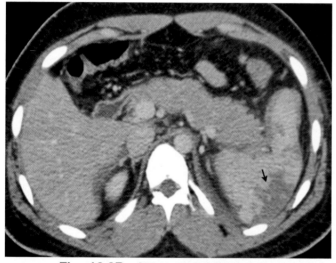

Fig. 18.2B: CT grade II splenic injury

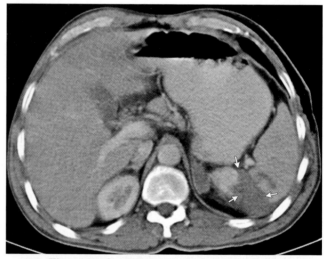

Fig. 18.2C: CT grade III splenic injury

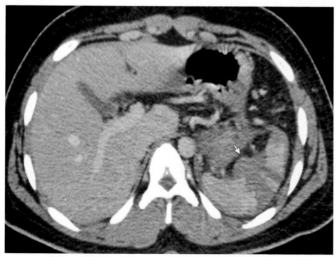

Fig. 18.2D: CT grade IV: Splenic injury

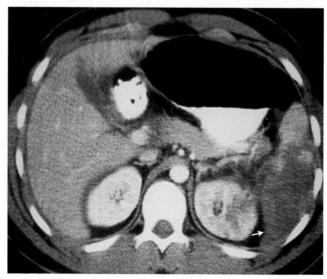

Fig. 18.2E: CT grade V: Splenic injury

18.3. Trauma

- CT shows non-enhanced lacerated splenic parenchyma and enhancing normal parenchyma (Fig. 18.3A).
- Caudal section shows the perisplenic hematoma (Fig. 18.3B).
- Post-splenectomy CT shows splenic fossa occupied by bowel loops (Fig. 18.3C).

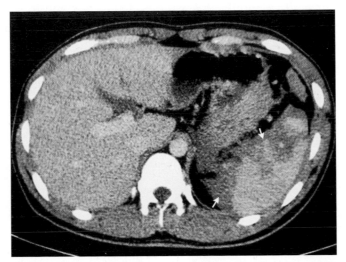

Fig. 18.3A: Plain CT shows lacerated splenic parenchyma

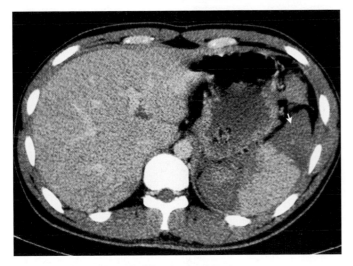

Fig. 18.3B: Plain CT shows perisplenic hematoma

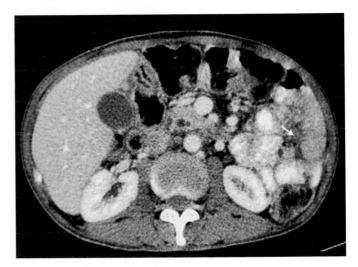

Fig. 18.3C: Plain CT shows splenic fossa occupied by bowel loops

19. ADRENALS

19.1 Adrenal Adenoma

Pre and post contrast images show a nonenhancing, solid, well-defined nonfunctioning left adrenal adenoma and normal appearing right adrenal (Figs 19.1A and B). This was detected incidentally.

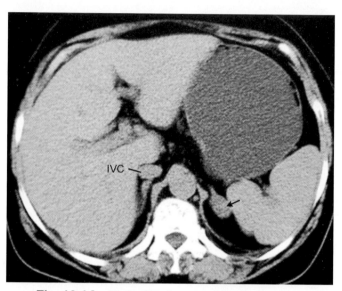

Fig. 19.1A: Plain CT shows adrenal adenoma

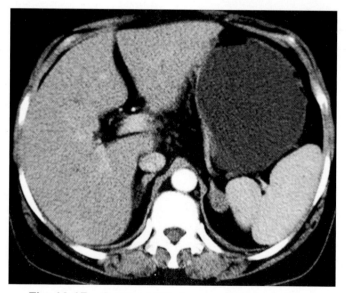

Fig. 19.1B: Contrast CT shows adrenal adenoma

19.2 Adrenal Leiomyosarcoma (Figs 19.2A to D)

Mass lesion is seen superomedial to left kidney in the region of adrenal gland. Fat planes between the mass, kidney, spleen and pancreas is intact. Mild enhancement is seen more in the periphery. No areas of necrosis or calcification seen within the lesion. Biochemical evaluation excluded a functional tumor of the adrenal gland. Histopathology confirmed adrenal leiomyosarcoma.

The diagnosis of leiomyosarcomas of the adrenal is one of exclusion and involves preoperative radiological and biochemical evaluation to exclude functional tumors of the adrenal gland. Aggressive surgical resection is associated with improved survival.

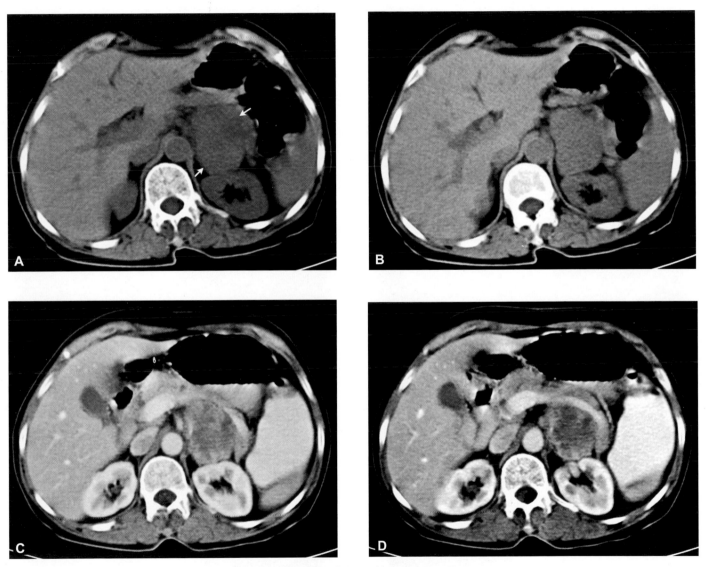

Figs 19.2A to D: Adrenal leiomyosarcoma

20. MISCELLANEOUS

20.1 Ascites

- Moderate ascites (Fig. 20.1A).
- Ascites with floating bowel loops (Figs 20.1B and C).
- Massive ascites (Fig. 20.1D)

   Ascites is a frequent finding on CT. Causes of ascites include congestive heart failure, hypoalbuminemia, cirrhosis, inflammation and neoplasm. In most cases the attenuation value of ascites is that of water, measuring 0-10 HU.

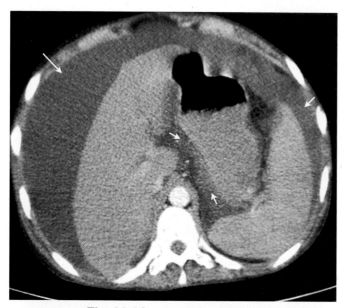

Fig. 20.1A: Moderate ascites

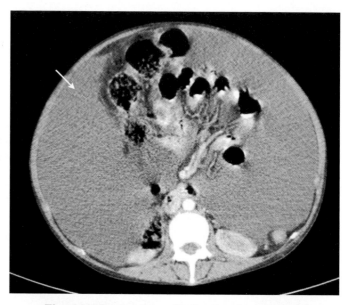

Fig. 20.1B: Ascites with floating bowel loops

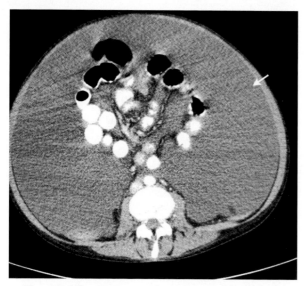

Fig. 20.1C: Ascites with floating bowel loops

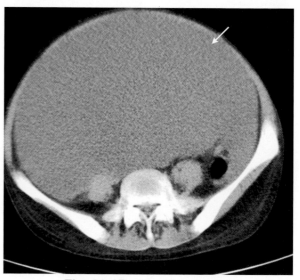

Fig. 20.1D: Massive ascites

20.2 Epigastric Hernia

Figures 20.2A and B CT images show a small out pouching of mesenteric fat with peritoneum through a small rent in anterior abdominal wall muscle layer into the epigastric soft tissues. No bowel loops have herniated.

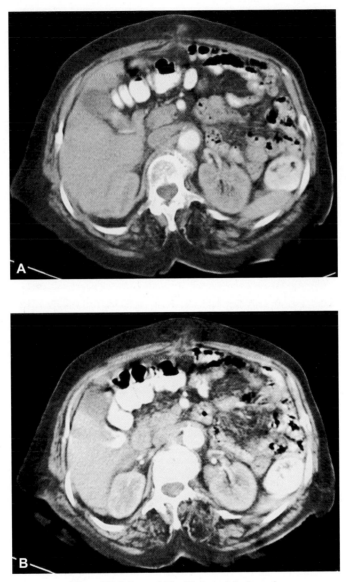

Figs 20.2A and B: Epigastric hernia

20.3 Lymphoma

Contrast CT abdomen shows multiple non enhancing round lesions in liver, spleen, pancreas and kidneys (Fig. 20.3).

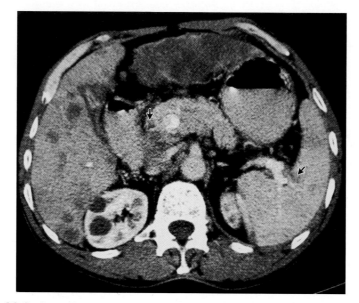

Fig. 20.3: Lymphoma deposits in liver, spleen, pancreas and kidneys

20.4 Portal Hypertension 1

Figures 20.4A and B are plain images and Figures 20.4C and D are post-contrast CT images in the portal phase of acquisition. Dilatation of splenic and portal veins is seen in association with splenomegaly and congestive hepatomegaly. Massive ascites and bilateral pleural effusion are noted. No varices are seen.

Portal hypertension is the build-up of pressure in the portal vein. Normally, the pressure is low compared with the arterial pressure, but slightly above the pressure in the other veins in the body system. The most common cause of portal hypertension is liver disease.

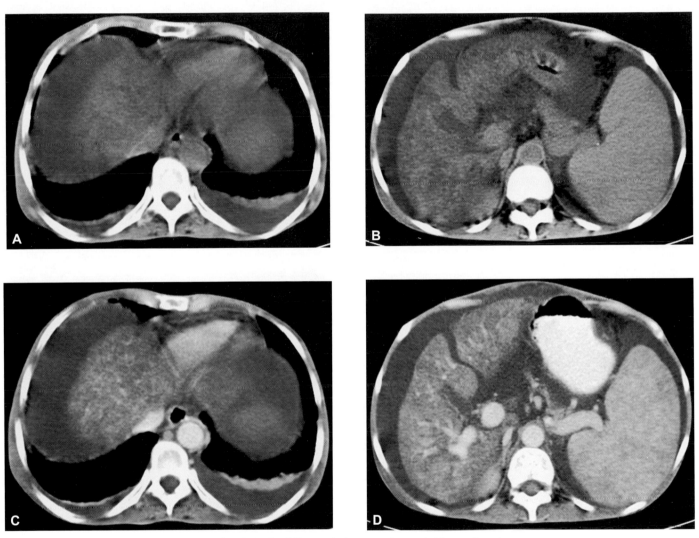

Figs 20.4A to D: Visceral changes in portal hypertension

20.5 Portal Hypertension 2

- CT shows esophageal varices (Fig. 20.5A).
- Shows cavernous transformation of portal vein (Fig. 20.5B).
- Shows splenic vein thromboses (Fig. 20.5C).
- Massive hepatosplenomegaly (Fig. 20.5D).

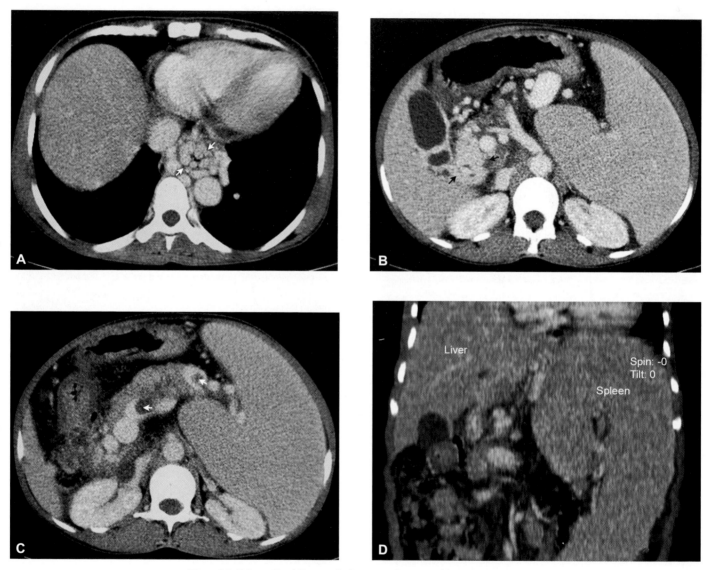

Figs 20.5A to D: Visceral changes in portal hypertension

20.6 Portal Hypertension 3

- Scout image shows massive splenomegaly (Fig. 20.6A).
- Splenomegaly and left pleural effusion (Fig. 20.6B).
- Splenomegaly and ascites (Fig. 20.6C).
- Spleno-renal collaterals (Fig. 20.6D).

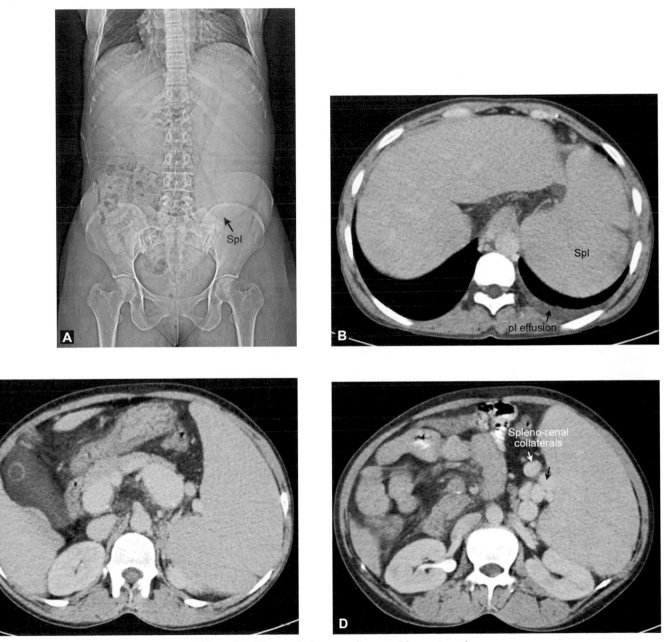

Figs 20.6A to D: Visceral changes in portal hypertension

Section 4

Genitourinary System

- Normal
- Congenital Disorders
- Trauma
- Infective-Inflammatory
- Neoplastic
- Miscellaneous

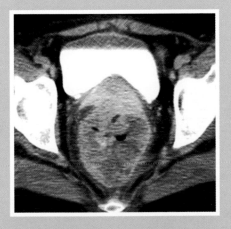
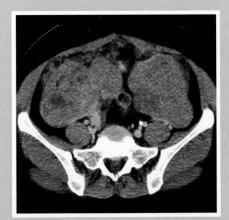
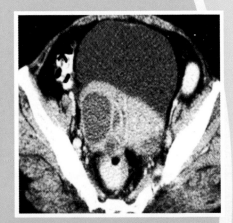

21. NORMAL

21.1 Normal Renal Anatomy

Figures 21.1A and B show normal renal anatomy and renal arteries respectively.

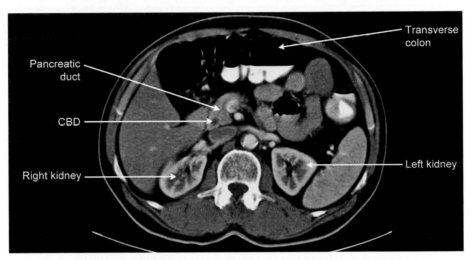

Fig. 21.1A: Normal renal anatomy

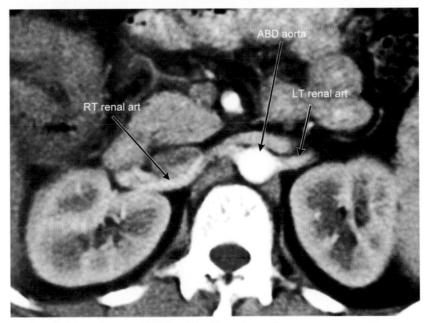

Fig. 21.1B: Renal arteries

Axial CT Sections of Male Pelvis (Figs 21.1C and 21.1D)

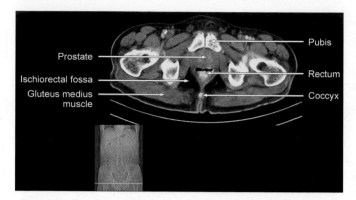

Fig. 21.1C: CT section of male pelvis through prostate

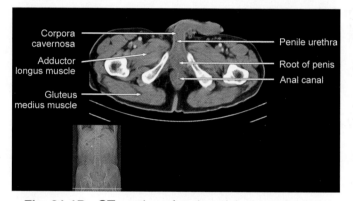

Fig. 21.1D: CT section of male pelvis through penis

Axial CT Sections of Female Pelvis (Figs 21.1E to 21.1I)

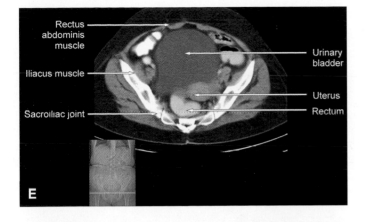

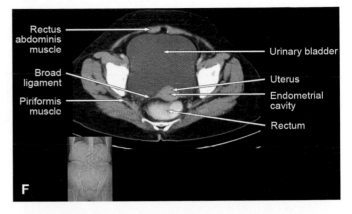

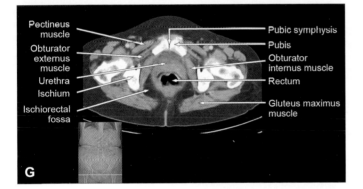

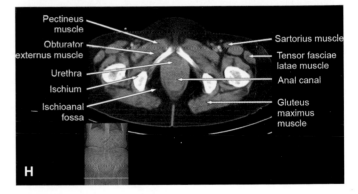

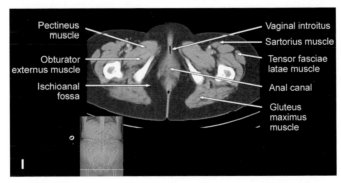

Figs 21.1E to I: Axial CT sections of female pelvis

21.2 Normal Seminal Vesicle

CT pelvis shows normal seminal vesicles as moustache-shaped structures (Fig. 21.2).

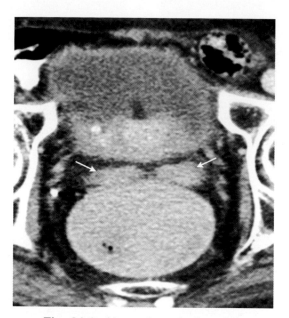

Fig. 21.2: Normal seminal vesicle

22. CONGENITAL DISORDERS

22.1 Renal Aplasia

Figures 22.1A (plain) and B (contrast) CT images show absence of left kidney. The left renal fossa is occupied by intestinal loops.

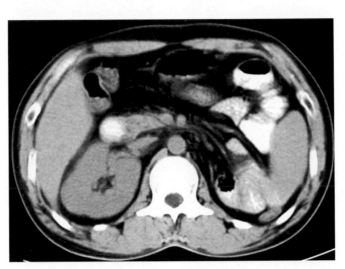

Fig. 22.1A: Plain CT image shows absence of left kidney

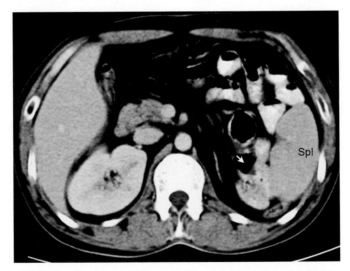

Fig. 22.1B: Contrast CT image shows absence of left kidney

22.2 Pelvi Ureteric Junction (PUJ) Obstruction 1

Gross hydronephrosis in left kidney with thinned out renal cortex reduced to 3 mm in thickness, pelvis is dilated and smoothly narrows down (Figs 22.2A to D).

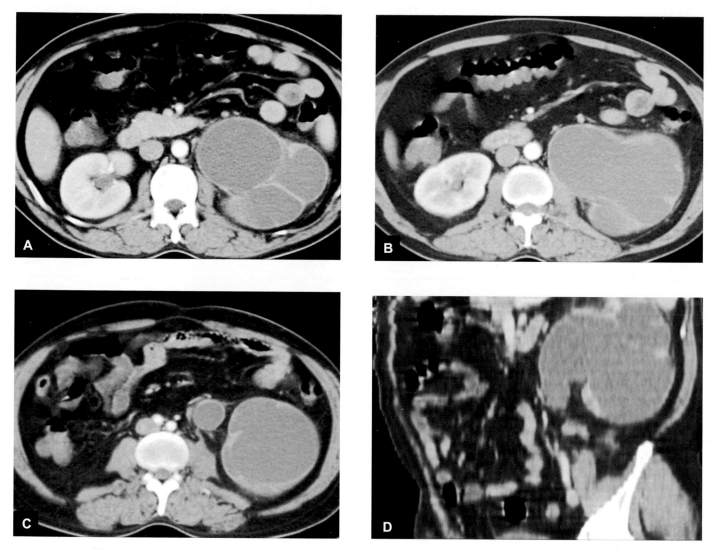

Figs 22.2A to D: Gross hydronephrosis in left kidney due to long standing PUJ obstruction

22.3 Pelvi Ureteric Junction (PUJ) Obstruction 2

- CT abdomen shows renal arteries and enhancement of left renal parenchyma. Right renal parenchyma does not show any enhancement except the capsule due to differential blood flow (Fig. 22.3A).
- Delayed CT shows contrast excretion in left renal pelvis and ureter. No contrast is excreted in the right renal pelvis which shows ballooning and sudden narrowing (Fig. 22.3B).
- CT shows excretion in left ureter. No contrast is seen in right ureter (Fig. 22.3C).
- Coronal image shows difference in size and excretion by the kidneys (Fig. 22.3D).

Non-excreting right kidney secondary to congenital pelvi-ureteic junction obstruction causing renal parenchymal damage.

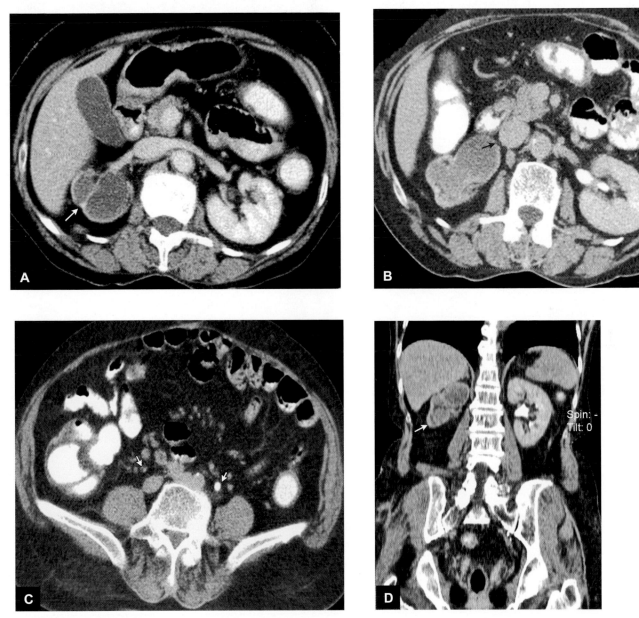

Figs 22.3A to D: Poorly excreting right kidney secondary to congenital pelvi-ureteric junction obstruction

22.4 PUJ Obstruction with Calculus

Calculus seen in proximal ureter with gross obstructive uropathy and renal cortex has become papery thin in a patient with PUJ Obstruction (Figs 22.4A to D).

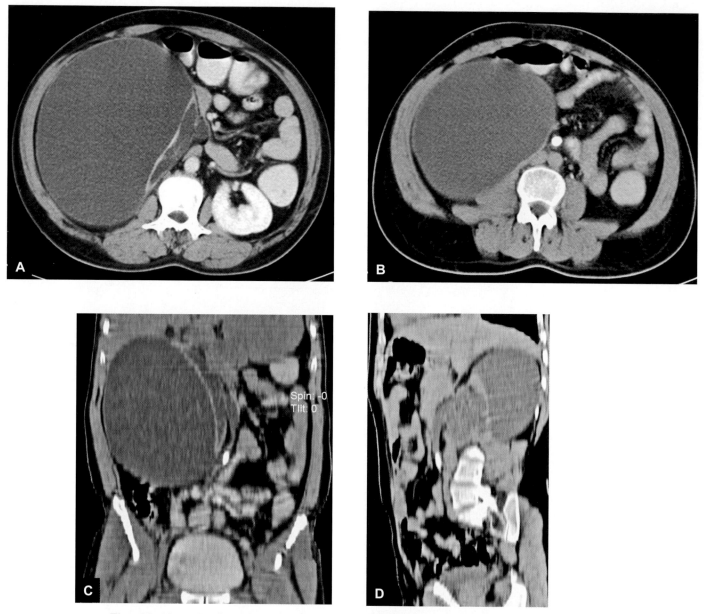

Figs 22.4A to D: Calculus seen in proximal ureter with gross obstructive uropathy

23. TRAUMA

23.1 Renal Trauma

In renal trauma 95% cases are minor in nature and hematuria is commonest manifestation.

But renal pedicle or vein injury may present without hematuria. Initial imaging is done at 60-70 sec post IV contrast injection for vascular enhancement and nephrogram. Delayed images (3-5 min) are taken to check for urine leak/urinoma.

- Contrast CT showing small right renal laceration (Fig. 23.1A).
- Contrast CT showing bigger right renal laceration (Fig. 23.1B).
- Contrast CT showing massive right renal laceration (Fig. 23.1C).
- Renal vascular injury (Figs 23.1D and E).

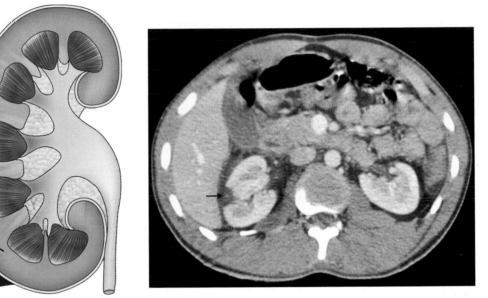

Fig. 23.1A: Renal small laceration

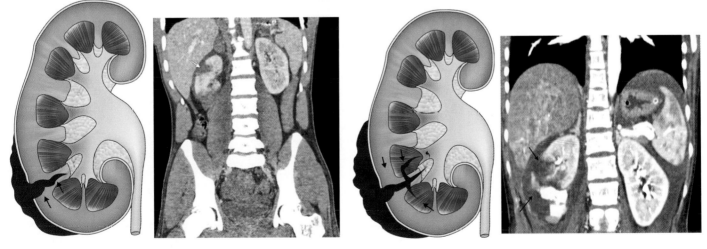

Fig. 23.1B: Renal bigger laceration   **Fig. 23.1C:** Renal massive tear

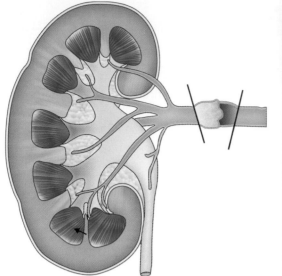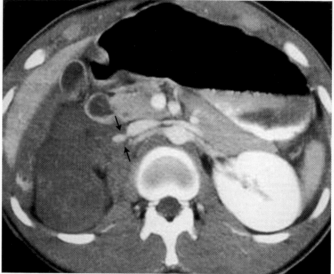

Fig. 23.1D: Renal vascular injury

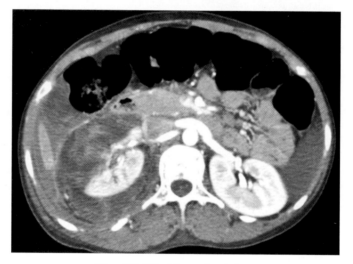

Fig. 23.1E: Vascular injury

23.2 Testicular Trauma

- Disrupted testis with loss of the normal testicular contour following trauma (Fig. 23.2A).
- Right post traumatic hematocele (Fig. 23.2B).

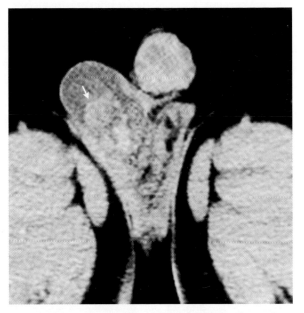

Fig. 23.2A: Traumatic right testicular disruption

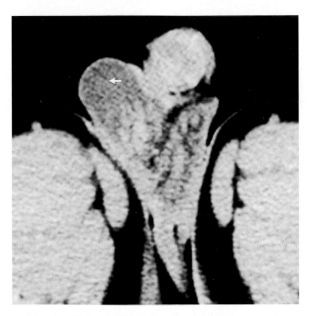

Fig. 23.2B: Post traumatic right hematocele

24. INFECTIVE-INFLAMMATORY

24.1 Emphysematous Pyelonephritis

Heterogeneously enhancing left renal enlargement is seen. Few air pockets are also seen in this lesion suggesting infection of renal parenchyma (Figs 24.1A to D).

Emphysematous pyelonephritis is an acute necrotizing parenchymal renal infiltration by gas producing uropathogens. This is a rare complication of diabetes mellitus with high mortality in severe cases.

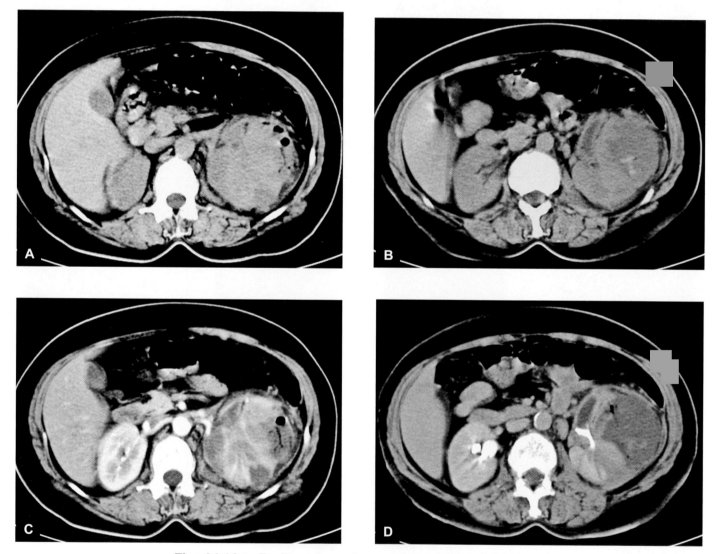

Figs 24.1A to D: Emphysematous pyelonephritis in left kidney

24.2 Pyelonephritis with Partially Thrombosed Renal Vein

Post-contrast CT images show enlarged left kidney with multiple hypodense non enhancing areas of collection and multiple air pockets (Figs 24.2A to D). Left renal vein is stretched and shows an intraluminal filling defect suggestive of thrombosis. Renal vein thrombosis occurring in association with acute pyelonephritis is rare.

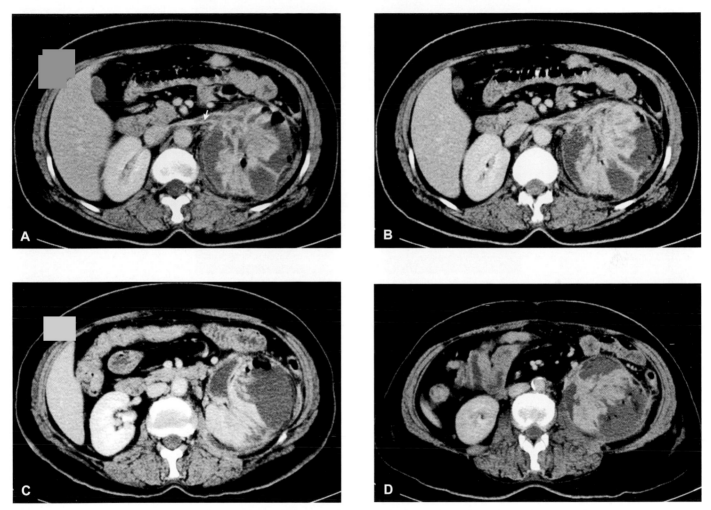

Figs 24.2A to D: Pyelonephritis in left kidney with partially thrombosed renal vein

24.3 Cystitis

CT image in cystitis shows thick irregular enhancing urinary bladder wall (Fig. 24.3).

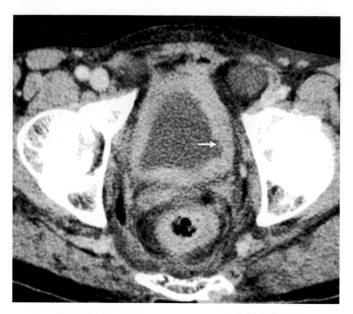

Fig. 24.3: Thick and irregular enhancing
urinary bladder wall due to cystitis

25. NEOPLASTIC

25.1 Renal Cell Carcinoma with Pulmonary Metastases

CT abdomen shows a heterogeneous enhancing left renal mass (Figs 25.1A and B) proved on histopathology as a renal cell carcinoma. Figures 25.1C to F show bilateral multiple lung metastases.

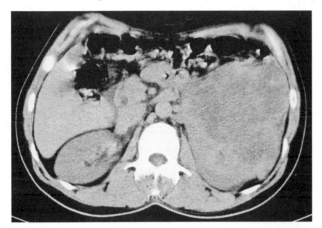

Fig. 25.1A: Plain CT shows left renal cell carcinoma

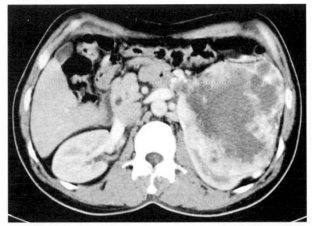

Fig. 25.1B: Contrast CT shows left renal cell carcinoma

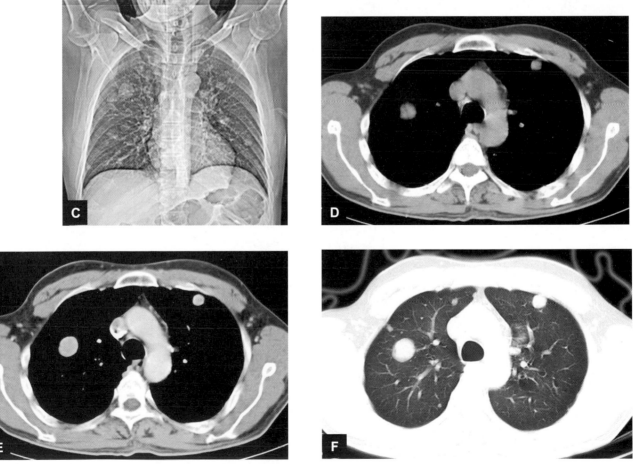

Figs 25.1C to F: Bilateral multiple lung metastases

25.2 Renal Cell Carcinoma

Contrast CT in 48 years old male shows heterogeneous enhancing left renal mass with areas of central necrosis (Figs 25.2A and B). Left renal vein and IVC do not show thrombosis (Figs 25.2C and D).

Bilateral pulmonary metastases are present (Fig. 25.2E). Bone metastasis is seen in the form of radio-opacities in left iliac bone (Fig. 25.2F).

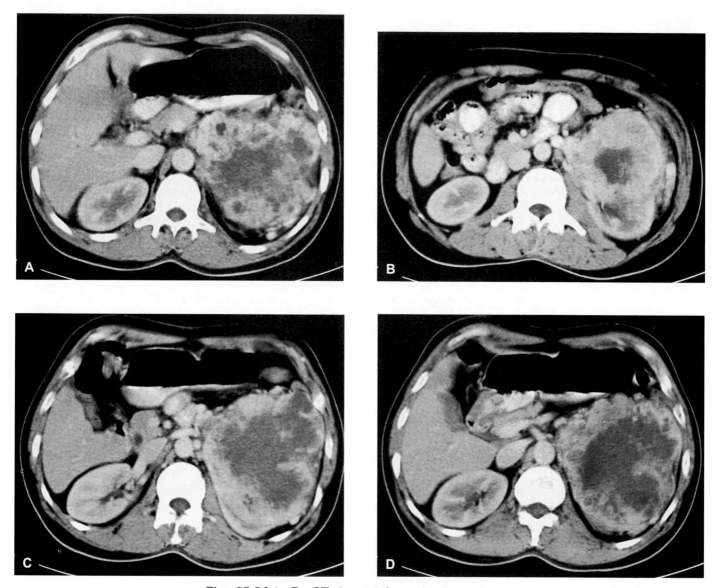

Figs 25.2A to D: CT shows left renal cell carcinoma

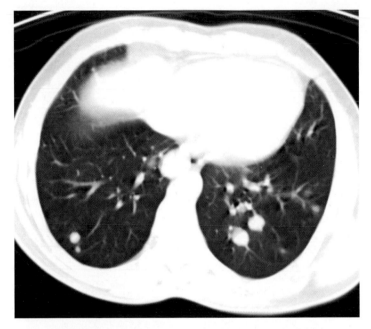

Fig. 25.2E: Bilateral multiple lung metastases

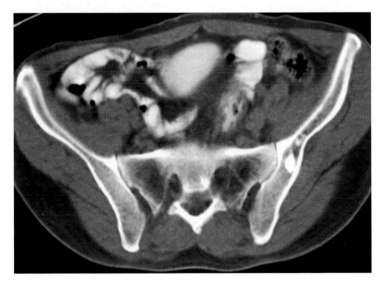

Fig. 25.2F: Bone metastasis

25.3 Renal Cell Carcinoma (RCC)

Solid peripherally calcified mass is seen on inferolateral aspect of right kidney (Figs 25.3A to D). The mass is predominantly located in the renal cortex. Kidney shows normal post contrast enhancement and excretion, the mass shows mild contrast enhancement.

The characteristic appearance of RCC (hypernephroma) is a solid renal lesion (may be cystic) which disturbs the renal contour. 10% of RCC will contain calcifications, RCC is the most common type of renal malignancy in adults responsible for approximately 80% of cases. It is also known to be the most lethal of all the genitourinary tumors.

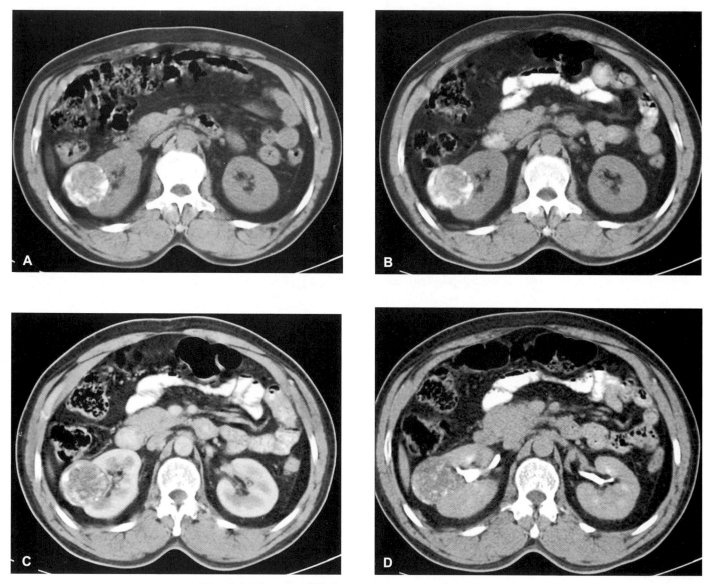

Figs 25.3A to D: CT shows right renal cell carcinoma

25.4 Carcinoma Bladder 1

55 years female presented with hematuria.
- Scout image shows staghorn calculus in right renal pelvis. Clamped urinary catheter is seen (Fig. 25.4A).
- Plain CT shows staghorn calculus with small renal calyceal calculi. A growth is seen within the bladder on right side (Figs 25.4B and C).
- Contrast CT shows uptake of contrast by renal parenchyma and excretion by both kidneys (Figs 25.4D and E).
- Delayed contrast CT shows contrast opacified right ureter coursing through the mass in urinary bladder (Fig. 25.4F). Histopathology proved this mass to be a low grade transitional cell carcinoma bladder.

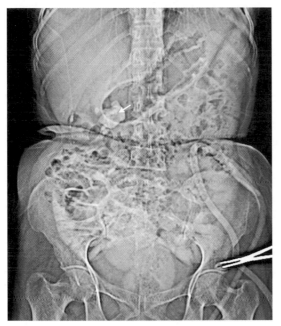

Fig. 25.4A: Scout image shows staghorn calculus in right renal pelvis

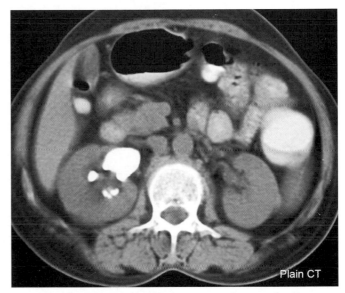

Fig. 25.4B: Plain CT shows staghorn calculus with small renal calyceal calculi

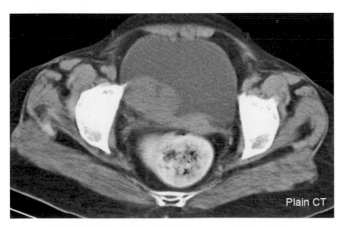

Fig. 25.4C: Plain CT shows growth within the bladder on right side

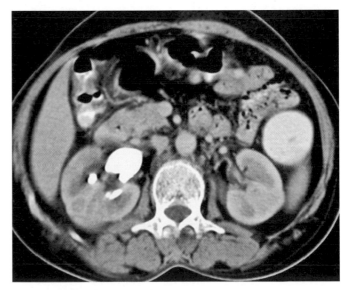

Fig. 25.4D: Contrast CT shows uptake of contrast by renal parenchyma and excretion by both kidneys

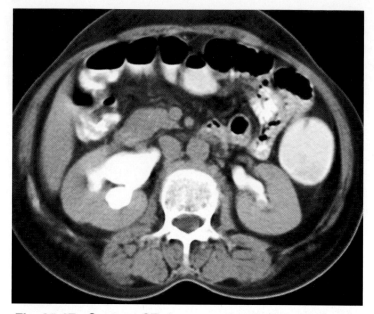

Fig. 25.4E: Contrast CT shows uptake of contrast by renal parenchyma and excretion by both kidneys

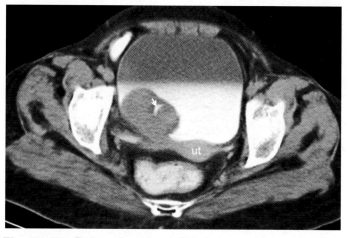

Fig. 25.4F: Delayed contrast CT shows contrast opacified right ureter coursing through the mass in urinary bladder

25.5 Carcinoma Bladder 2

Plain CT shows carcinoma of bladder (Fig. 25.5A). Posterior and right lateral wall of urinary bladder shows irregular wall thickening (Fig. 25.5B). Right vesicoureteric junction is involved. Fat plane with rectum is however preserved.

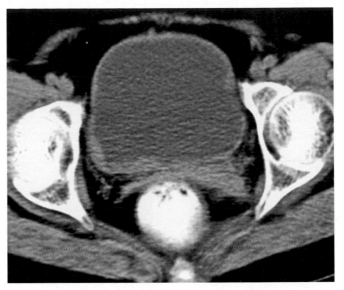

Fig. 25.5A: Plain CT in carcinoma of bladder

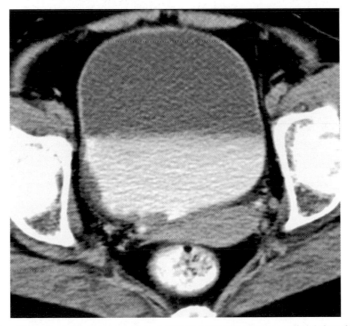

Fig. 25.5B: Delayed contrast CT shows irregular wall thickening
in region of right lateral wall of urinary bladder

25.6 Intradiverticular Bladder Carcinoma

Diverticulum is seen communicating with bladder in plain (Figs 25.6A and B) and delayed post-contrast images (Figs 25.6C and D). Neoplastic growth is seen in the diverticulum (Figs 25.6A, C, E and F).

Imaging plays an important role in identifying bladder diverticula as a potential site for neoplasm. Carcinoma arising within urinary bladder diverticula has a poorer prognosis than the neoplasms that originate within the main bladder lumen as a result of early transmural tumor infiltration.

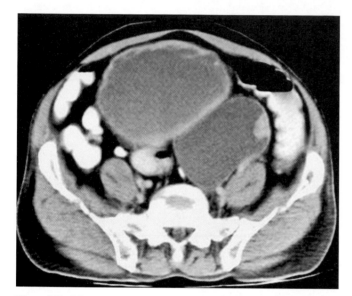

Fig. 25.6A: Contrast CT shows a large bladder diverticulum. Neoplastic growth is seen in the diverticulum

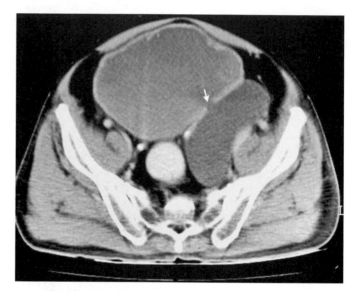

Fig. 25.6B: Contrast CT shows a diverticulum communicating with bladder

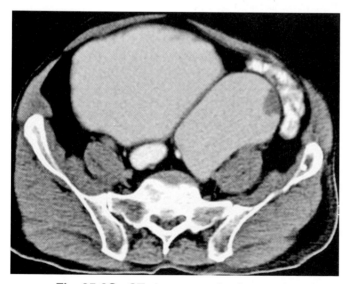

Fig. 25.6C: CT shows neoplastic growth in the diverticulum

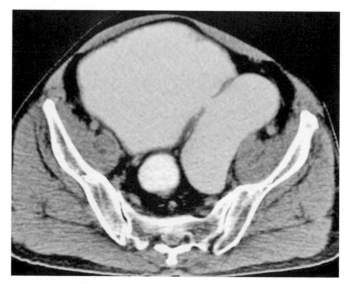

Fig. 25.6D: Delayed contrast CT shows a diverticulum communicating with bladder

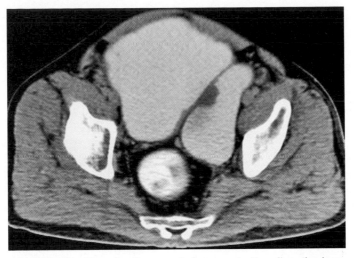

Fig. 25.6E: Neoplastic growth is seen in the diverticulum

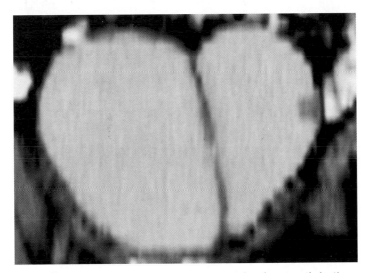

Fig. 25.6F: Recon image shows neoplastic growth in the
diverticulum and communication of diverticulum with bladder

25.7 Carcinoma Prostate

Prostate is enlarged with irregular contours (Figs 25.7A and B). The fat plane with urinary bladder is lost (Figs 25.7A and B). Enhancing metastasis is seen in liver (Fig. 25.7C). Small cyst is seen in right kidney (Figs 25.7C). Malignant left pleural effusion is present. The spine shows degenerative changes (Fig. 25.7D).

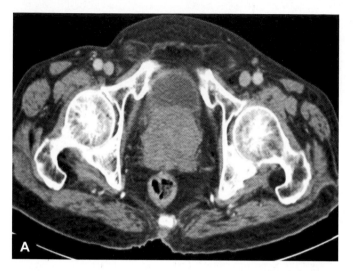
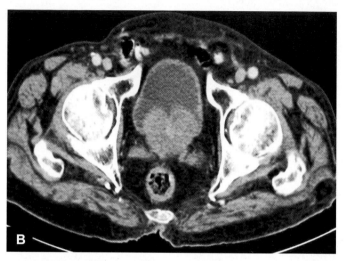

Figs 25.7A and B: Carcinoma prostate

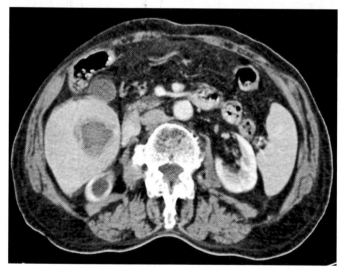

Fig. 25.7C: Metastasis in liver

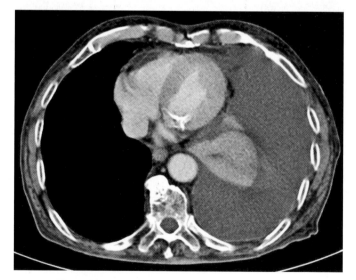

Fig. 25.7D: Malignant left pleural effusion

25.8 Carcinoma Prostate with Metastases

Prostate shows enlargement and surface irregularity and ill-defined margins protruding into the bladder base (Figs 25.8A and B). Para-aortic lymphadenopathy is seen (Fig. 25.8C). Sclerotic metastases are seen in the vertebral body (Fig. 25.8D) and ala of sacrum (Fig. 25.8E) on the left.

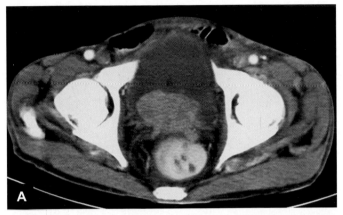
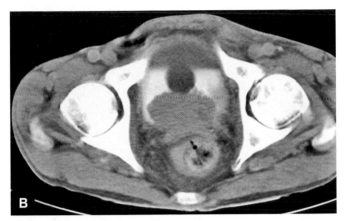

Figs 25.8A and B: Carcinoma prostate

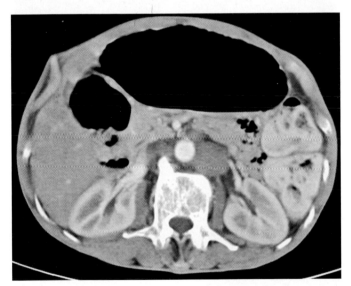
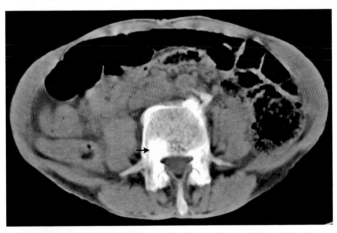

Fig. 25.8C: Para-aortic lymphadenopathy

Fig. 25.8D: Sclerotic metastases in vertebral body

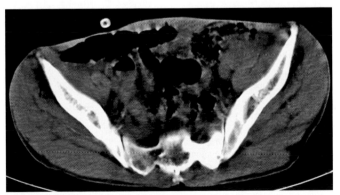

Fig. 25.8E: Sclerotic metastases in left ala of sacrum

25.9 Seminoma Testis

28 years old male with history of painless progressive swelling in left testis.

   Plain (Fig. 25.9A) and contrast CT (Fig. 25.9B) shows a solid enhancing left testicular mass. Metastatic lesions were noted in right lung (Fig. 25.9C) and intra-abdominal lymph node (Fig. 25.9D). FNAC proved it to be a seminoma.

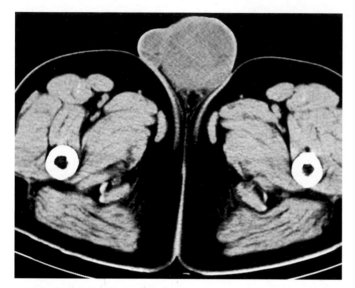

Fig. 25.9A: Plain CT shows a left testicular mass

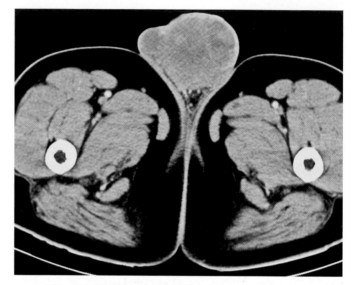

Fig. 25.9B: Contrast CT shows an enhancing left testicular mass

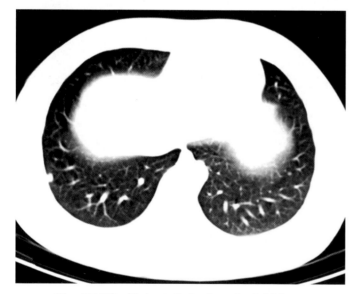

Fig. 25.9C: Metastatic lesions in right lung

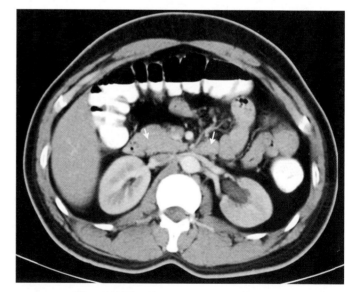

Fig. 25.9D: Metastatic lymph nodes

25.10 Metastases from Seminoma Testis

- CT Abdomen in a patient with history of 'burnt out' seminoma of testis shows a metastatic retroperitoneal conglomerate mass of adenopathy encasing the aorta and left renal hilum (Fig. 25.10A).
- Post-chemotherapy CT abdomen shows resolution however some residual non-enhancing soft tissue at left renal hilum is still seen (Fig. 25.10B).

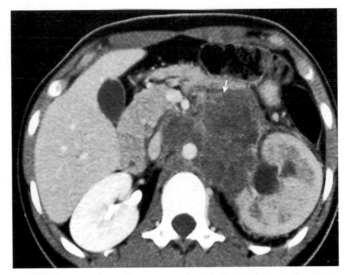

Fig. 25.10A: Metastatic retroperitoneal conglomerate mass of adenopathy encasing the aorta and left renal hilum

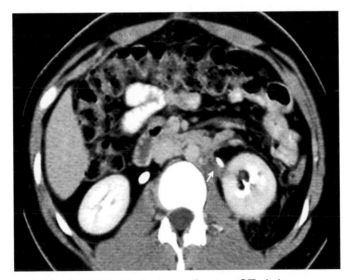

Fig. 25.10B: Post-chemotherapy CT abdomen shows significant resolution

25.11 Carcinoma Penis

Plain (Fig. 25.11A) and contrast (Fig. 25.11B) CT show an enhancing mass involving the penis with loss of penile architecture.

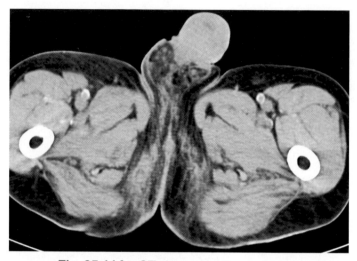

Fig. 25.11A: CT shows penile carcinoma

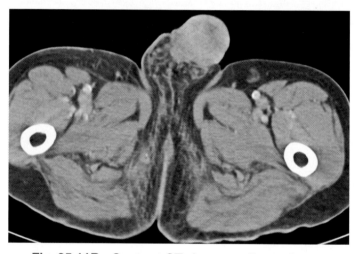

Fig. 25.11B: Contrast CT shows penile carcinoma

25.12 Broad Ligament Fibroid

CT images show a moderately enhancing soft tissue density mass in left adnexa attached to superolateral aspect of uterus. Left ovary is seen separately from the mass (Figs 25.12A to D).

This turned out to be a broad ligament fibroid on surgery.

Extrauterine fibroids though do occur, but are rare. Among the extrauterine fibroids, broad ligament fibroids are the most common and because of its rarity it poses specific diagnostic difficulties.

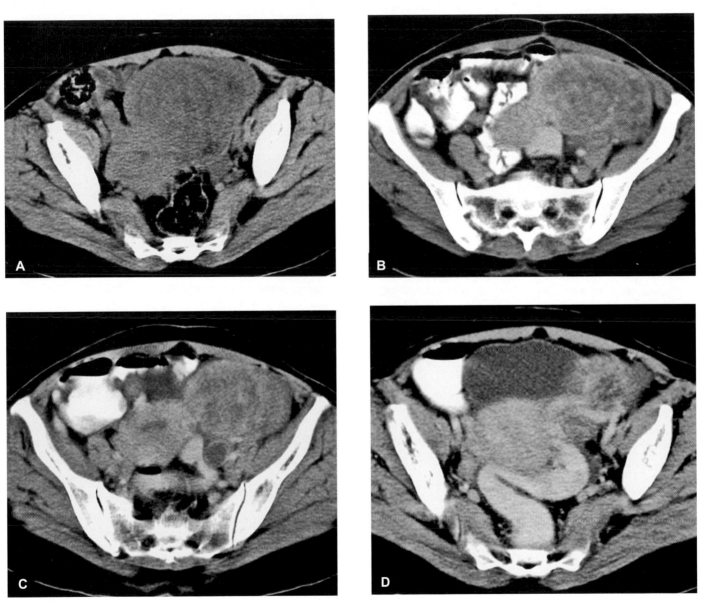

Figs 25.12A to D: Broad ligament fibroid

25.13 Endometrial Carcinoma

There is irregularity and thickening of endometrial wall associated with collection in the uterine cavity (Figs 25.13A to D). Biopsy proved this to be a high grade carcinoma of endometrium.

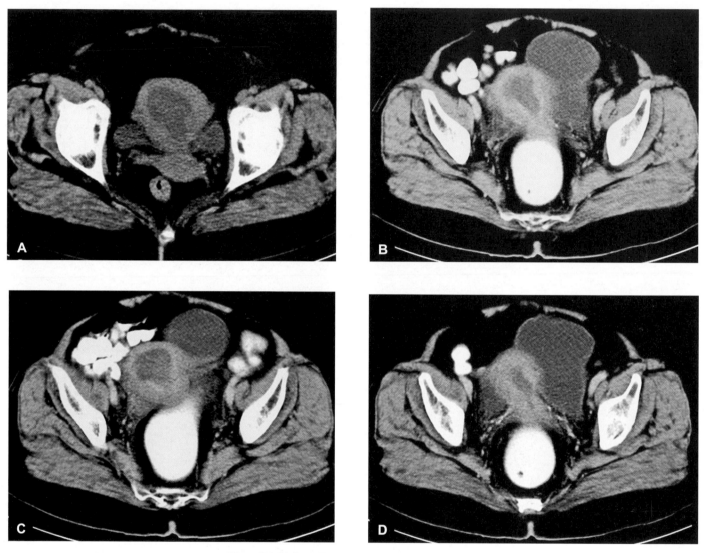

Figs 25.13A to D: Endometrial carcinoma

25.14 Carcinoma Cervix 1

Figures 25.14A and B show a cervical mass extending into bladder anteriorly (vertical arrow) and rectum posteriorly (horizontal arrow) in a patient with cervical carcinoma.

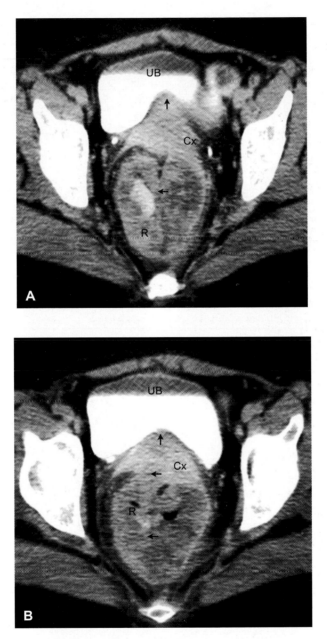

Figs 25.14A and B: Carcinoma cervix

25.15 Carcinoma Cervix 2

- Plain CT abdomen-pelvis shows a hyperdense cervical mass with loss of fat plane anteriorly with urinary bladder and posteriorly with rectum (Fig. 25.15A).
- Immediate post-contrast CT shows normal contrast uptake by left kidney. Right kidney shows gross hydronephrosis (Fig. 25.15B).
- Shows invasion of the uterus, urinary bladder, rectum and right lower ureter (Figs 25.15C to E).

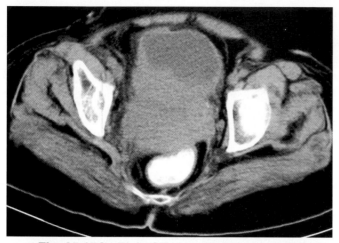

Fig. 25.15A: Plain CT shows cervical growth

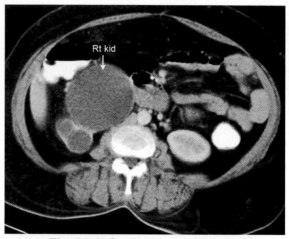

Fig. 25.15B: Contrast CT shows hydronephrotic right kidney

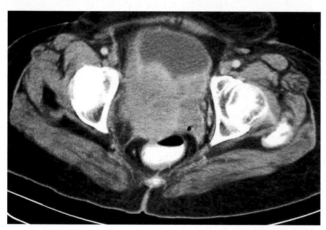

Fig. 25.15C: Contrast CT shows cervical growth

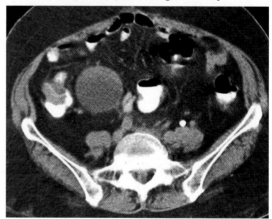

Fig. 25.15D: Contrast CT shows hydronephrotic right kidney

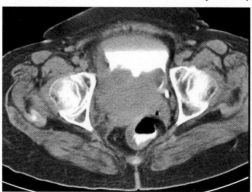

Fig. 25.15E: Contrast CT shows cervical growth invading the uterus, urinary bladder, rectum and right lower ureter

25.16 Carcinoma Cervix 3

Immediate (Figs 25.16A and B) and delayed (Figs 25.16C and D) post-contrast CT images show a solid enhancing mass in the cervix. Fat stranding and few sub centimeter sized lymph nodes are seen in the left adnexa. The fat plane between the mass and rectum is lost. However, the fat plane between the mass and bladder is maintained. The course and caliber of ureter is intact on either sides. Biopsy confirmed squamous cell carcinoma of cervix.

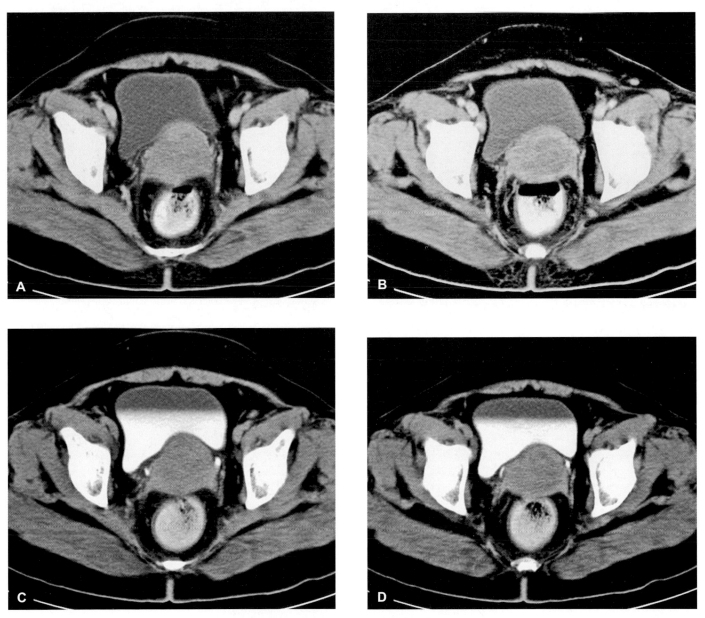

Figs 25.16A to D: Carcinoma cervix

25.17 Pyometra following Radiotherapy

Patient was earlier treated with radiotherapy for carcinoma of cervix.
- No obvious pelvic mass is seen. However the cervical canal is stenosed (Fig. 25.17A).
- Massive fluid collection is seen in the uterus (Figs 25.17B to D).

  This was due to stenosis of cervix following radiotherapy.

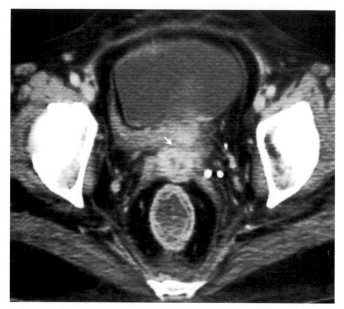

Fig. 25.17A: Stenosed cervical canal

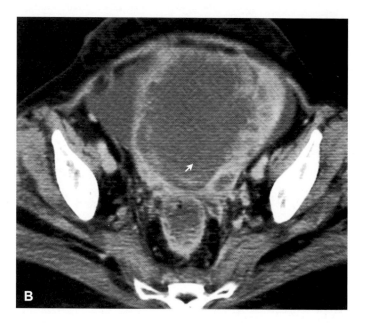

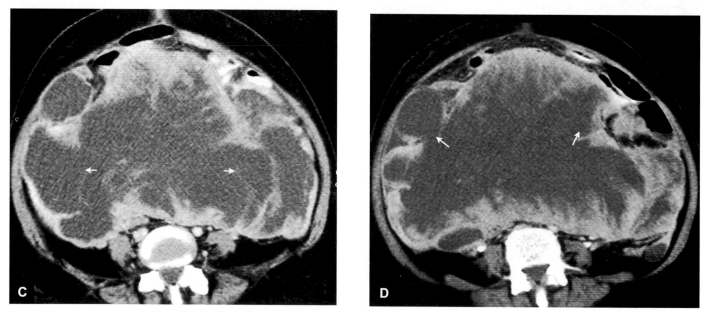

Figs 25.17B to D: Massive fluid collection is in the uterus (pyometra)

25.18 Cystic Ovarian Tumor

Contrast CT shows a large cystic lesion with enhancing thick septae and enhancing mural nodules arising from right ovary (Figs 25.18A to D).

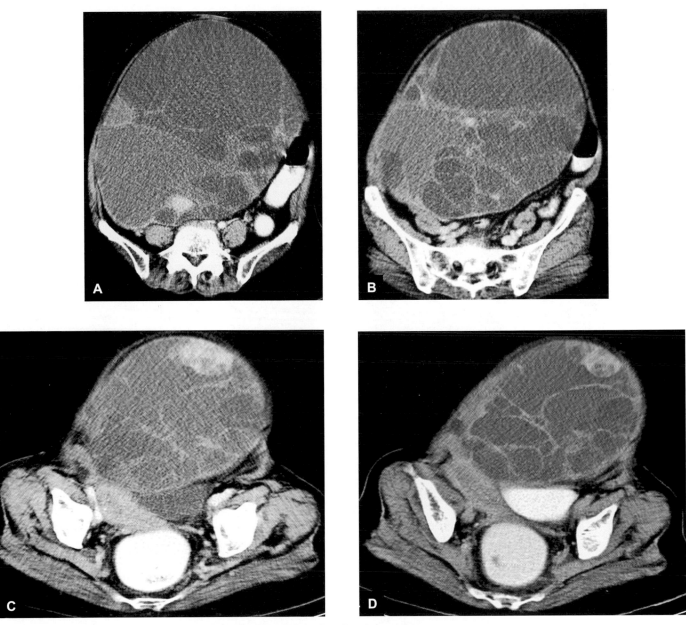

Figs 25.18A to D: Cystic ovarian tumor

25.19 Solid Ovarian Tumor 1

Bilateral Solid Ovarian Tumor

- Adnexal masses are seen bilaterally (Fig. 25.19A).
- Adnexal masses show mild enhancement (Fig. 25.19B).

  Bilateral solid ovarian enlargement may be benign or malignant. Benign ovarian enlargement includes mature cystic teratomas, cystadenomas and fibrothecomas.

  Ovarian malignancies include epithelial, stromal, germ-cell tumors and metastases from gastrointestinal tract, breast and lymphoma.

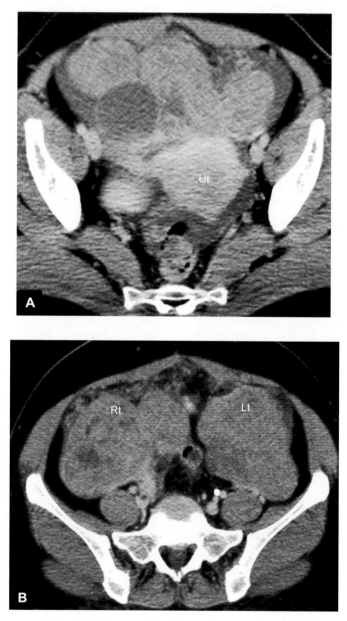

Figs 25.19A and B: Bilateral ovarian tumors

25.20 Solid Ovarian Tumor 2

Plain (Fig. 25.20A) and post contrast (Fig. 25.20B) CT images show a feeding vessel entering the right ovarian mass which turned out to be an undifferentiated epithelial ovarian malignancy.

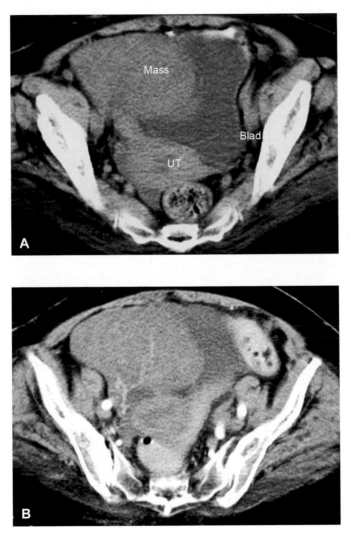

Fig. 25.20A and B: Ovarian tumor

25.21 Vulvar Carcinoma (Figs 25.21A and B)

Asymmetric soft tissue density lesion is seen in vulva on right side in this 65 years female. No local or distant intraabdominal metastases were seen on contrast CT abdomen. Biopsy showed it to be a squamous cell carcinoma of vulva.

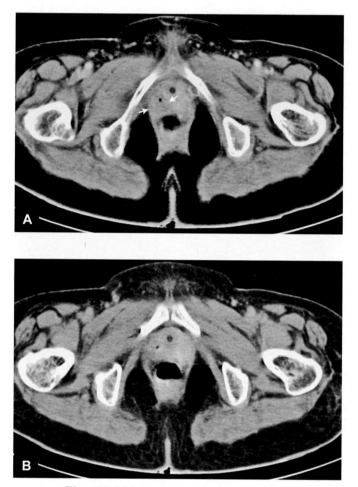

Figs 25.21A and B: Vulvar carcinoma

26. MISCELLANEOUS

26.1 Renal Pelvis Calculus

Partially obstructing left renal pelvic calculus:
- Scout image shows a left paravertebral calculus (Fig. 26.1A).
- Plain CT confirms that calculus is located in left renal pelvis causing obstructive uropathy as seen from dilatation of renal pelvis and calyces (Fig. 26.1B).
- Medullary phase shows enhancement of renal parenchyma. Stagnated urine does not enhance (Fig. 26.1C).
- Excretory phase shows contrast in dilated renal pelvis and calyces. Contrast density obscures the calculus (Fig. 26.1D).

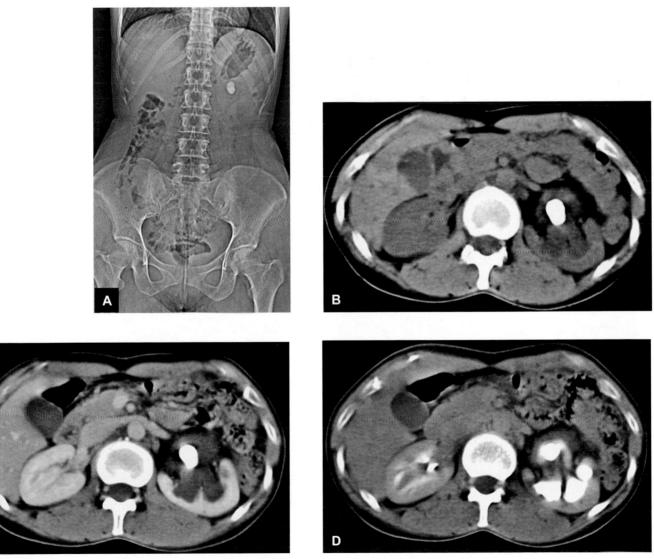

Figs 26.1A to D: Left renal calculus causing obstructive uropathy

26.2 Ureteric Calculus

Coronal recon image of plain CT abdomen and pelvis shows obstructive uropathy on left secondary to left lower ureteric calculus as seen in NCCT abdomen and pelvis (Fig. 26.2).

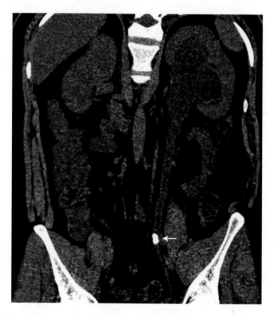

Fig. 26.2: Obstructive uropathy secondary to left lower ureteric calculus

26.3 Obstructive Uropathy

Plain CT Abdomen Images Show

- Mild dilatation of pelvicalyceal system of right kidney (Fig. 26.3A) is seen.
- Few small calculi in the dilated right pelvicalyceal system with dilated ureter (arrow) (Figs 26.3B and C).
- Right upper ureteric calculus (Fig. 26.3D). Atherosclerotic calcification is seen in the abdominal aorta.

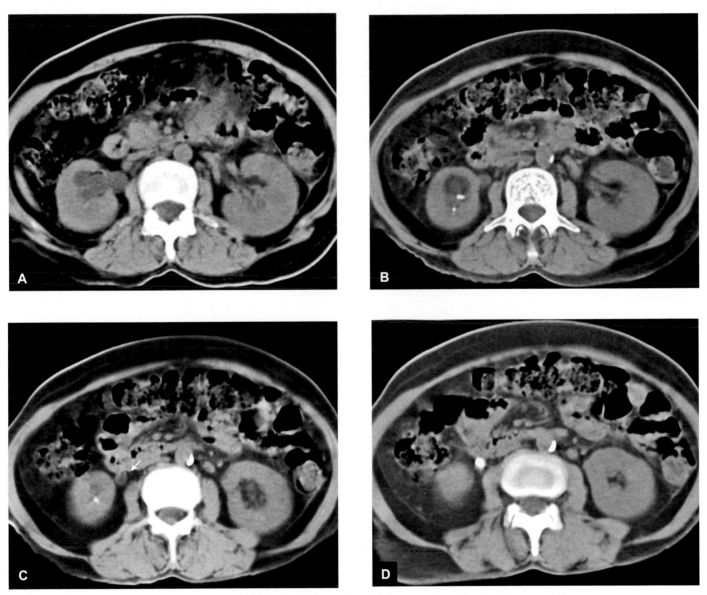

Figs 26.3A to D: Right upper ureteric calculus causing obstructive uropathy

26.4 VU Junction Calculus

Plain CT study shows bilateral hydronephrosis (Fig. 26.4A) secondary to vesicoureteric (VU) junction calculi (Fig. 26.4B).

In ureteric colic intravenous urography has traditionally been used as the means of investigation, but has been superseded by CT urography which gives more information and may detect alternative or additional pathology which would otherwise be missed on intravenous urography. The use of non-contrast CT urography is recommended as the initial investigation for patients with ureteric colic.

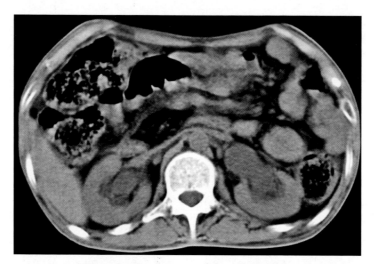

Fig. 26.4A: Bilateral hydronephrosis

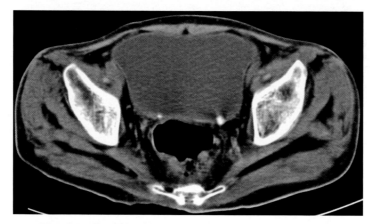

Fig. 26.4B: Bilateral vesicoureteric junction calculi

26.5 Vesicle Calculus

CT scan shows urinary bladder calculus with irregular margins (Fig. 26.5).

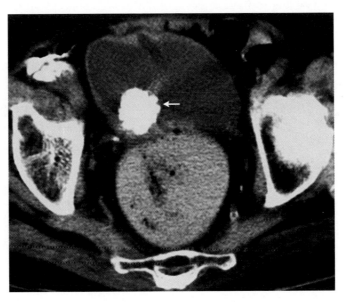

Fig. 26.5: Vesicle calculus

26.6 Hydrocele

CT Scan Shows Bilateral Hydrocele (Fig. 26.6)

Hydrocele is the accumulation of fluid around a testicle. It is the fluid secreted from remnant piece of peritoneum wrapped around the testis, called the tunica vaginalis.

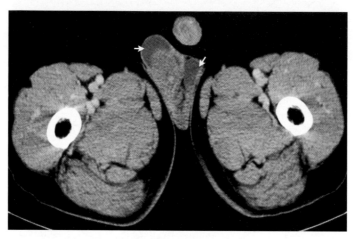

Fig. 26.6: Bilateral hydrocele

26.7 Follicular Cyst

CT shows follicular cysts in right ovary (Fig. 26.7).

A follicle is a fluid-filled sac containing an egg. Follicular cysts form when the follicle grows larger than normal during the menstrual cycle and does not release the egg. They usually, resolve spontaneously over the course of weeks to months.

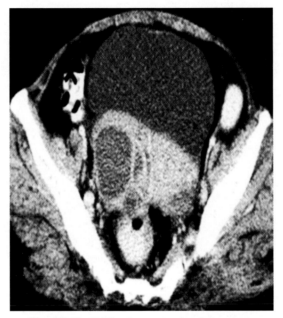

Fig. 26.7: Follicular cysts in right ovary

26.8 Simple Ovarian Cyst

Plain and contrast CT shows thin walled bilateral simple ovarian cysts (Figs 26.8A and B).

    A simple ovarian cyst is a fluid-filled sac. Graafian follicular cysts and corpus luteum cysts are functional simple cysts.

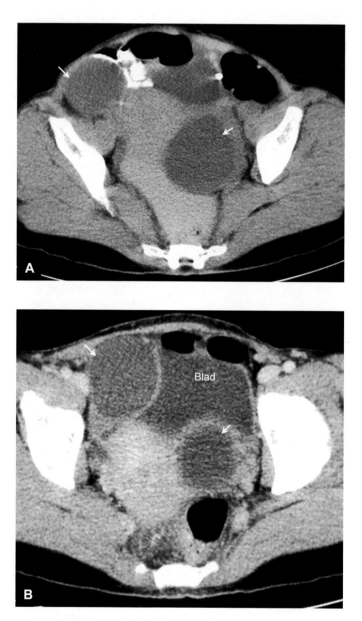

Figs 26.8A and B: Bilateral simple ovarian cysts

26.9 Ovarian Vein Thrombosis

Contrast-enhanced CT-scan images show bilateral intravascular filling defect in the ovarian veins (Figs 26.9A and B).

Postpartum ovarian vein thrombosis is an uncommon complication. CT angiography is the investigation of choice.

The severity of this disease is related to the extension of the thrombus into the inferior cava vein and the hazard of pulmonary embolism (13%).

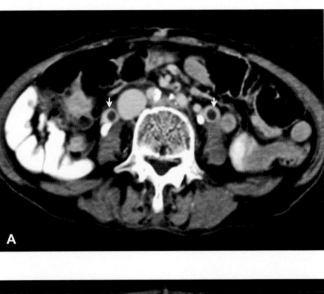

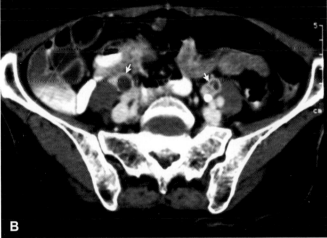

Figs 26.9A and B: Bilateral intravascular filling defect in the ovarian veins

Section 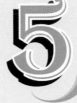

Musculoskeletal System

- Trauma
- Infective-Inflammatory
- Neoplastic
- Miscellaneous

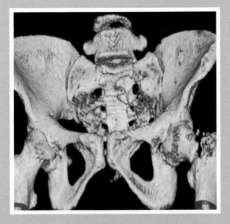

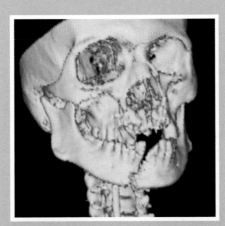

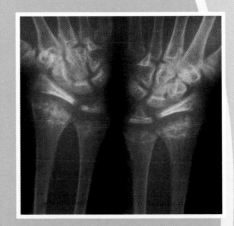

27. TRAUMA

Fractures

1. Depressed Fracture Frontal Bone

CT brain shows depressed fracture of frontal bone (Fig. 27.1).

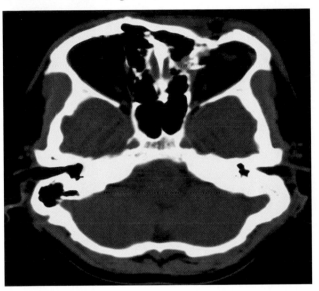

Fig. 27.1: Depressed fracture frontal bone

2. Pneumocranium

- Bone window shows comminuted depressed fracture of frontal bone. Hypodensities in neuroparenchyma indicate pneumocephalus (Fig. 27.2A).
- Brain window shows hypodensities in neuroparenchyma, pneumocephalous having CT value (-) 300 to (-) 900 HU. Air is also seen in the ventricular system (Pneumoventricle) (Fig. 27.2B).

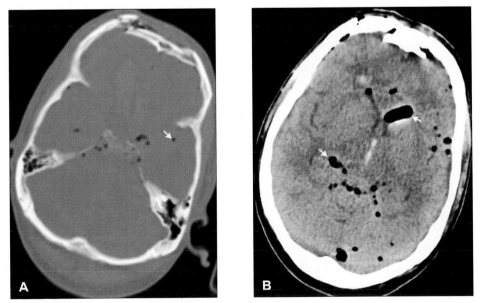

Figs 27.2A and B: Comminuted depressed fracture of frontal bone with pneumocephalus and pneumoventricle

3. Fracture of Parietal Bone

- CT image shows liner undisplaced fracture of right parietal bone (Fig. 27.3A).
- CT image shows comminuted depressed fracture of left parietal bone (Fig. 27.3B).

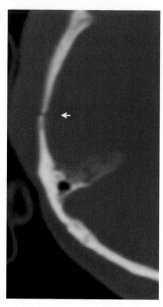

Fig. 27.3A: Fracture of
right parietal bone

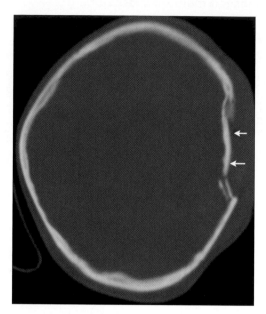

Fig. 27.3B: Fracture of left parietal bone

4. Fracture of Occipital Bone

- CT head bone window shows fracture on the right side of occipital bone (Fig. 27.4A).
- CT head brain window shows left frontal hemorrhagic contusion (Fig. 27.4B).

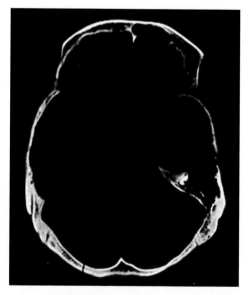

Fig. 27.4A: Fracture of occipital bone

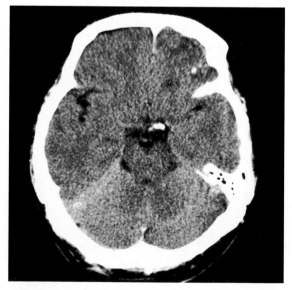

Fig. 27.4B: Left frontal hemorrhagic contusion

5. Fracture Temporal Bone

HRCT of temporal bone shows fracture line involving right mastoid air cells, extending from external auditory canal up to the middle ear (Figs 27.5A and B).

The evaluation of trauma patients with routine CT scans for brain is inadequate for temporal bone fractures. The characteristic fracture extends from the petrotympanic fissure at the glenoid fossa to the anterior inferior aspect of the medial bony external auditory canal. The high resolution CT scan is essential to identify fracture of the temporal bone in every patient with facial nerve injury.

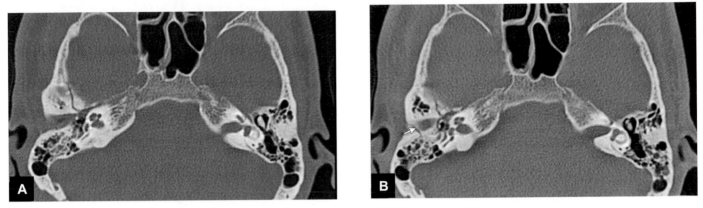

Figs 27.5A and B: Fracture of right temporal bone

6. Fracture Orbital Walls

Fracture of lateral, medial and inferior wall of left orbit, fracture of left zygomatic arch, medial and posterolateral wall of left maxillary sinus with maxillary hemosinus (Figs 27.6A to D).

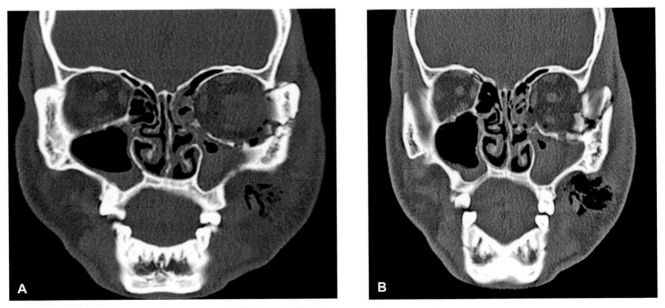

Figs 27.6A and B: Fracture of left orbital walls

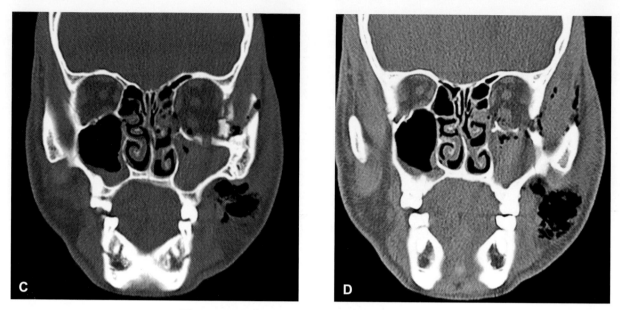

Figs 27.6C and D: Fracture of left orbital walls

7. Fracture of Orbital Floor

Coronal CT image shows fracture of floor of right orbit and herniation of orbital fat (Fig. 27.7).

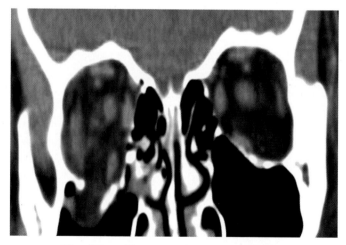

Fig. 27.7: Fracture of right orbital floor

8. Fracture of Mandible

Reconstructed 3D CT images of mandibular fracture, which helps to plan surgery better (Fig. 27.8).

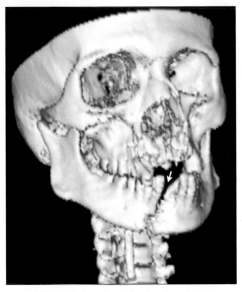

Fig. 27.8: Mandibular fracture

9. Fracture Facial Bones

Facial Fractures

- Mandible on left side (Fig. 27.9A).
- Hard palate on left side (Fig. 27.9B).
- Walls of left maxillary sinus and hemosinus (Fig. 27.9C).
- Left zygomatic arch and walls of left maxillary sinus (Fig. 27.9D).
- Left lateral orbital floor (Fig. 27.9E).
- Reconstructed 3D CT image shows most of the fractures (Fig. 27.9F).

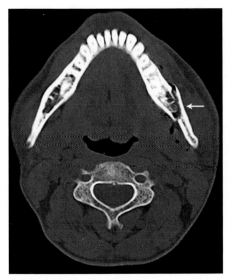 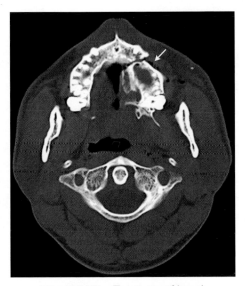 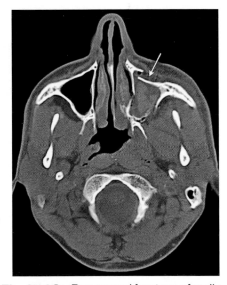

Fig. 27.9A: Fracture of mandible on left side

Fig. 27.9B: Fracture of hard palate on left side

Fig. 27.9C: Depressed fracture of walls of left maxillary sinus and hemosinus

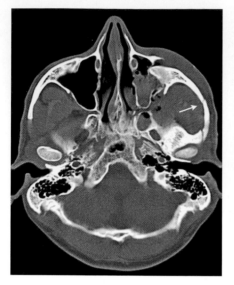

Fig. 27.9D: Fracture of left zygomatic arch and walls of left maxillary sinus

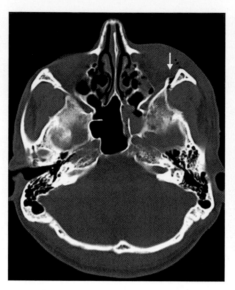

Fig. 27.9E: Fracture of left lateral orbital floor

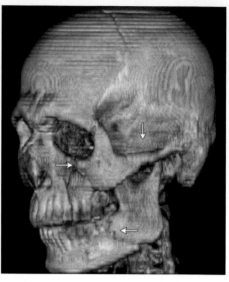

Fig. 27.9F: Reconstructed 3D CT image shows most of the fractures

10. Fracture of Mandible and Frontal Bone

Fracture of body of mandible and frontal bone (Figs 27.10A to D).

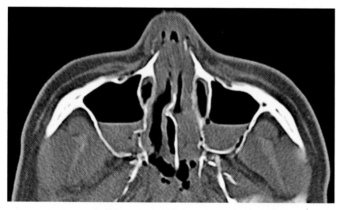

Fig. 27.10A: Multiple fractures involving maxillary sinuses and nasal septum

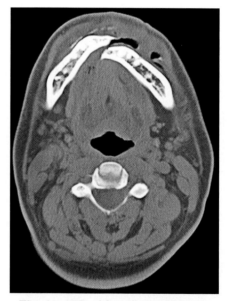

Fig. 27.10B: Mandibular fracture with overriding

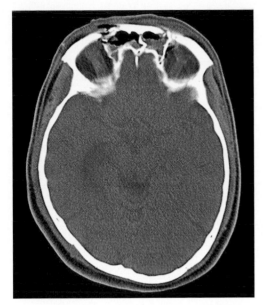

Fig. 27.10C: Fracture frontal bone

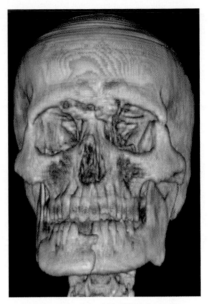

Fig. 27.10D: 3D CT showing multiple fractures

11. Fracture Symphysis Menti

CT shows undisplaced fracture of symphysis menti in a 9 years male child (Figs 27.11A and B).

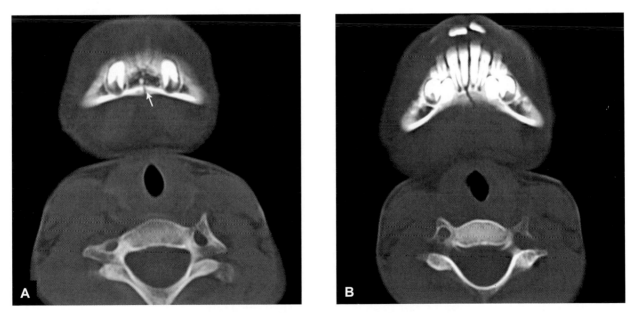

Figs 27.11A and B: Fracture of symphysis menti

12. Fracture Dens and Body of Axis

Figures 27.12A and B axial images, Figures 27.12C and D sagittal images and Figure 27.12E is coronal reformatted image. Figure 27.12F is a volume rendered image.

Fracture of the Dens is seen. The fracture line is seen to extend into the body of axis (second cervical vertebra) up to the right foramen transversarium. Reformatted images give a better view.

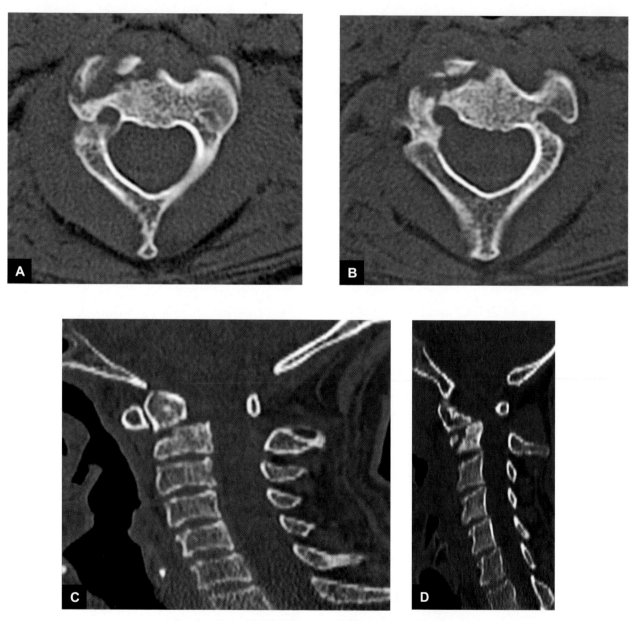

Figs 27.12A to D: Fracture of dens and body of axis

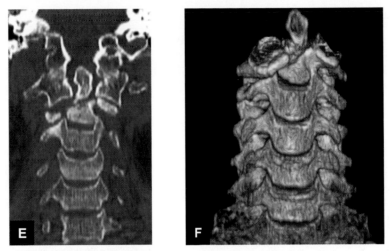

Figs 27.12E and F: Fracture of dens and body of axis

13. Fracture Destruction Odontoid Process (Figs 27.13A to D)

Fracture and destruction of odontoid process of C-2 vertebra is seen with retropulsion of body of C-2 vertebra and narrowing of cervical canal. Sclerosis and irregularity of lateral masses of C-2 is seen. These are features of post-infective sequelae.

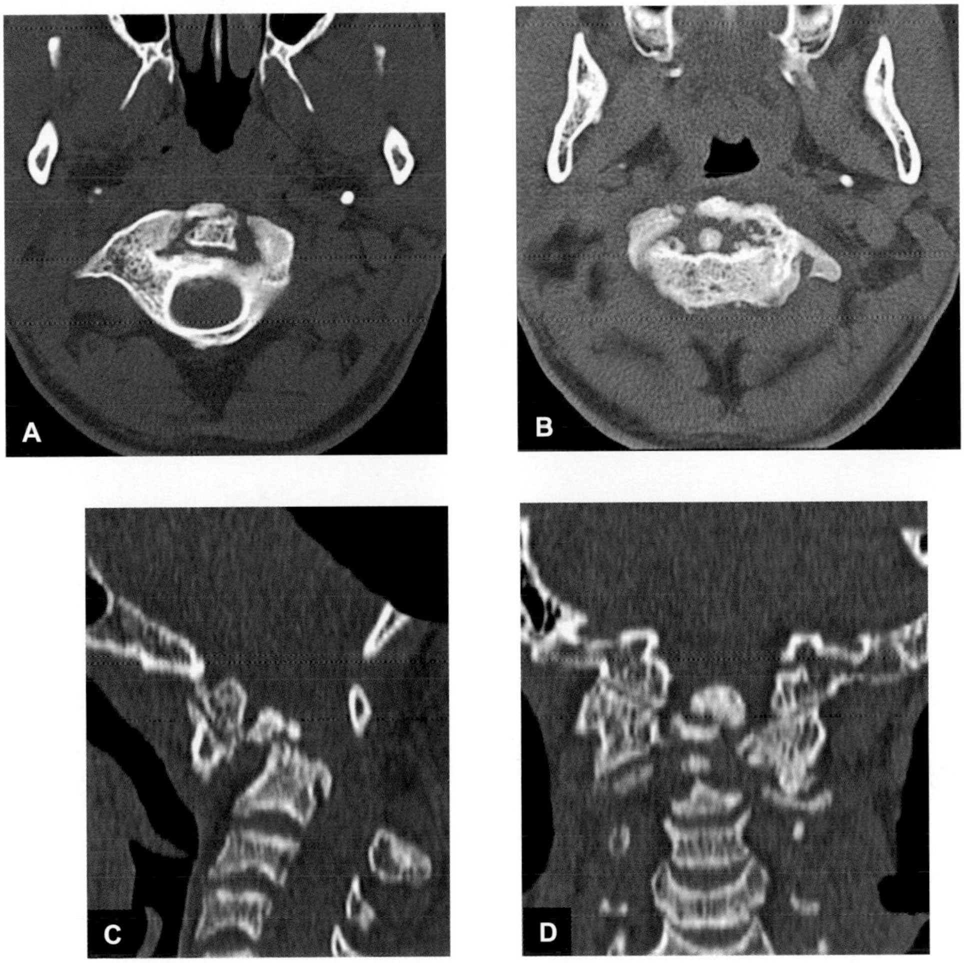

Figs 27.13A to D: Fracture and destruction of odontoid process of C2 vertebra

14. Compression Fracture Vertebral Body

Axial (Fig. 27.14A), sagittal reformatted (Fig. 27.14B), volume rendered (Figs 27.14C and D) CT images in a patient with history of fall from height.

Wedge compression fracture of body of L1 vertebra is seen with retropulsion of the body. Bony fragment is seen encroaching on the spinal canal. In addition, L2 and L3 vertebrae are also fractured.

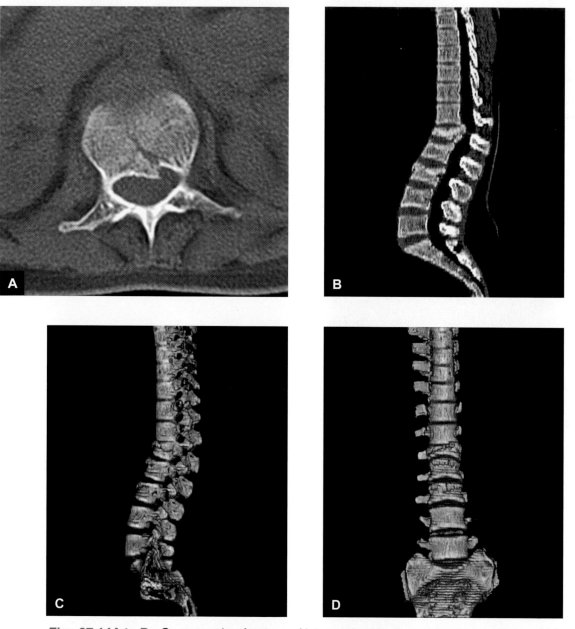

Figs 27.14A to D: Compression fracture of L1 vertebral body and fractures of L2 and L3

15. Fracture Scapula

- Fracture of scapula at junction of body, neck and spine (Fig. 27.15A).
- Fracture at tip of acromion and coracoid processes (Figs 27.15B to D).

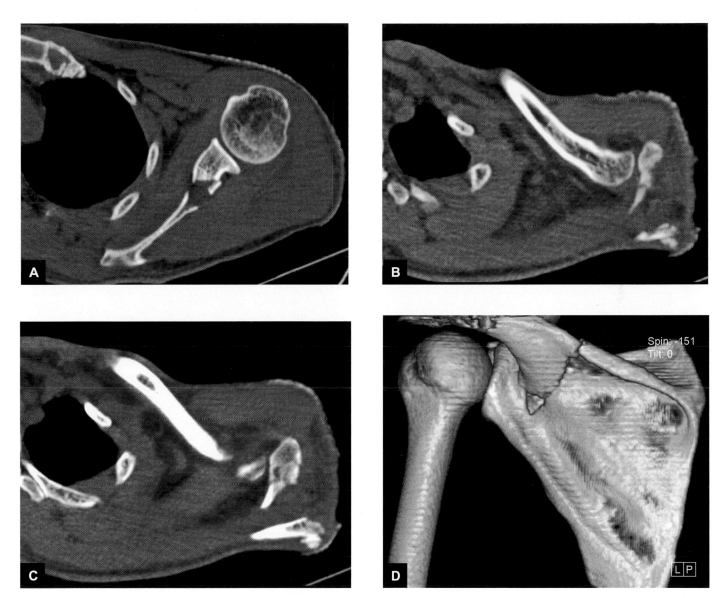

Figs 27.15A to D: Fracture of scapula

16. Fracture Right Acetabulum (Figs 27.16A to D)

Multidimensional joint fractures are seen best by CT scan and various reconstructions as shown here. These subtle fractures can be missed on plain radiographs.

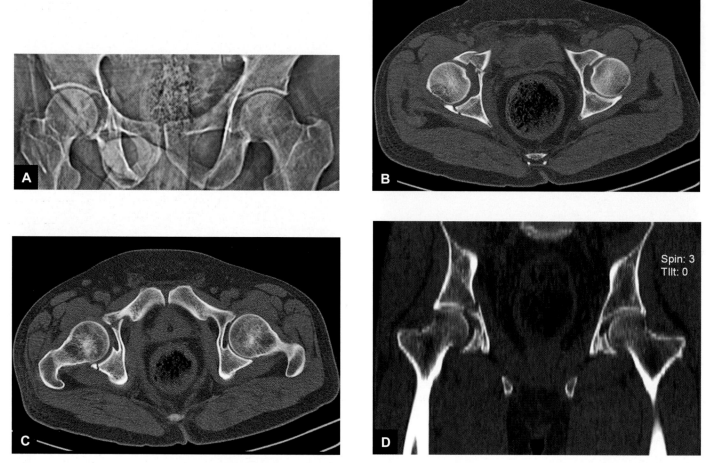

Figs 27.16A to D: Fracture of right acetabulum

17. Fracture Neck Femur

- Axial image of CT pelvis in bone window and reformatted 3D CT image shows fracture of neck of left femur (Figs 27.17A and B).

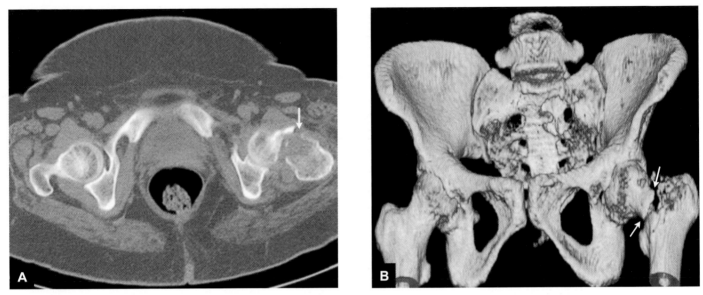

Figs 27.17A and B: Fracture of neck of left femur

18. Fracture Patella

Comminuted fracture of left patella (Figs 27.18A and B).

X-rays are usually sufficient to diagnose a patellar fracture. CT scan may be necessary for more difficult cases where X-rays are not definitive.

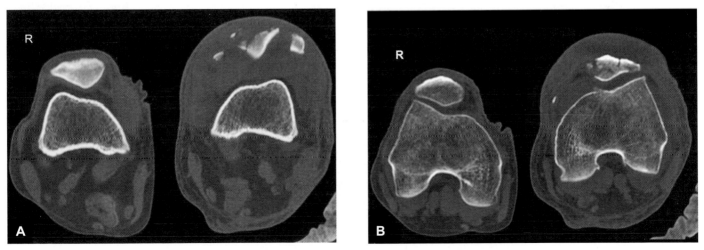

Figs 27.18A and B: Comminuted fracture of left patella

19. Fracture Tibia-Fibula

Depressed fracture of left tibial plateau with communited fracture of proximal diaphysis of tibia and fibula (Figs 27.19A to F).

Although some fractures of tibial plateau can be seen on plain radiograph, CT scan with reconstruction is the investigation of choice.

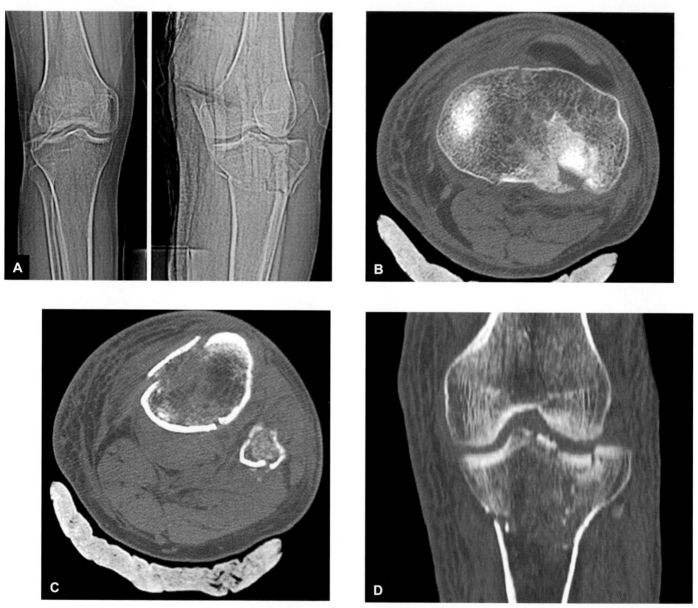

Figs 27.19A to D: Fracture of tibia-fibula

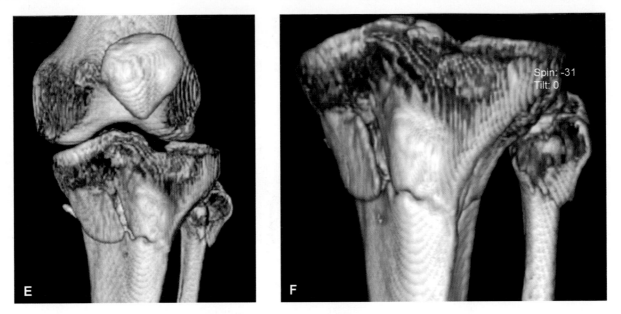

Figs 27.19E and F: Fracture of tibia-fibula

20. Fracture Calcaneum

The "Lover's fracture" is an intra-articular fracture of calcaneum (Fig. 27.20) as a result of axial loading force produced by a leap from a height and landing on heels. It is called "lover's fracture" because it is the type of fracture that can presumably be produced by a lover jumping out of the bedroom window of his beloved to escape from her surprised and enraged spouse or parents.

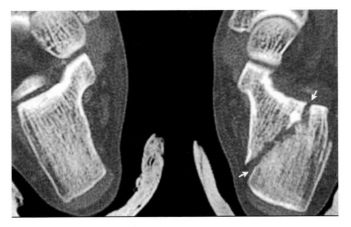

Fig. 27.20: Fracture of calcaneum

28. INFECTIVE - INFLAMMATORY

28.1. Cold Abscess

- CT shows hypodense area (abscess) in muscles – psoas and gluteus medius (Figs 28.1A and B).

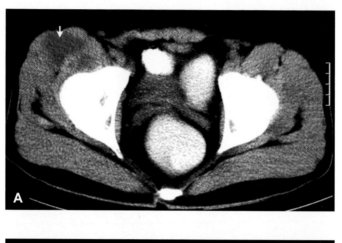

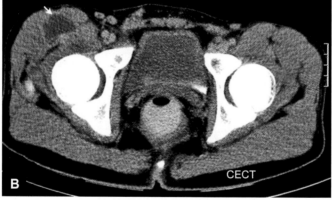

Figs 28.1A and B: Cold abscess

28.2. Iliacus Cold Abscess

- CT scan shows hypodense areas in right iliacus muscle, the muscle is edematous and underlying iliac bone shows scalloping (Figs 28.2A and B).

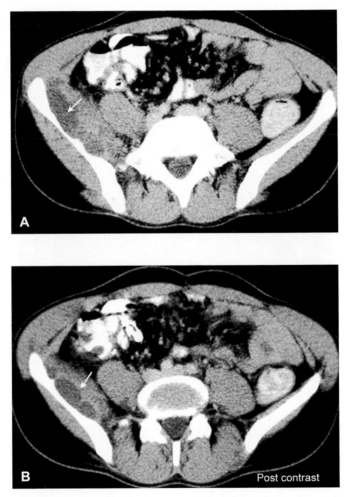

Figs 28.2A and B: Cold abscess involving iliacus muscle

29. NEOPLASTIC

29.1 Bone Island or Enostosis

Scout image (Fig. 29.1A) and axial CT images (Figs 29.1B and C) show two focal densely sclerotic compact bones in the spongiosa with thorny or brush borders. When the lesion is more than 20 mm it is known as giant bone island.

Bone island or enostosis represents a focus of mature compact (cortical) bone within the cancellous bone (spongiosa). Typically asymptomatic, this benign lesion is usually an incidental finding, with a preference for the pelvis, femur, and other long bones. On radiography it is seen as a homogeneously dense, sclerotic focus in the cancellous bone and on CT scan, a bone island appears as a high attenuation focus.

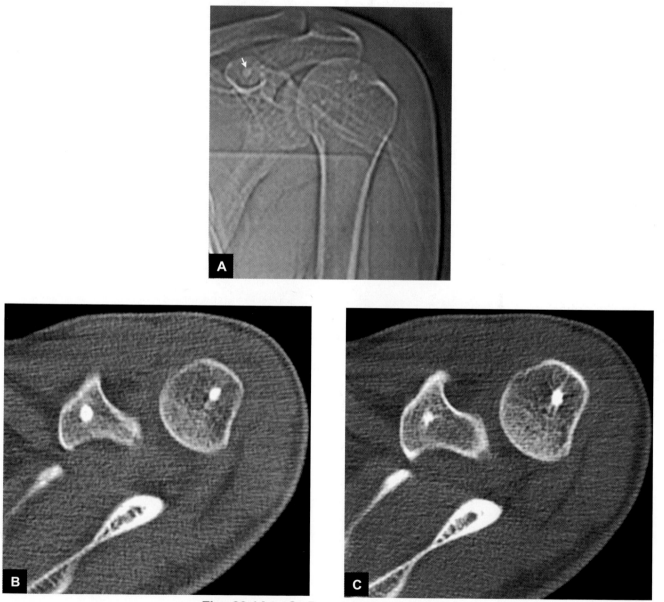

Figs 29.1A to C: Bone island or enostosis

29.2 Femoral Osteoid Osteoma 1

- Scanogram left femur shows a round radiolucent area with sclerosed margins 10 mm in diameter (Fig. 29.2A).
- Coronal image shows a hyperdense central focus (nidus) thereby confirming the lesion to be osteoid osteoma (Fig. 29.2B).
- Sagittal and axial image also demonstrates the osteoid osteoma (Figs 29.2C and D).

Osteoid osteoma is a benign osteoblastic tumor consisting of a central core of vascular osteoid tissue (the nidus) surrounded by a peripheral zone of sclerotic bone. The hallmark of osteoid osteoma is dull or aching pain relieved by NSAIDS.

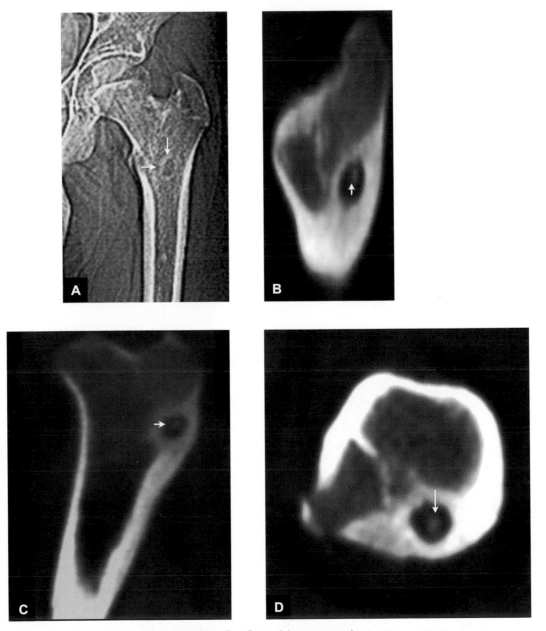

Fig. 29.2A to D: Osteoid osteoma 1

29.3 Femoral Osteoid Osteoma 2

- Scanogram left femur shows a diffuse ill-defined sclerosed area measuring 11 mm (arrow) (Fig. 29.3A).
- Coronal image shows a hyperdense central focus (nidus) thereby confirming the lesion to be osteoid osteoma (Fig. 29.3B).
- Coronal and sagittal image demonstrate the osteoid osteoma (Figs 29.3C and D).

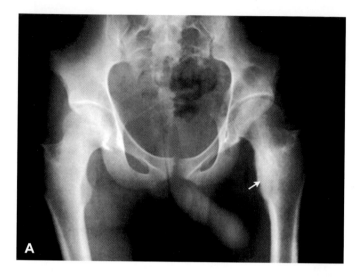

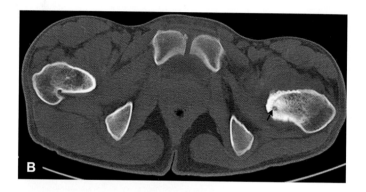

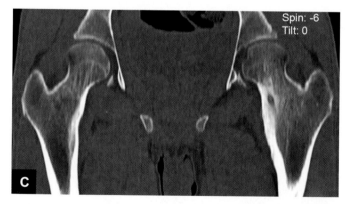

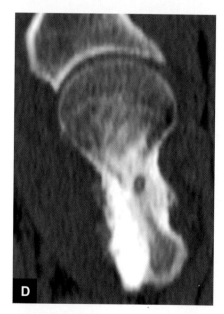

Figs 29.3A to D: Osteoid osteoma 2

29.4 Spinal Osteoma

Osteoid Osteoma

- Plain radiograph of spine shows mild sclerosis of lamina of T1 vertebra (Fig. 29.4A).
- Plain CT at that level reveals a rounded low attenuation area with central hyperdense nidus in the lamina of T1 vertebra. This is 10 mm in diameter. Diagnosis: osteoid osteoma (Fig. 29.4B).
- Nuclear scan of the same patient shows a hot spot at the site of lesion due to increased vascularity (Fig. 29.4C).

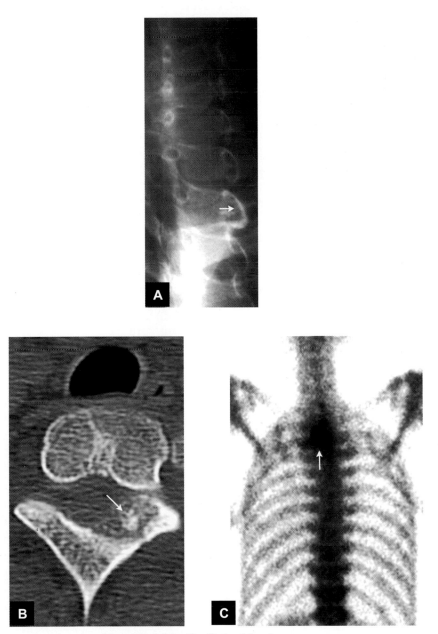

Figs 29.4A to C: Osteoid osteoma

30. MISCELLANEOUS

30.1 Aneurysmal Bone Cyst

A 16 years male had history of painful swelling near right ankle.

Scanogram (Fig. 30.1A), axial images (Figs 30.1B and C), coronal reformatted image (Fig. 30.1D), sagittal reformatted image (Fig. 30.1E). Volume rendered image (Fig. 30.1F).

An eccentric expansile lytic lesion is seen in the distal diaphysis and metaphysis region of right tibia. Multiple septae are seen. The inner portion is sclerotic. No periosteal reaction is seen. The lesion does not cross the epiphyseal plate.

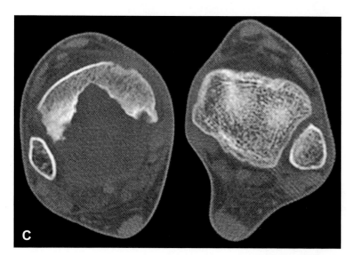
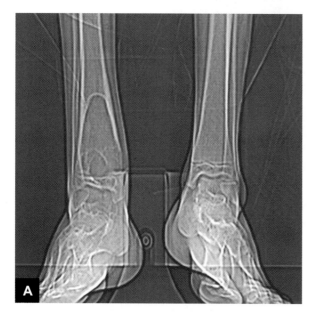
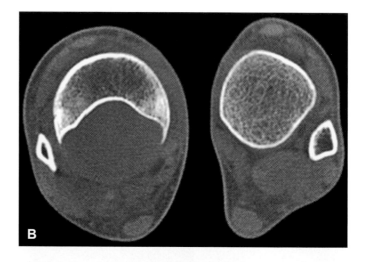
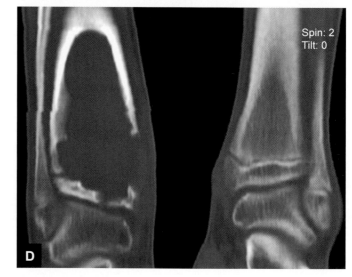

Figs 30.1A to D: Aneurysmal bone cyst

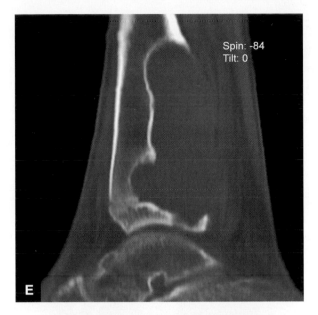

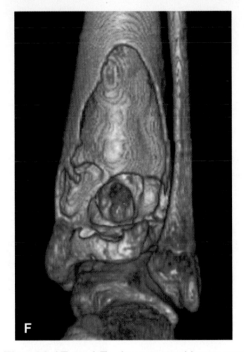

Figs 30.1E and F: Aneurysmal bone cyst

30.2 Avascular Necrosis (AVN) Femur

38 years female had pain in left hip.

CT images show partial destruction of inferomedial aspect of femoral head, acetabular remodeling and superolateral migration of remnant of femoral head forming pseudoarthrosis with false acetabulum formed by left iliac blade (Figs 30.2A to F).

AVN results from loss of the blood supply to an area of the bone, the bone tissue dies and the bone collapses. If it involves the bones of a joint, it often leads to destruction of the articular surfaces.

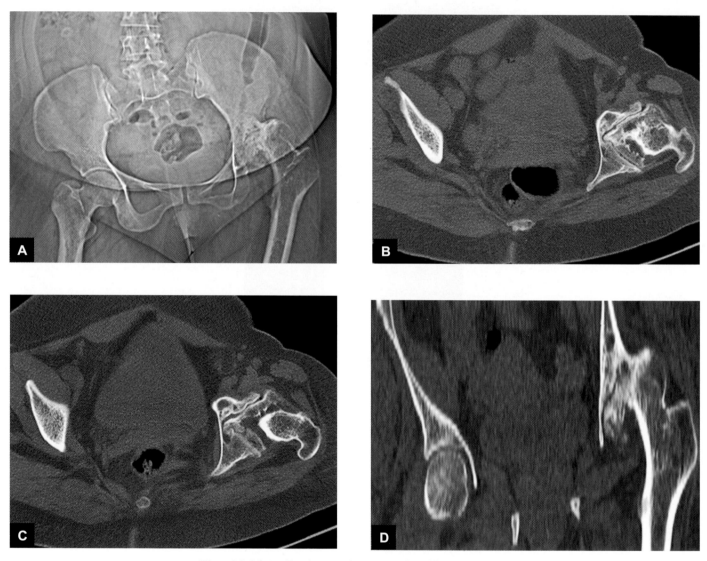

Figs 30.2A to D: Avascular necrosis of femoral head

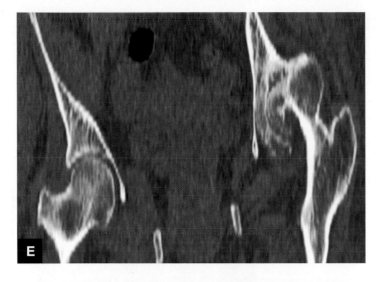

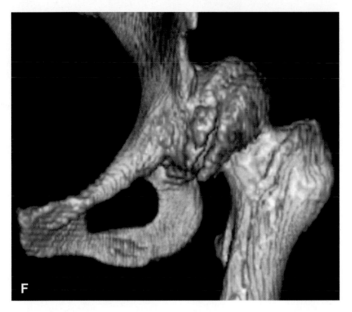

Figs 30.2E and F: Avascular necrosis of femoral head

30.3 Osteochondritis Dissecans

Osteochondritis Dissecans of Tibial Plafond

- Coronal CT scan shows osteochondral lesion with loose body at lateral aspect of tibial plafond (distal articular surface of tibia) (Fig. 30.3A).
- Sagittal reconstructed image shows osteolysis at lateral aspect of tibial plafond in a case of osteochondritis dissecans (Fig. 30.3B).
- Axial image shows osteolysis at lateral aspect of tibial plafond (Fig. 30.3C).

On conventional radiographs, osteochondritis dissecans of the tibial plafond appears lucent and may contain a loose bony fragment. CT and MR imaging are able to show the exact location and extent of the lesion.

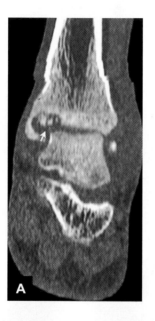

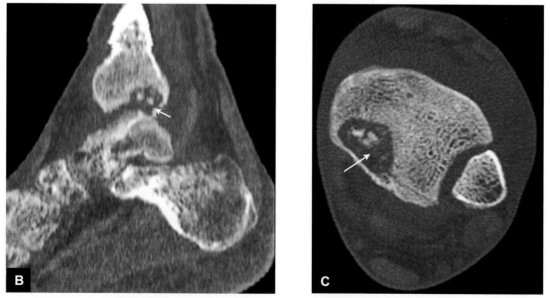

Figs 30.3A to C: Osteochondritis dissecans of tibial plafond

30.4 Rickets

- X-ray of both hands in a patients with rickets shows osteomalacia with widening of growth plate, splaying and cupping of distal metaphysis of radius and ulna with irregular metaphyseal margins (Fig. 30.4A).
- CT axial and coronal reconstructed images confirm the X-ray findings of defective mineralization of osteoid tissue in cortical and cancellous bone (Figs 30.4B to D).

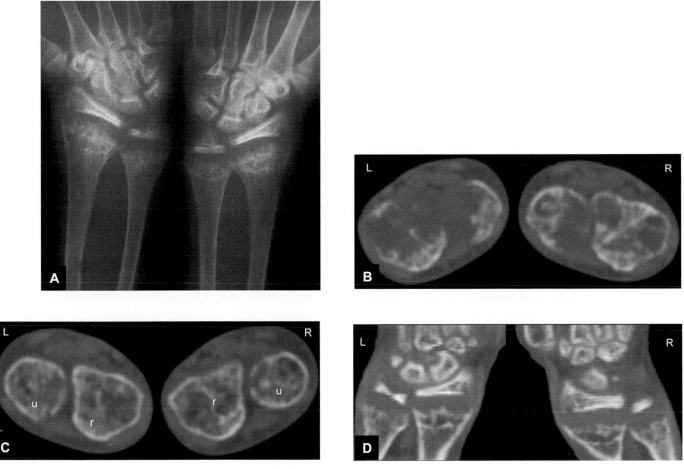

Figs 30.4A to D: Rickets

30.5 Loose Bodies in Shoulder Joint

CT scan of left shoulder shows two loose bodies in the joint (Fig. 30.5). These on becoming symptomatic can cause painful joint movement and delimit range of movement.

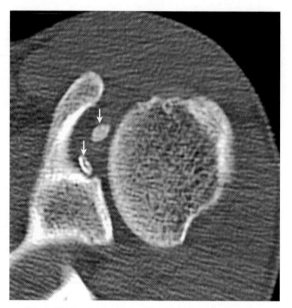

Fig. 30.5: Loose bodies in shoulder joint

Section 6

Central Nervous System

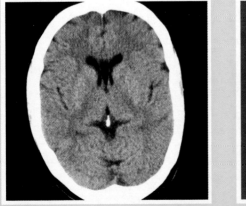
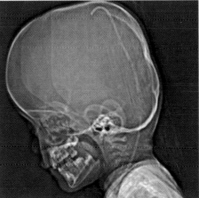
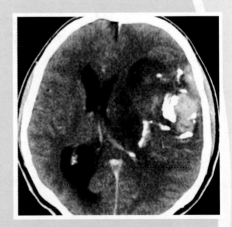

31. NORMAL BRAIN ANATOMY

31.1 Axial CT sections of Brain (Figs 31.1A to J)

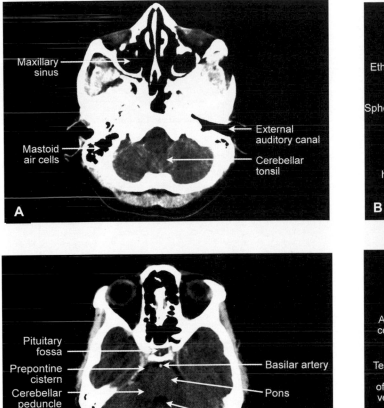

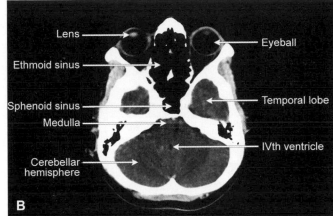

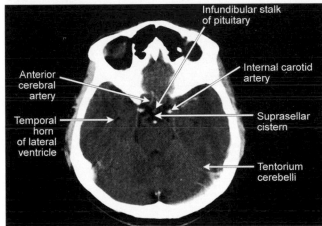

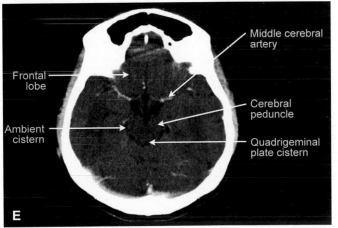

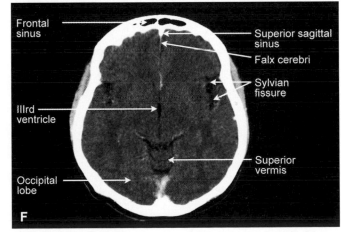

Figs 31.1A to F: Axial CT sections of brain

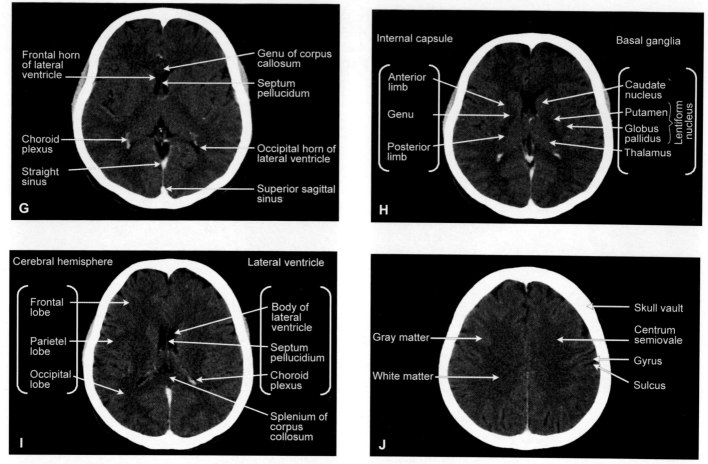

Figs 31.1G to J: Axial CT sections of brain

32. CONGENITAL DISORDERS

32.1 Cavum Septum Pellucidum

• CT brain shows persistent cavum septum pellucidum at various levels (Figs 32.1A to C).

The septum pellucidum has a cavity of 1 to 2 mm in width. When this cavity is larger, it is cavum septum pellucidum or fifth ventricle, a normal variant. The term fifth ventricle is a misnomer because unlike ventricular cavities it does not contain cerebrospinal fluid nor is it lined by ependyma.

Cavum vergae (VIth ventricle) is the continuation of cavum septi in midline posteriorly and is located posterior to fornix.

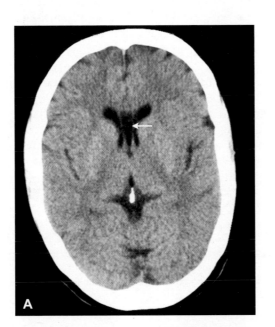

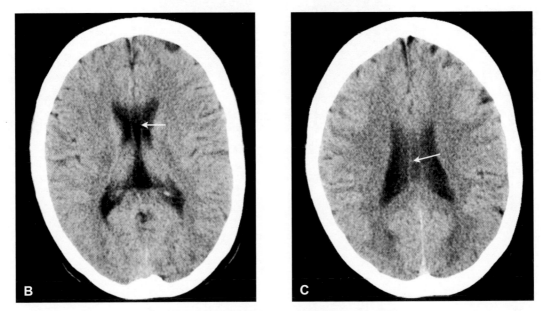

Figs 32.1A to C: Cavum septum pellucidum

32.2 Arnold-Chiari Malformations

8 years male child operated two years ago for lumbar meningomyelocele with shunt tube for hydrocephalous. Follow up CT (Figs 32.2A to H) shows Chiari II malformation with malposition of shunt tube. Posterior fossa is small, peg-shaped cerebellar tonsils are low placed and are lying below the widened foramen magnum. Hydrocephalous is present and the tip of the shunt tube is seen in the brain parenchyma.

Chiari I Malformation – Cerebellar tonsils herniate below foramen magnum > 5 mm, clinical symptoms in form of cranial nerve dysfunctions and/or sensory or motor disturbances in the extremities. Posterior fossa is usually small. This is never associated with meningomyelocele but basilar impression can be present.

Chiari II Malformation – There is dysgenesis of hindbrain associated with caudal displacement of brainstem and fourth ventricle. Cerebellar tonsils and vermis are herniated below foramen magnum. May be associated with lumbar meningomyelocele but never associated with basilar impression. Hydrocephalous may be present due to dysfunction of aqueduct of Sylvius.

Chiari III Malformation – Characterized by low occipital or high cervical meningomyeloencephalocele.

Chiari IV Malformation – Posterior fossa is small funnel-shaped with cerebellar agenesis and pontine hypoplasia.

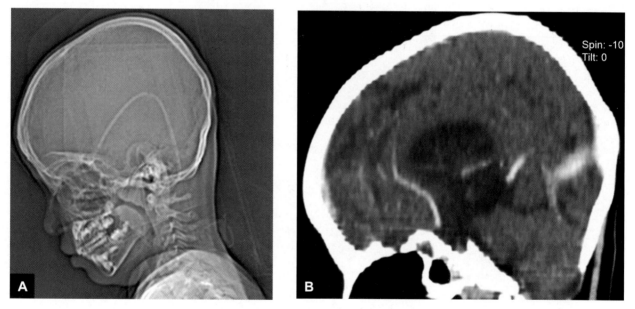

Figs 32.2A and B: Arnold-Chiari malformation

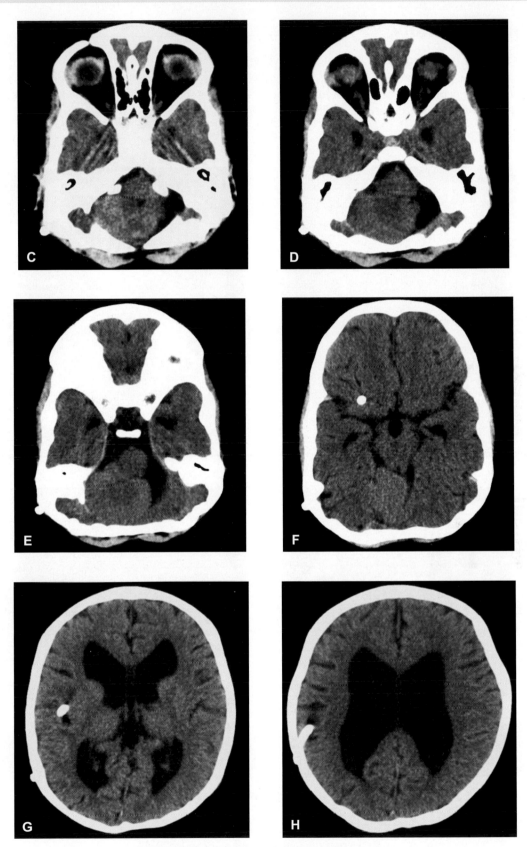

Figs 32.2C to H: Arnold-Chiari malformation

32.3 Schizencephaly

Open lip schizencephaly occupying the left hemicranium (Figs 32.3B to D).

Schizencephaly means split brain. CSF filled cleft extends from the ependymal surface of ventricles to the pia mater. Differential diagnosis of schizencephaly is porencephalic cyst in which the CSF cleft is lined by gliotic white matter, whereas in schizencephaly the cleft is lined by heterotopic gray matter.

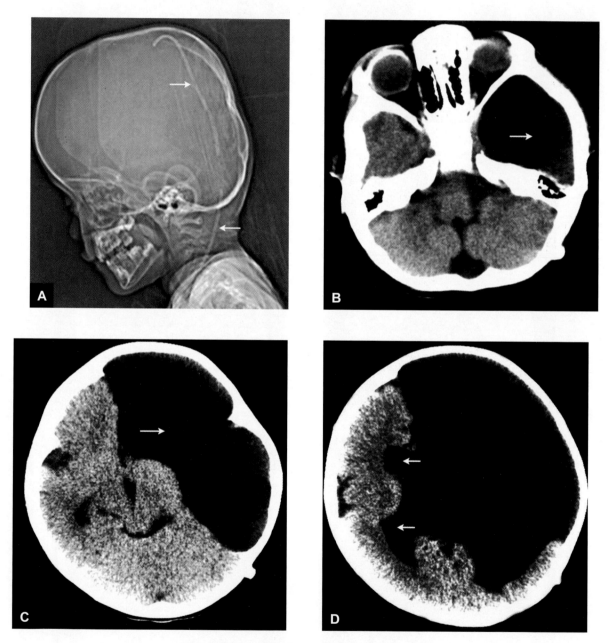

Figs 32.3A to D: Open lip schizencephaly

32.4 Cranial Meningocele

Meningocele of anterior cranial vault in a newborn (Fig. 32.4).

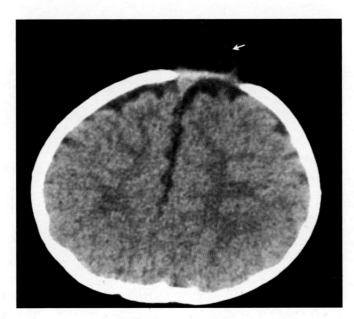

Fig. 32.4: Cranial meningocele

32.5 Dolichoectatic Basilar Artery

Prominent tortuous dilated basilar artery is seen (Figs 32.5A to D).

    The dolichoectatic basilar artery is associated with various consequences especially in relation to the pathogenesis of brainstem infarction. When this anomaly is diagnosed on CT, even if it is clinically asymptomatic, patients may be subjected to medical therapy to prevent ischemic stroke.

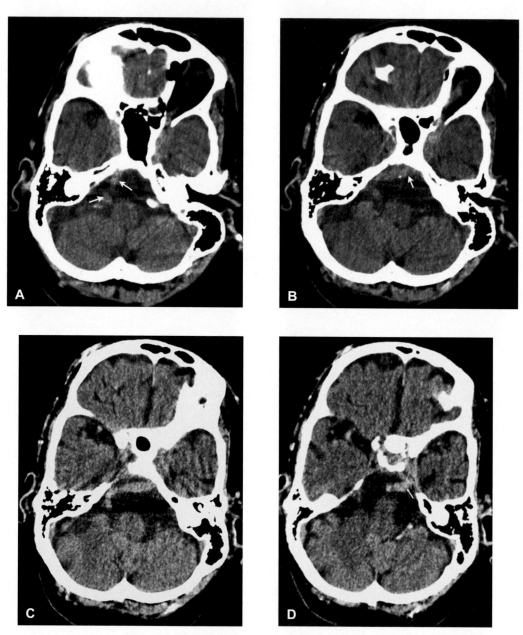

Figs 32.5A to D: Dolichoectatic basilar artery

33. TRAUMA AND VASCULAR INSULT

33.1 Cerebral Contusion (Fig. 33.1)

Cerebral contusion due to traumatic brain injury. 'Salt and pepper lesion' appearance seen is due to mixture of edema, infarcted and injured brain tissue with small hemorrhagic component.

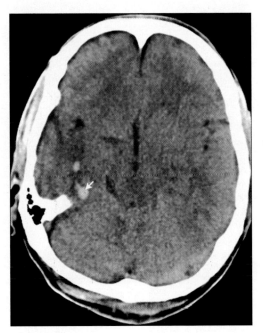

Fig. 33.1: Cerebral contusion

33.2 Extradural Hematoma

- CT bone window and brain window show a small linear undisplaced fracture of middle cranial fossa and extradural hematoma in vicinity. Black spot in the hematoma is due to loculated air (Fig. 33.2A).
- CT Brain shows right biconvex extradural hematoma with small loculated air inside (Fig. 33.2B).
- CT Brain shows left biconvex extradural hematoma (Fig. 33.2C).

Extradural or epidural hematoma occurs due to accumulation of blood in the space between inner table of skull and dura. This is usually associated with fracture of cranial vault. It has a biconvex shape and is due to the rupture of branches of middle meningeal artery. It does not cross the suture line.

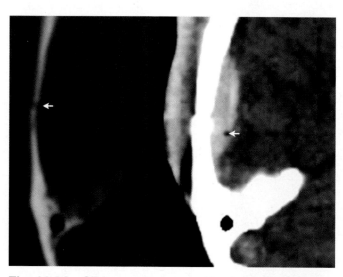

Fig. 33.2A: CT bone window and brain window show a fracture of temporal bone and extradural hematoma in vicinity

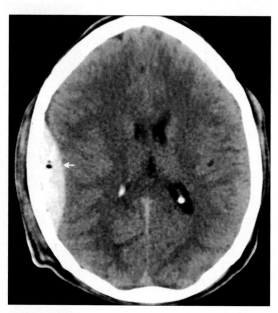

Fig. 33.2B: CT brain shows right biconvex extradural hematoma

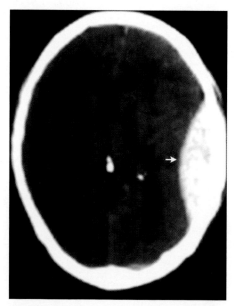

Fig. 33.2C: CT brain shows left biconvex extradural hematoma

33.3 Diffuse Cerebral Edema

CT brain shows diffuse areas of hypodensity, more in white matter (Fig. 33.3). Due to the mass effect the gyri are flattened and CSF containing structures are effaced.

Diffuse cerebral edema is either due to cytotoxic origin, i.e. due to cell damage as in ischemia/infarct or it might be of vasogenic origin as in hemorrhage, neoplasm or inflammation. Traumatic head injury causes congestive brain edema due to sudden increase in extracellular water.

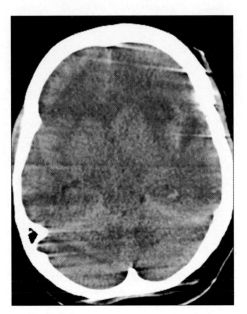

Fig. 33.3: Diffuse cerebral edema

33.4 Diffuse Axonal Injury

CT shows a diffuse axonal injury (DAI) caused by shearing injuries and is seen as petechial hemorrhages at grey white matter junction, basal ganglia and pons (Fig. 33.4).

Diffuse axonal injury (DAI) is a result of traumatic deceleration injuries and is a frequent cause for persistent vegetative state in patients. DAI typically consists of several focal white-matter lesions measuring 1-15 mm size.

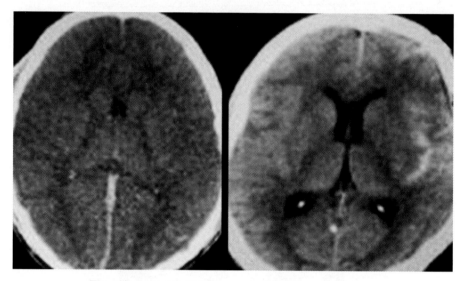

Fig. 33.4: Axial CT shows a diffuse axonal injury

33.5 Post-traumatic Subarachnoid Hemorrhage

Plain CT shows a post-traumatic subarachnoid hemorrhage along the left tentorial leaflet (Fig. 33.5). Linear and an undisplaced fracture of right parietal bone (arrow) with an extra cranial soft tissue swelling seen adjacent to the fracture.

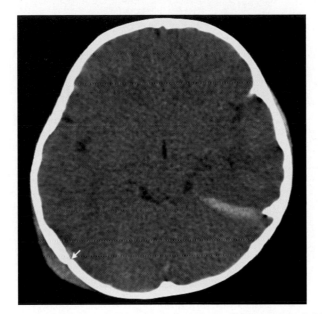

Fig. 33.5: Subarachnoid hemorrhage along the left tentorial leaflet

33.6 Subarachnoid Hemorrhage 1

Subarachnoid hemorrhage is usually due to ruptured aneurysm or AV malformations (Fig. 33.6).

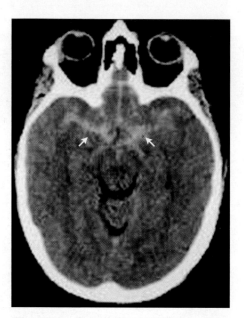

Fig. 33.6: Subarachnoid hemorrhage

33.7 Thalamic Bleed

Non hypertensive patient presented with sudden weakness in right upper limb and right lower limb. Intracranial bleed seen in left thalamus, measuring 9 mm in diameter (Fig. 33.7).

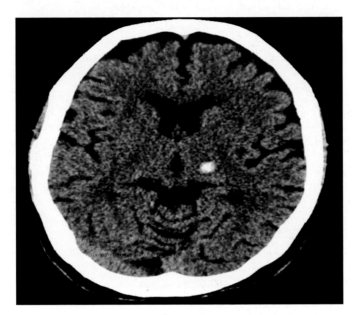

Fig. 33.7: Intracranial bleed seen in left thalamus

33.8 Cerebral Hemorrhage

Plain CT brain shows fresh hemorrhage as hyperdense lesion in left parafalcine parietal cortex (Fig. 33.8).

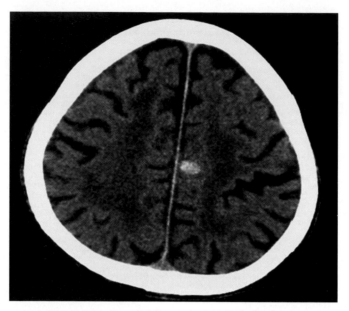

Fig. 33.8: Parafalcine cerebral hemorrhage

33.9 Subarachnoid Hemorrhage 2

- Diffuse SAH along the cisterns (Fig. 33.9A).
- SAH in the interhemispheric fissure and in the left cerebral sulcus (Fig. 33.9B).
- SAH in left cerebellopontine angle cistern and hemorrhagic contusion in left temporal lobe (Figs 33.9C and D).

SAH is bleeding into the subarachnoid space, the area between the arachnoid membrane and the pia mater surrounding the brain. This may occur spontaneously, usually from a ruptured cerebral aneurysm or may result from head injury. Symptoms of SAH include thunderclap headache (severe headache of rapid onset), vomiting, confusion, lowered level of consciousness and/or seizures. The diagnosis is confirmed on CT scan.

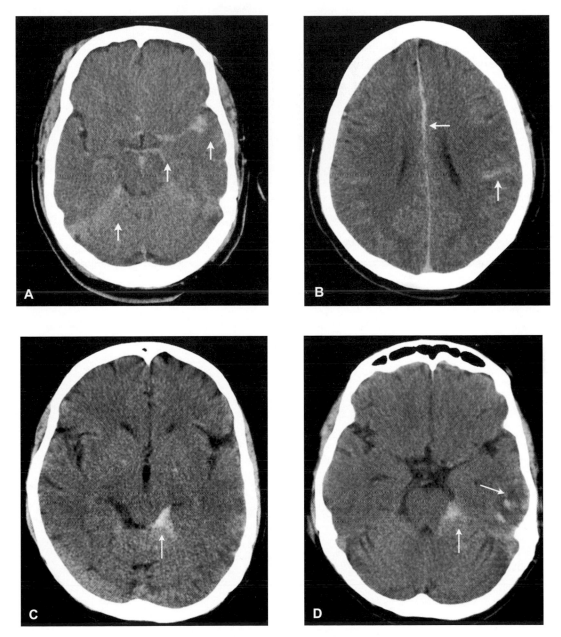

Figs 33.9A to D: Subarachnoid hemorrhage

33.10 Mixed Patterns of Hemorrhage

CT scan brain shows mixed/combined patterns of post-traumatic intracranial hemorrhage seen as EDH-Extradural hematoma, SDH-Subdural hematoma, SAH-Subarachnoid Hemorrhage and C-Parenchymal contusion (Fig. 33.10).

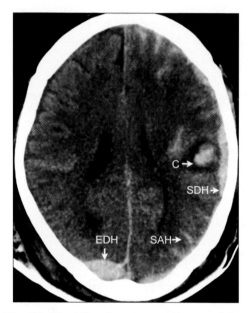

Fig. 33.10: Mixed patterns of hemorrhage

33.11 Epidural or Extradural Hemorrhage with Active Bleeding

- CT brain shows acute extradural hemorrhage as hyperdense collection extending to interhemispheric fissure (Figs 33.11A and B). Hypodense areas in it suggest fresh bleed into the extradural hematoma due to swirling of blood and is called 'the Swirl Sign'.

The swirl sign is an ominous sign of epidural or extradural hemorrhage and has two components, an active component and a relatively earlier bleed. The active component is usually a small rounded lesion that is isoattenuating to the brain and that represents actively extravasating unclotted blood. The earlier component is the hyperattenuating extraaxial hematoma collection, which typically measures 50 - 70 HU. We prefer to call it 'Black in white sign.'

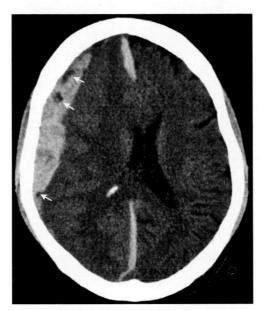

Fig. 33.11A: Extradural hemorrhagic with active bleeding

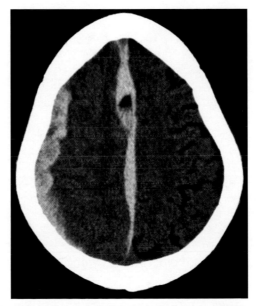

Fig. 33.11B: Extradural hemorrhagic with bleed extending to interhemispheric fissure

33.12 Subdural Hematoma 1

58 years old male presented with headache since one month and weakness on left side of body since 10 days. Plain CT Brain (Figs 33.12A to D) shows chronic (hypodense) right subdural hematoma causing mass effect in the form of compression of right lateral ventricle and contralateral shift of midline structures. The hyperdensities seen in this subdural hematoma suggests fresh bleed, i.e. acute on chronic hematoma.

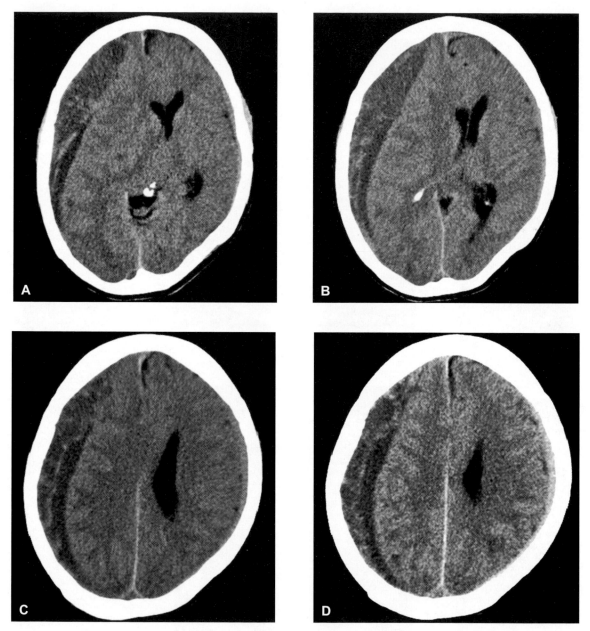

Figs 33.12A to D: Plain CT brain shows chronic right subdural hematoma

33.13 Subdural Hematoma 2

Intracranial hemorrhage occurring between dura and arachnoid matter it is called subdural hemorrhage. It has a concavo-convex appearance and does not cross the midline. It occurs due to injury to bridging cortical veins. Various phases of subdural hematoma can be differentiated by the CT appearance of blood.

- Acute subdural hematoma, the blood appears hyperdense and has CT value of 50-70 HU. This phase lasts for around one week (Fig. 33.13A).
- Subacute hematoma it is less brighter (dull bright) and at places hypodensities are seen in it due to the beginning of liquefaction. This phase lasts for 1-2 weeks and the isodense blood has a density of 25-40 HU (Fig. 33.13B).
- In chronic subdural hematoma, the blood has liquefied completely and looks hypodense. This phase starts after 3 weeks of primary insult. The hypodense blood has a density of < 25 HU (Fig. 33.13C).
- Interhemispheric acute subdural hematoma. This is commonly seen in battered baby syndrome (Fig. 33.13D).

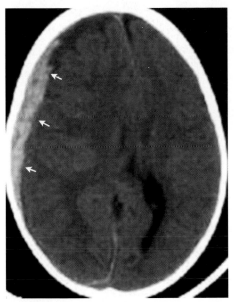

Fig. 33.13A: Plain CT brain shows acute subdural hematoma

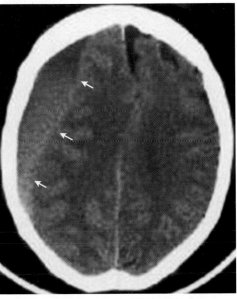

Fig. 33.13B: Plain CT brain shows subacute subdural hematoma

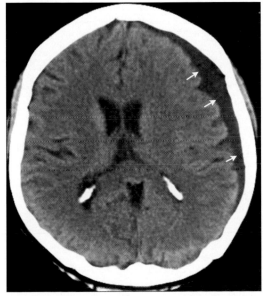

Fig. 33.13C: Plain CT brain shows chronic subdural hematoma

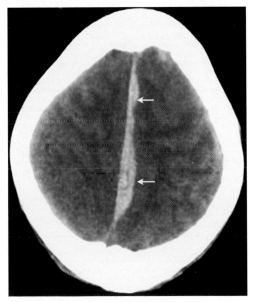

Fig. 33.13D: Plain CT brain shows interhemispheric acute subdural hematoma

33.14 Chronic Extradural Hematoma

Left anterior extra axial hypodense (20 HU) crescenteric collection (Fig. 33.14) causing mass effect in form of compression of frontal and temporal horns of left lateral ventricle with shift of midline structures to the right.

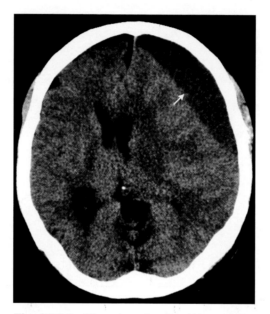

Fig. 33.14: Chronic extradural hematoma

33.15 Extradural Hemorrhage

Massive extradural hemorrhage on right side. There is mass effect in form of obliterating compression of right lateral ventricle, contralateral shift of falx cerebri and left lateral ventricle which is compressed and narrowed (Fig. 33.15).

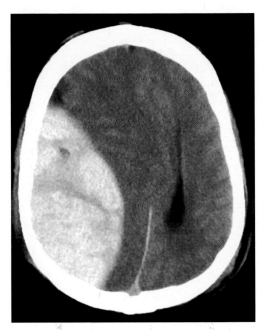

Fig. 33.15: Plain CT brain shows a
large extradural hemorrhage

33.16 Cerebrovascular Accident – Early Sign

- Plain CT shows hyperdense appearance of MCA-'Hyperdense MCA' sign (Fig. 33.16A), which is the earliest indicator of impending cerebral ischemia/infarct. This patient had left hemi-paresis of sudden onset.
- CT brain shows that a frank infarct has not yet set in (Fig. 33.16B).

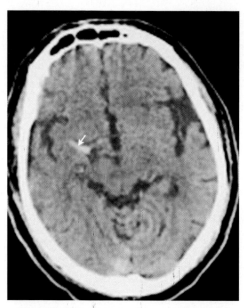

Fig. 33.16A: Hyperdense MCA sign

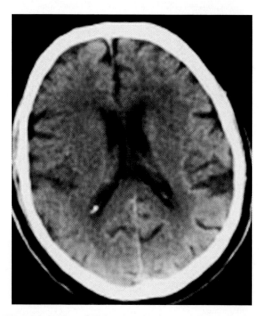

Fig. 33.16B: CT brain shows no frank infarct

33.17 Infarcts 1

Ischemia or infarction causes tissue damage which occurs due to reduced blood supply to an organ or area. Most common cause is occlusion of an artery supplying that region. This is more common in organ like brain which has areas of only single end arterial supply.

Once the brain tissue is infracted the dead neurons slowly undergo gliotic change. Normal brain has a CT attenuation value of more than 30HU. A fresh infarct has CT value 25-30 HU. An old infarct has a further reduction in CT value to 10-15 HU. Old infarct ultimately undergoes gliotic change, volume loss and is finally replaced by CSF density fluid and is then known as cystic encephalomalacia/porencephalic cyst.

Fresh Infarcts

- Left anterior frontal cortex (Fig. 33.17A)
- Left gangliocapsular region (Fig. 33.17B)
- Posterior temporal cortex near the midline (Fig. 33.17C)
- Right caudate nucleus (Fig. 33.17D)
- Right parietal cortex. Post-contrast (E2) CT image shows gyriform enhancement due to increased reperfusion vascularity (Fig. 33.17E)
- Right cerebellar region (Fig. 33.17F)
- Left posterior parietal cortex (Fig. 33.17G)
- Anterior limb of right internal capsule (Fig. 33.17H)
- Left external capsule (Fig. 33.17I)
- Right anterior high frontal cortex (Fig. 33.17J)
- Left anterior cortex near midline- gyrus rectus region (Fig. 33.17K).

Old Infarct

- Old infarct right fronto-temporal region, gliotic change is seen and is progressing towards cystic encephalomalacia (Fig. 33.17L).
- Old infarct left posterior parietal region (a). In post contrast image (b) there is no enhancement (Fig. 33.17M).

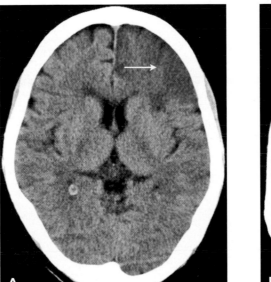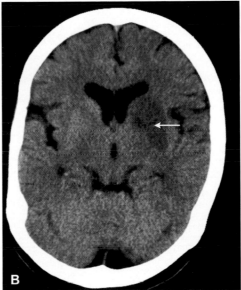

Figs 33.17A and B: Infarcts

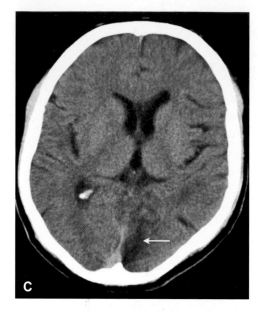

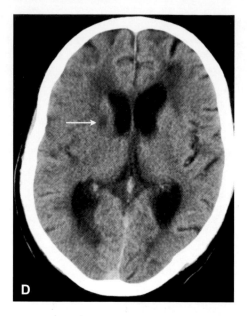

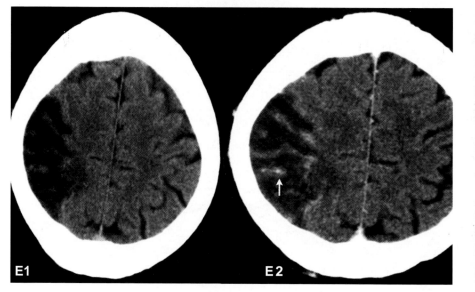

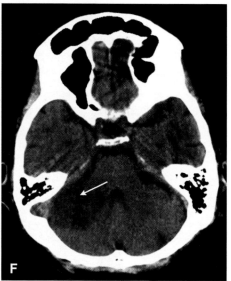

Figs 33.17C to F: Infarcts

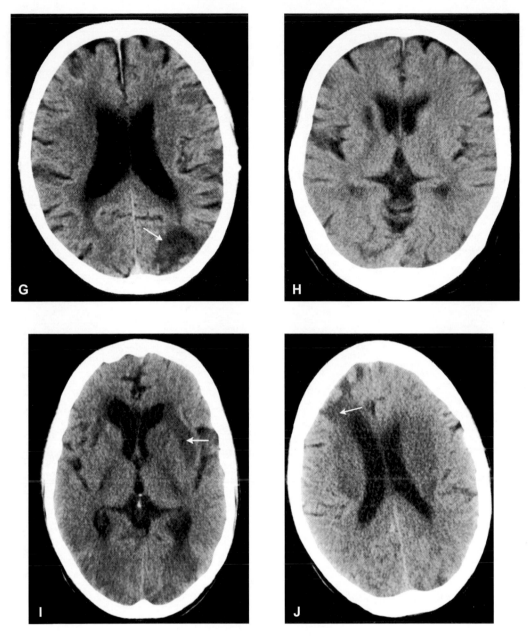

Figs 33.17G to J: Infarcts

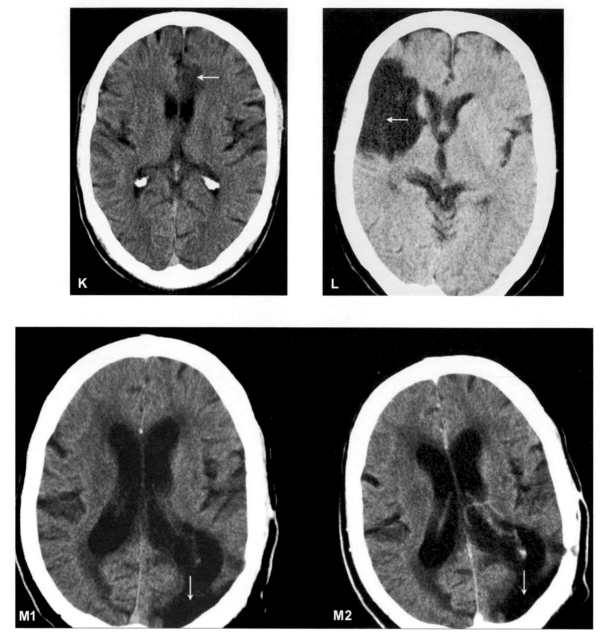

Figs 33.17K to M: Infarcts

33.18 Infarcts 2

1. Temporal Lobe Infarct (Fig. 33.18A)

Sudden weakness in left upper and lower limbs resulting from acute infarct in right temporoparietal region.

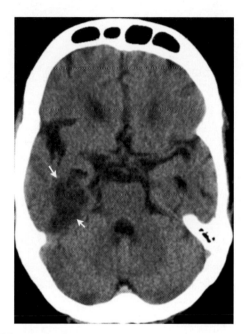

Fig. 33.18A: Plain CT brain shows right temporal lobe infarct

2. Middle Cerebral Artery (MCA) Territory Infarct-1 (Figs 33.18B and C)

Right MCA infarct is seen as hypodense area in right cerebral hemisphere. The mass effect has caused compression on ipsilateral lateral ventricle with minimal shift of midline structures.

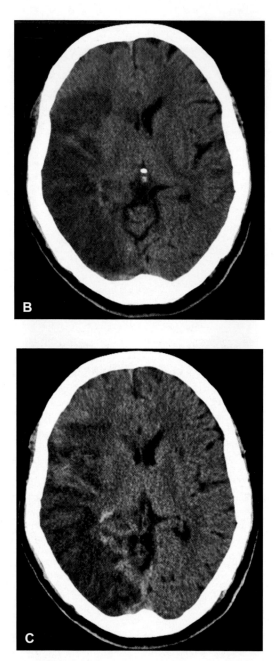

Figs 33.18B and C: Right middle cerebral artery territory infarct

3. MCA Territory Infarct-2

Plain (Fig. 33.18D) and contrast CT (Fig. 33.18E) shows nonenhancing hypodense left MCA territory infarct. The mass effect of edema is causing compression of left lateral ventricle and mild shift of midline structures to contralateral side.

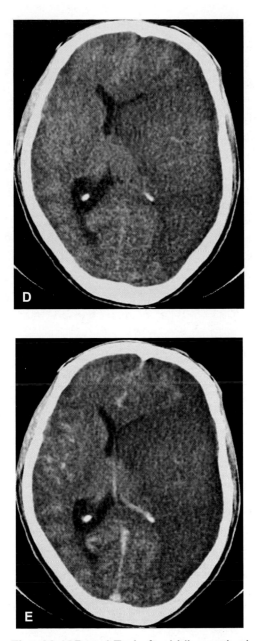

Figs 33.18D and E: Left middle cerebral artery territory infarct

4. Posterior Cerebral Infarct

Axial CT show left posterior cerebral infarct (Fig. 33.18F).

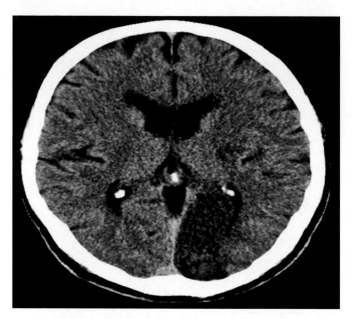

Fig. 33.18F: Left posterior cerebral infarct

5. Posterior Parietal Infarct

Left posterior parietal infarct (Fig. 33.18G).

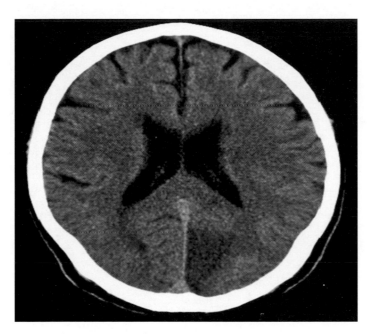

Fig. 33.18G: Posterior parietal infarct

6. Pontine Infarct

Plain CT brain shows an infarct in pons as a hypodense area (Figs 33.18H and I).

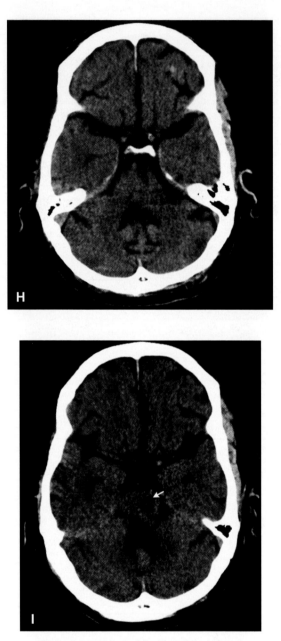

Figs 33.18H and I: Pontine infarct

7. Thalamic Infarct (Fig. 33.18J)

Left thalamic infarct, patient presented with sudden onset of weakness of the right side of the body.

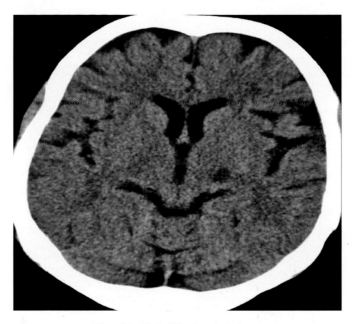

Fig. 33.18J: Thalamic infarct

33.19 Gliosis as Sequelae to Infarct

Plain CT images show hypodense area (2 to 7 HU value similar to that of CSF) in the region of old right temporoparietal infarct due to gliosis as a sequele (Figs 33.19A to D).

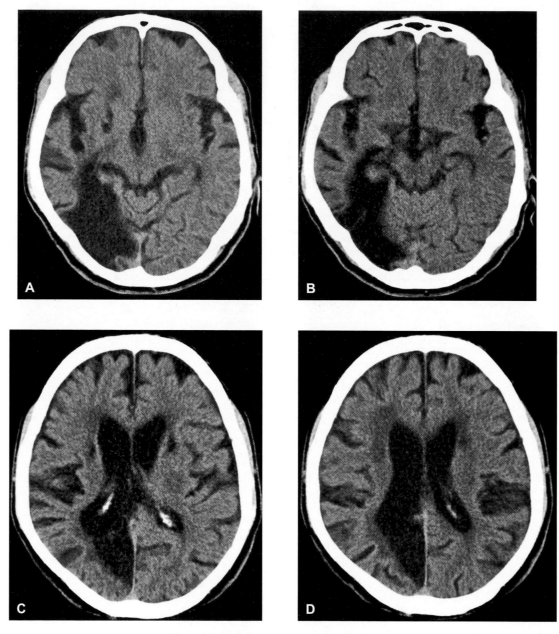

Figs 33.19A to D: Post infarct gliosis

33.20 Hemorrhagic Venous Infarct

Plain CT brain shows multiple hemorrhagic lesions in the brain parenchyma with perilesional edema and mass effect in a 20 years old female brought with sudden unconsciousness (Fig. 33.20).

Hemorrhagic venous infarct are visible as large subcortical hematomas or fluffy petechial hemorrhages within the area of hypodensity. The large hemorrhages are subcortical and multifocal with irregular margins.

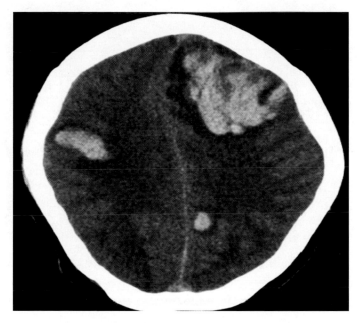

Fig. 33.20: Hemorrhagic venous infarct

33.21 Post-infarct Gliosis (Figs 33.21A and B)

Plain CT brain shows gliosis in left fronto-parietal region following an old infarct. The resultant volume loss has caused the focal dilatation of left lateral ventricle.

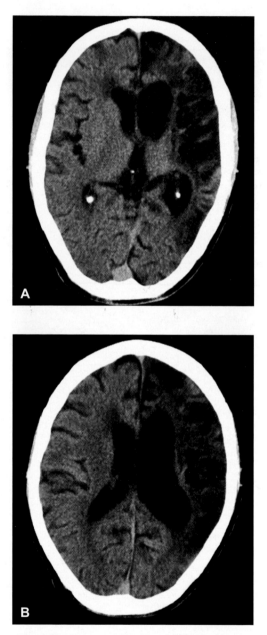

Figs 33.21A and B: Post-infarct gliosis

34. INFECTIVE-INFLAMMATORY

34.1 Ring Enhancing Lesions

Ring enhancing lesions in brain are due to following causes:
- Infective : Bacterial –tuberculosis, pyogenic abscesses, fungal – histoplasmosis, parasitic- cysticercosis.
- Inflammatory/demyelinating : Multiple sclerosis, radiation necrosis, leukoencephalopathies.
- Neoplastic : Primary tumors like high grade glioma, leukemia, craniopharyngioma, metastasis.
- Miscellaneous : Resolving infarct/hematoma, partially thrombosed aneurysm and post surgery.
  Ring enhancing lesions that can cross corpus callosum are: lymphoma glioblastoma multiforme and astrocytoma.

The radiological differential diagnoses of a ring-enhancing lesion in the brain would include granuloma, tuberculoma, cysticercus, pyogenic abscess, metastatic disease and a high-grade glioma. Tuberculomas generally have an irregular margin and have significant perilesional edema. Cysticercus granuloma has smooth regular margin and a central nidus.

- Plain CT brain show edema as hypodensities (Fig. 34.1A1).
- Contrast CT shows ring enhancing lesion in right fronto-parietal region with surrounding edema (Fig. 34.1A2).
- Plain CT brain showing star-shaped hypo-density due to edema (Fig. 34.1B1).
- Contrast CT shows ring enhancing lesion in right high parietal region (Fig. 34.1B2).
- Plain CT brain shows edema as hypodensities (Fig. 34.1C1).
- Contrast CT brain showing multiple ring enhancing lesions in high parietal region, some of them have a central hyperdense nidus (neurocysticercosis) (Fig. 34.1C2).
- Plain CT brain showing edema as hypo density in right high parietal region (Fig. 34.1D1).
- Contrast CT brain showing thick walled enhancing lesion with surrounding edema (glioma/metastasis) (Fig. 34.1D2).

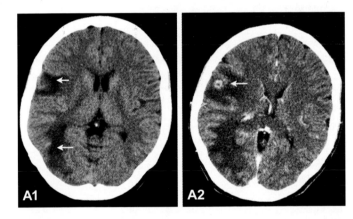

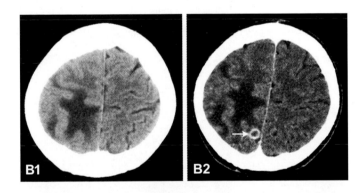

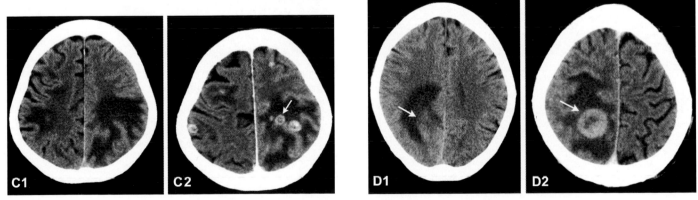

Figs 34.1A1 to D2: Ring enhancing lesions

34.2 Ring Enhancing Intracranial Granulomas (Figs 34.2A to E)

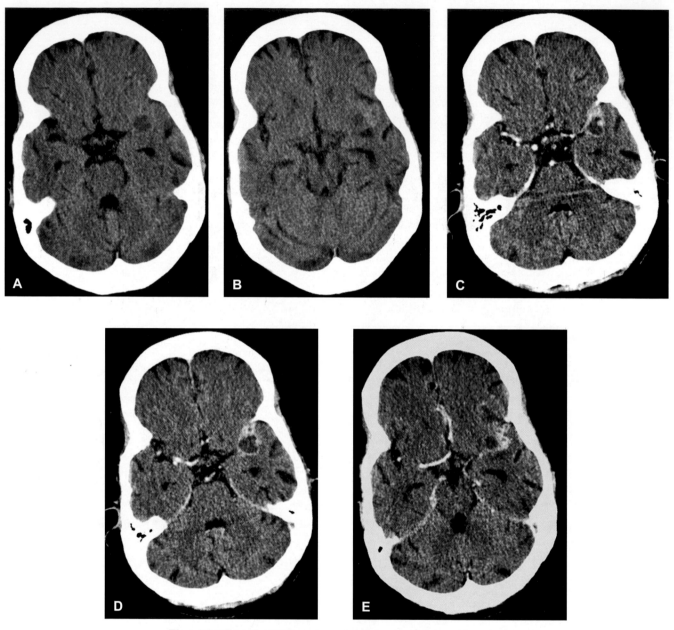

Figs 34.2A to E: Ring enhancing intracranial granulomas

34.3 Tuberculoma

Pre (Figs 34.3A and B) and post-contrast (Figs 34.3C and D) CT brain images show conglomeration of intensely enhancing ring lesions with perilesional edema in right frontal lobe.

Tuberculoma is usually formed by conglomeration of several miliary tubercles, which form around the outer sheaths of the small cerebral blood vessels. The center of the conglomeration becomes caseous, inspissated and sometimes liquified. A thick capsule may form around these lesions.

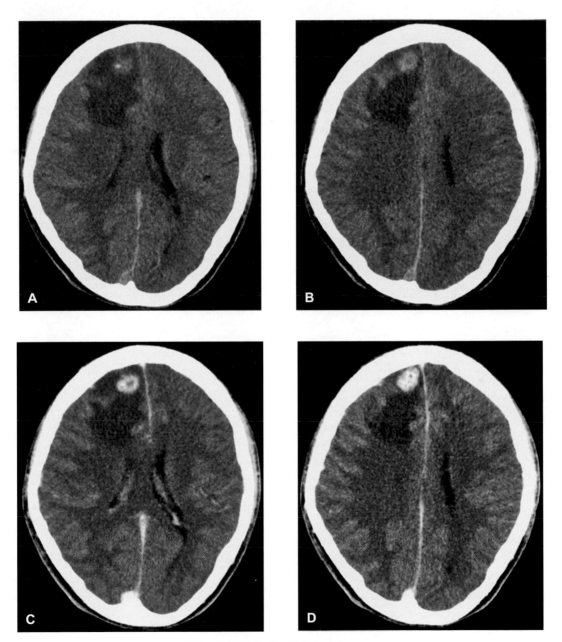

Figs 34.3A to D: Tuberculomas

34.4 Cerebral Abscess

- Plain CT scan of head shows right frontal hypodense area (Fig. 34.4A).
- Post-contrast CT shows subtle enhancement of its walls (Fig. 34.4B).

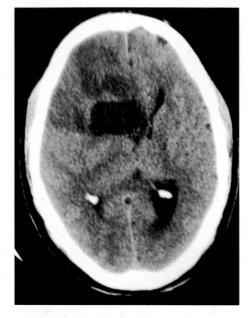 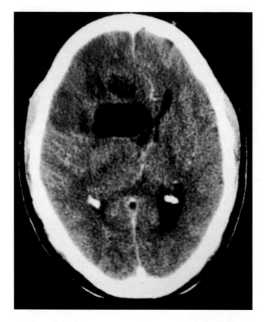

Fig. 34.4A: Plain CT shows right frontal hypodense area

Fig. 34.4B: Post-contrast CT shows subtle enhancement of its walls

34.5 Temporal Lobe Abscess

- Scout image of CT brain shows loculated air in the cranium suggesting air fluid level (Fig. 34.5A).
- CT brain shows right temporal abscess with air-fluid level (Fig. 34.5B).
- Contrast CT shows minimal enhancement of wall of the abscess (Fig. 34.5C).
- CT temporal bone shows right otomastoiditis with breach of dural plate of petrous temporal bone (Fig. 34.5D) which was the etiology factor.

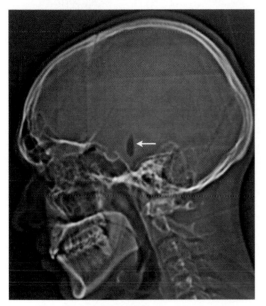

Fig. 34.5A: Scout image shows loculated air in the cranium with air fluid level

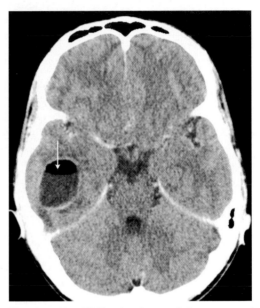

Fig. 34.5B: CT brain shows right temporal abscess with air-fluid level

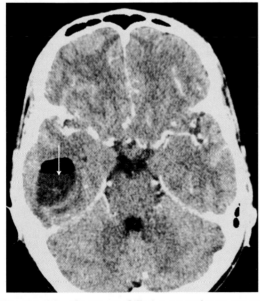

Fig. 34.5C: Contrast CT shows enhancement of wall of the abscess

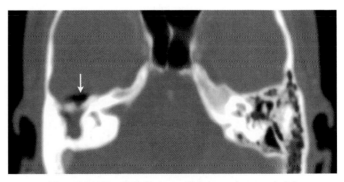

Fig. 34.5D: CT temporal bone shows right otomastoiditis with breach of petrous temporal bone

34.6 Meningitis (Figs 34.6A to D)

17 years female with high grade fever, headache, nausea, altered sensorium and presence of neck stiffness.
Contrast CT brain shows abnormal enhancement along the cerebral sulci, right sylvian fissure and tentorial leaflet suggestive of meningitis.

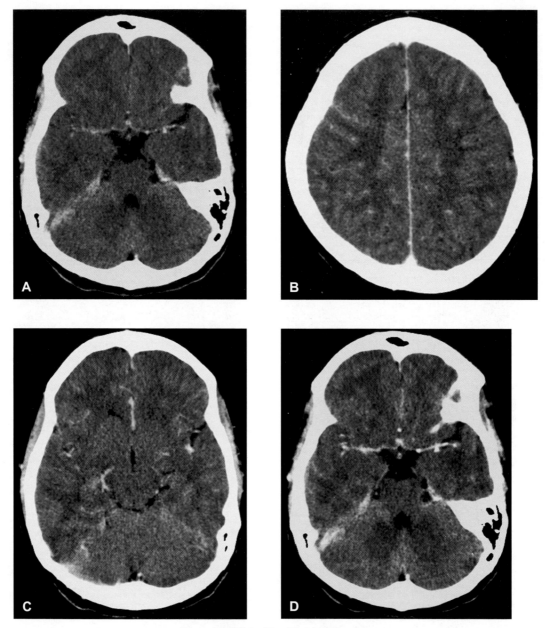

Figs 34.6A to D: Meningitis

35. NEOPLASTIC

35.1 Intraventricular Lipoma (Figs 35.1A to D)

CT images show a massive left MCA territory infarct. Careful viewing shows asymmetric focal bulge in posterior horn of right lateral ventricle that is not explainable with mass effect due to edema. The intraventricular CT value in this region of the bulge was (-)40 to (-)50 HU (confirms tissue as fat) as against 2-10 HU for CSF. It was diagnosed as infarct with intraventricular lipoma.

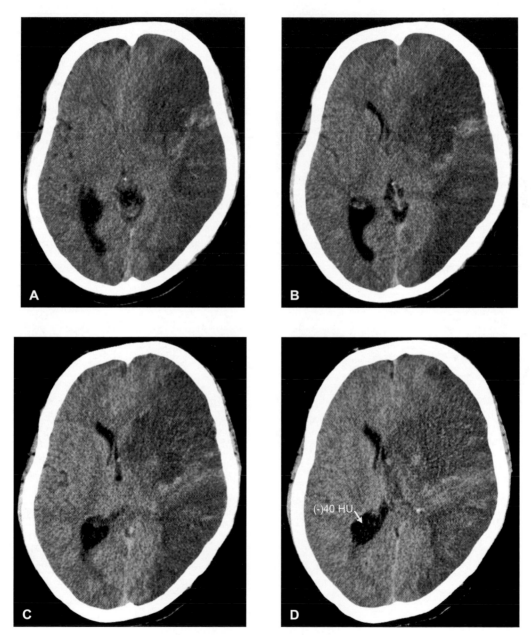

Figs 35.1A to D: Intraventricular lipoma

35.2 Glioblastoma Multiforme

- CT shows a mass with hyperdense areas of calcification in left parietal lobe (Fig. 35.2A). It is causing mass effect in the form of compression of left lateral ventricle and a significant shift of midline structures to contralateral side.
- Contrast CT shows the enhancing components of the mass and the mass effect caused by it (Fig. 35.2B).

This was found to be a glioblastoma multiforme on histopathology. Glioblastoma multiforme rarely calcifies. It is one of the most malignant forms of glioma and is the most common primary brain tumors. 5% of glioblastoma multiforme have multifocal origin.

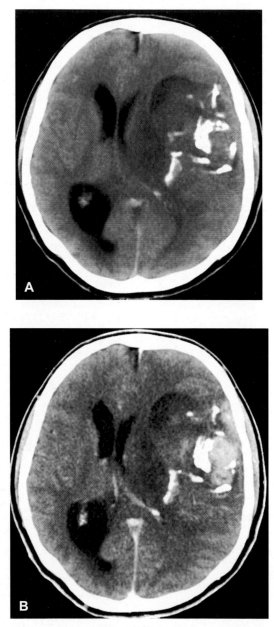

Figs 35.2A and B: Glioblastoma multiforme

35.3 Metastases from Lung

Contrast CT brain show multiple enhancing metastases with primary being a solitary pulmonary nodule in right lung (Fig. 35.3A).

Brain metastases are usually located at corticomedullary junction. They are hypo to isodense on plain CT and enhance after contrast administration. They are usually multiple and of different sizes (Fig. 35.3B). They may be associated with edema.

90-95% of brain metastases arise from bronchus, breast, gastrointestinal tract, renal tumors, melanoma and choriocarcinoma.

Metastases from leukemia, lymphoma and neuroblastomas are more common in children.

Calcified brain metastasis arise from neoplasms of breast, gastrointestinal tract and bone tumors. Cystic/solid brain metastases arise from lung tumors. Hemorrhagic brain metastasis is seen to arise from renal cell carcinoma, melanoma, thyroid carcinoma and choriocarcinoma.

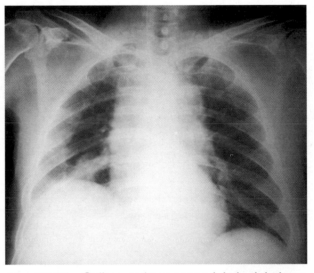

Fig. 35.3A: Solitary pulmonary nodule in right lung

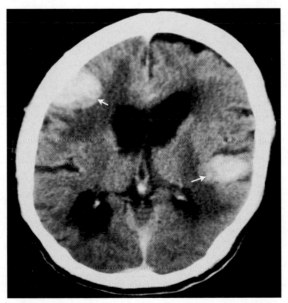

Fig. 35.3B: Contrast CT brain show multiple enhancing metastases

36. MISCELLANEOUS

36.1 Intracranial Calcifications

Intracranial Physiological Calcification

- Falx cerebri anteriorly (Fig. 36.1A).
- Tip of lentiform nuclei bilaterally (Fig. 36.1B).
- Pineal body (Fig. 36.1C).
- Choroid plexuses (Fig. 36.1D).

Intracranial physiological calcifications are unaccompanied by any evidence of disease and have no demonstrable pathological cause. They are often due to calcium and sometimes iron deposition in the blood vessels of different structures of the brain, CT is the most sensitive means of detection of these calcifications.

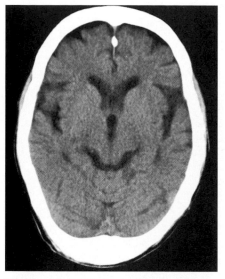

Fig. 36.1A: Plain CT brain shows calcification of falx cerebri anteriorly

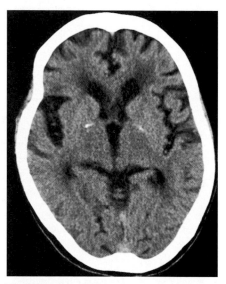

Fig. 36.1B: Plain CT brain shows calci-fication of tip of lentiform nuclei bilaterally

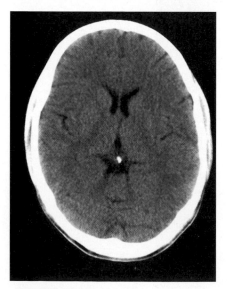

Fig. 36.1C: Plain CT brain shows calcification of pineal body

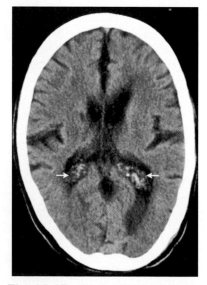

Fig. 36.1D: Plain CT brain shows calcification of choroid plexuses

36.2 Basal Ganglion Calcification

Figures 36.2A and B are plain CT images which show the dense calcification of basal ganglia seen in a 45 years male, chronic tobacco chewer and hypertensive on irregular treatment with history of giddiness on and off.

Basal ganglia calcification causes are physiological due to aging.

Endocrinal disorders like hypo or hyper parathyroidism.

Metabolic disorders like leigh disease, fahr disease and mitochondrial cytopathies.

Familial disorders like cockayne syndrome and lipoid proteinosis.

TORCHES infection. The acronym has also been listed as TORCHES, for TOxoplasmosis, Rubella, Cytomegalovirus, HErpes simplex, Syphilis.

Lead or carbon monoxide poisoning.

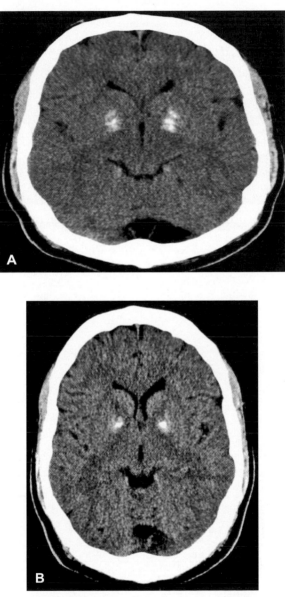

Figs 36.2A and B: Plain CT brain shows bilateral dense calcification of basal ganglia

36.3 Calcification Putamen

Plain CT shows calcification at the tip of putamen bilaterally (Fig. 36.3). This is a normal physiological finding and is seen more often in elderly. This patient was 65 years old.

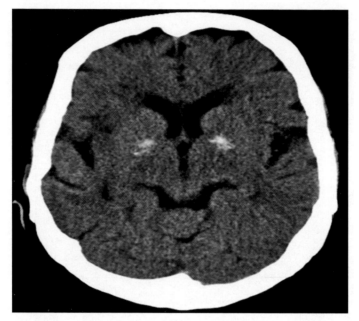

Fig. 36.3: Plain CT brain shows calcification of putamen

36.4 Choroid Plexus Calcification

Plain CT brain shows calcification in choroid plexus and pineal body (Fig. 36.4).

The choroid plexus consists of many capillaries, separated from the ventricles by choroid epithelial cells. Fluid filters through these cells from blood to become CSF fluid with active transport of substances into, and out of, the cerebrospinal fluid.

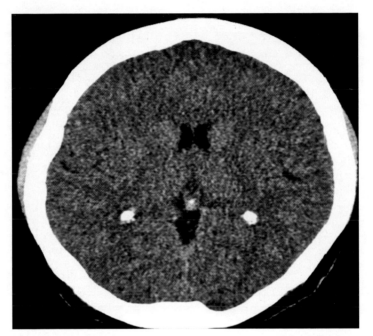

Fig. 36.4: Plain CT brain shows calcification of choroid plexus

36.5 Craniotomy

Craniotomy seen as a bone defect in the scanogram (Fig. 36.5A). Craniotomy with gliosis (Fig. 36.5B). Old infarct with gliotic change in right gangliocapsular region (Fig. 36.5C). Craniotomy in bone window (Fig. 36.5D).

Craniotomy is an opening made into the cranium. It is performed for brain tumor removal, removal of blood clot, to control hemorrhage from a leaking blood vessel, to repair arteriovenous malformations, to drain a brain abscess, to relieve pressure inside, to perform a biopsy or to inspect the brain.

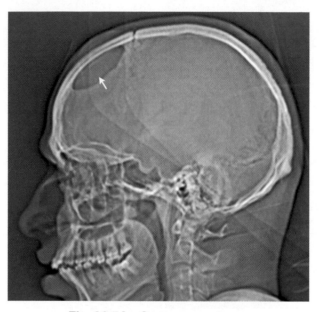

Fig. 36.5A: Scanogram shows craniotomy as a bone defect

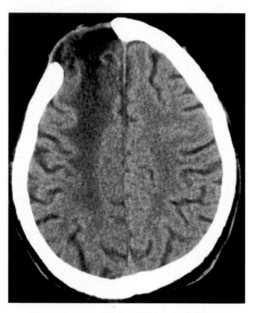

Fig. 36.5B: Plain CT brain shows craniotomy with gliosis

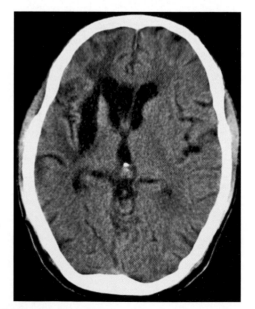

Fig. 36.5C: Plain CT brain shows old infarct with gliotic change in right gangliocapsular region

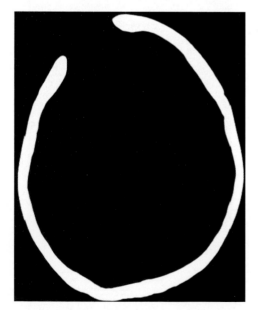

Fig. 36.5D: Plain CT brain shows craniotomy in bone window

36.6 VP Shunt

VP shunt in a 78 year old male. The shunt tube is seen to enter through the burr hole into the occipital horn (Figs 36.6A and B) of right lateral ventricle, however, the tip of the shunt is seen to lie in the thalamocapsular region outside the ventricular system (Figs 36.6C and D) with resultant poor function of the shunt.

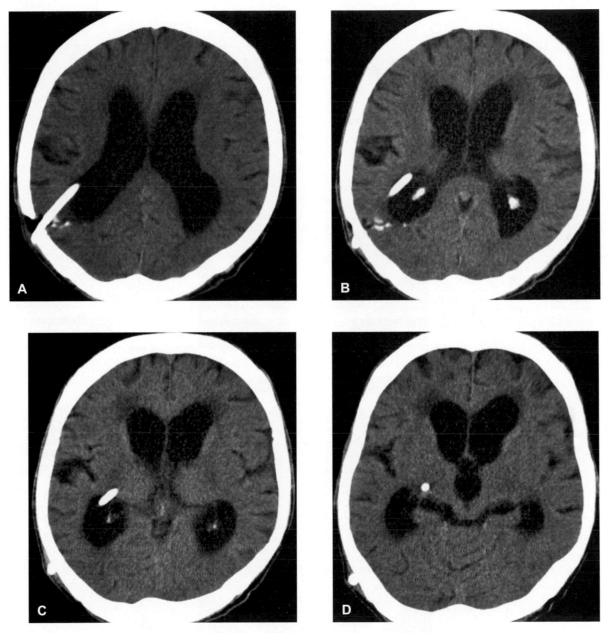

Figs 36.6A to D: Plain CT brain shows the position of VP shunt

36.7 Normal Pressure Hydrocephalus (NPH)

In 66 years old male with ataxia, gait imbalance and urinary incontinence, plain CT brain shows disproportionate dilatation of ventricular system as compared to parenchymal atrophy (Figs 36.7A and B).

NPH is an acquired hydrocephalus that most often occurs in people over the age of 60 years. NPH is different from typical hydrocephalus in that it may not cause an obvious increase of pressure, but may have fluctuations in CSF pressure from high to normal to low. The three classic symptoms of NPH are difficulty in walking, dementia and problems with bladder control.

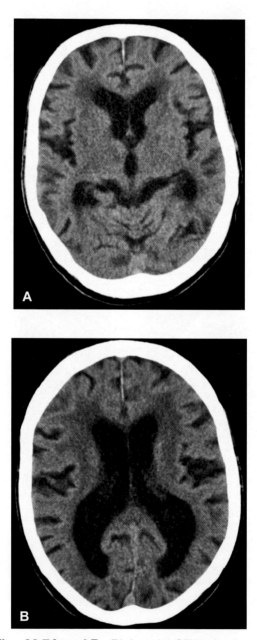

Figs 36.7A and B: Plain axial CT brain shows
normal pressure hydrocephalus

36.8 Benign Enlargement of Subarachnoid Spaces (BESS)

- CT brain shows prominent subarachnoid spaces in a child (Figs 36.8A and B).

Patients who have BESS have long been suspected of having an increased propensity for subdural hematomas either spontaneously or as a result of accidental injury. Subdural hematomas in infants are often equated with non accidental trauma (NAT). Caution must be exercised when investigating for NAT based on the sole presence of subdural hematomas, especially in children who are otherwise well and who have BESS.

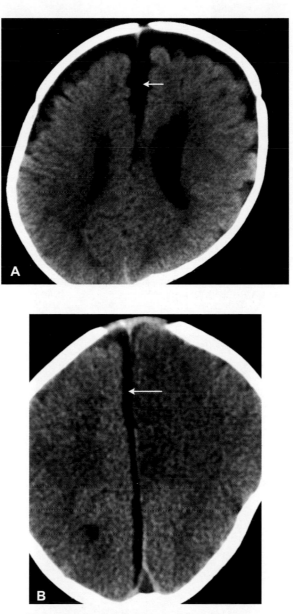

Figs 36.8A and B: Plain CT brain shows prominent subarachnoid spaces

36.9 Atrophy

- CT brain shows prominent sulci consistent with atrophy of frontal parenchyma (Fig. 36.9A).
- CT brain shows prominent cerebellar folia suggesting cerebellar atrophy (Fig. 36.9B).
- CT brain shows cerebral and cerebellar parenchymal atrophy (Fig. 36.9C).

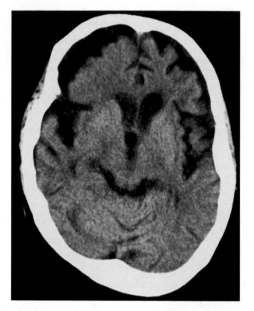

Fig. 36.9A: CT brain shows prominent sulci consistent with atrophy of frontal parenchyma

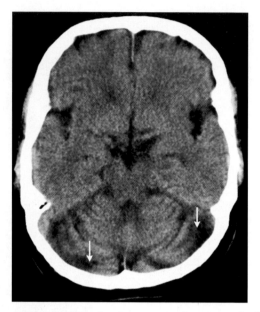

Fig. 36.9B: CT brain shows prominent cerebellar folia suggesting cerebellar atrophy

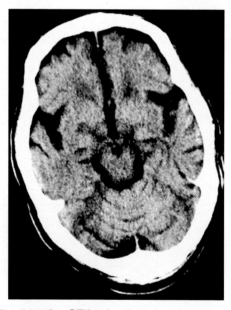

Fig. 36.9C: CT brain shows cerebral and cerebellar atrophy

36.10 Hepatic Encephalopathy

55 years male with hepatic encephalopathy, CT head shows effacement of cerebral sulci and chinking of ventricles suggestive of diffuse cerebral edema. In addition there is bilateral basal ganglion calcification (Figs 36.10A and B).

Hepatic encephalopathy is brain damage that occurs as a complication of liver disorders like cirrhosis or hepatitis or any condition resulting in alkalosis. The exact cause of hepatic encephalopathy is unknown.

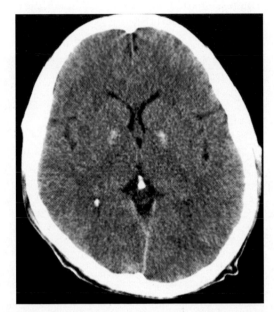

Fig. 36.10A: CT brain shows effacement of cerebral sulci and chinking of ventricles with bilateral basal ganglion calcification

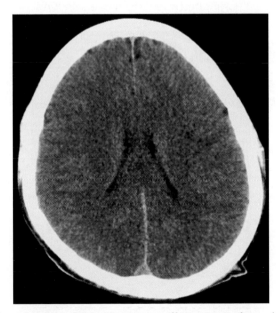

Fig. 36.10B: CT brain shows effacement of cerebral sulci and chinking of body of lateral ventricles

36.11 Lipoid Proteinosis (LP)

CT brain shows bilateral comma-shaped calcifications in amygdala diagnostic of intracranial manifestation of lipoid proteinosis.

Lipoid proteinosis is a rare entity with an insidious onset and affects the entire body and predominantly manifests through lesions of skin, mucous membrane and brain. It is characterized by deposition of hyaline-like material at the level of the basement membrane. Radiological hallmark is the presence of bean to comma-shaped intracranial calcifications in the temporal lobes in amygdale.

Lateral radiograph of skull shows open C-shaped suprasellar calcification (Fig. 36.11A). CT brain shows bilateral comma-shaped calcifications in both amygdale (Fig. 36.11B).

LP has a chronic course and a potential to affect quality of life adversely.

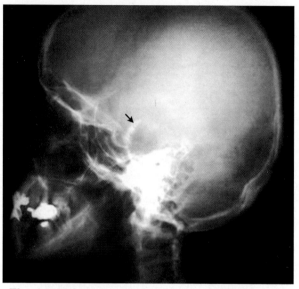

Fig. 36.11A: Lateral radiography of skull shows C-shaped suprasellar calcification

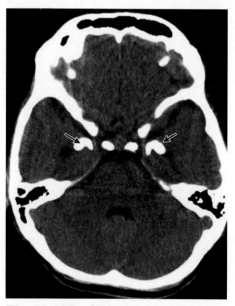

Fig. 36.11B: CT brain shows bilateral comma-shaped calcifications in both amygdale

37. SPINE

37.1 Normal Anatomy of Spine (Figs 37.1A to L)

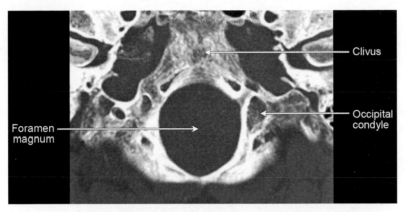

Fig. 37.1A: Occipital condyle

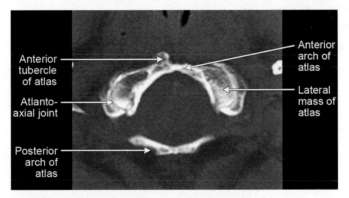

Fig. 37.1B: C1 vertebra (atlas)

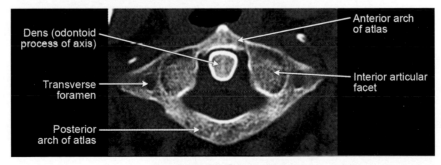

Fig. 37.1C: C1 vertebra

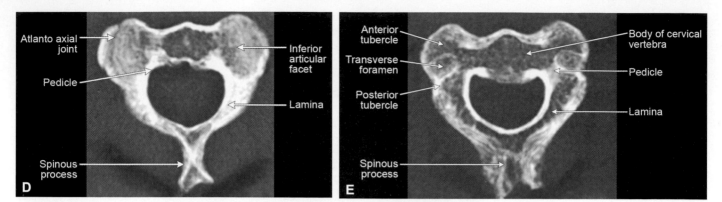

Figs 37.1D and E: C2 vertebra

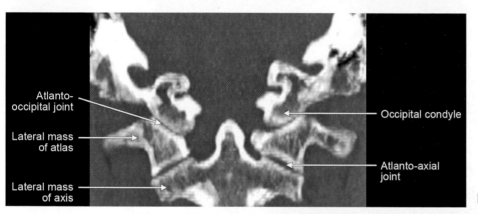

Fig. 37.1F: C1 – C2 coronal recon

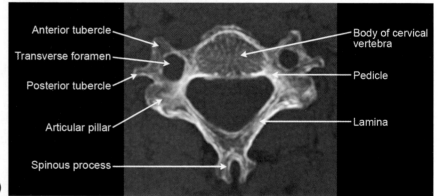

Fig. 37.1G: Typical cervical vertebra (3–7)

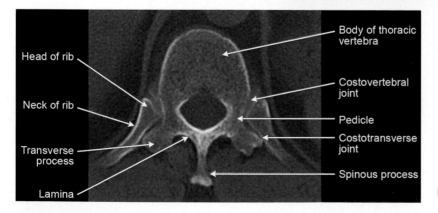

Fig. 37.1H: Typical thoracic vertebra

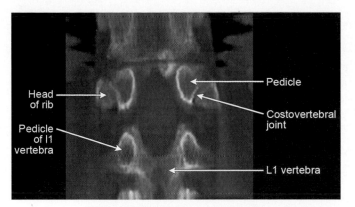

Head of rib

Pedicle of l1 vertebra

Pedicle

Costovertebral joint

L1 vertebra

Fig. 37.1I: T12 – L1 coronal

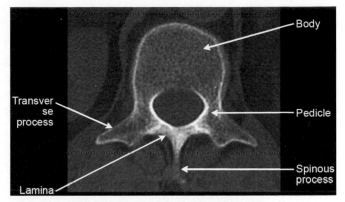

Body

Transverse process

Pedicle

Lamina

Spinous process

Fig. 37.1J: Typical lumbar vertebra

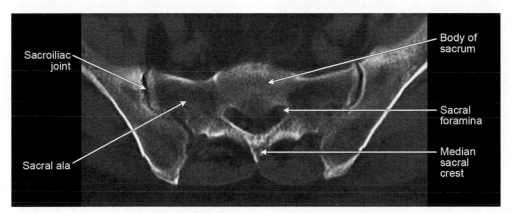

Sacroiliac joint

Sacral ala

Body of sacrum

Sacral foramina

Median sacral crest

Fig. 37.1K: S1 vertebra and sacroiliac joint

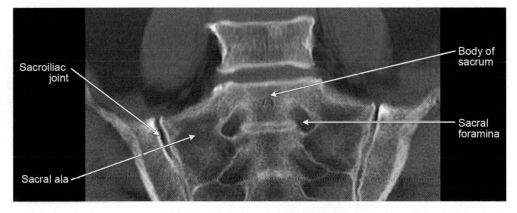

Sacroiliac joint

Sacral ala

Body of sacrum

Sacral foramina

Fig. 37.1L: L5 – S1-3 coronal recon

37.2 Fracture Vertebral Body

History of fall from height. Distension of abdomen. Plain CT shows traumatic burst fracture of body of LV 4 with hemo-pneumoperitoneum (arrow) (Figs 37.2A to D). Figure 37.2E shows pre and paravertebral collection.

Burst fracture is a traumatic spinal injury in which a vertebra breaks from a high-energy axial load, with pieces of the vertebra shattering into surrounding tissues and sometimes into the spinal canal. They are most often caused by car accidents or by falls. Burst fractures are categorized by the severity of the deformity, canal compromise, loss of vertebral body height and neurological deficit.

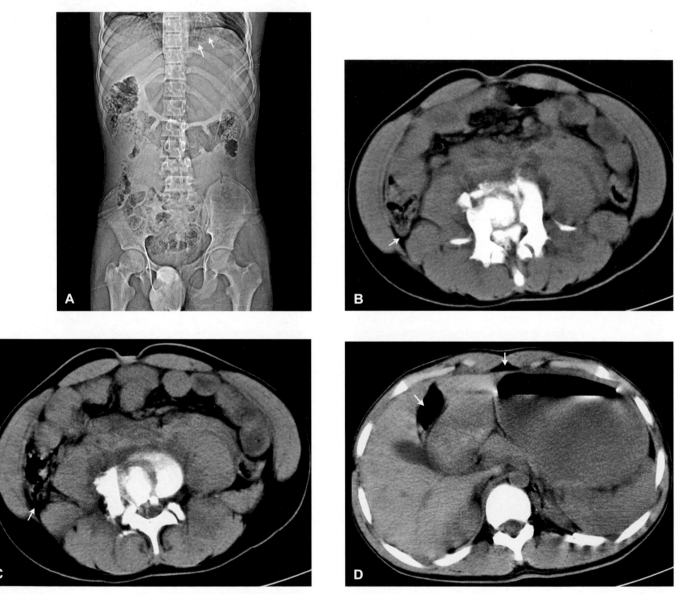

Figs 37.2A to D: Plain CT images shows traumatic burst fracture of body of LV4 with hemopneumoperitoneum (arrow)

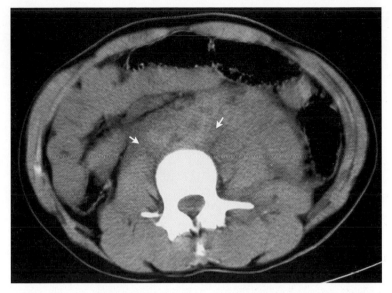

Fig. 37.2E: Plain CT shows pre and paravertebral collection

37.3 Cervical Spondylosis

Sagittal reformatted CT shows height of C5-C6 intervertebral disc is significantly reduced. Small osteophytes are seen at this level, projecting posteriorly into the spinal canal. Small anterior osteophytes are also seen (Figs 37.3A and B).

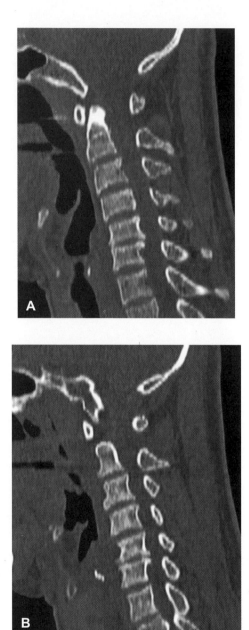

Figs 37.3A and B: Sagittal reformatted CT shows reduced height of C5-C6 intervertebral disc with osteophytosis

37.4 Craniovertebral Anomaly

Occipitalization of atlas with bony fusion of odontoid process and arch of atlas on right side (Figs 37.4A to E).

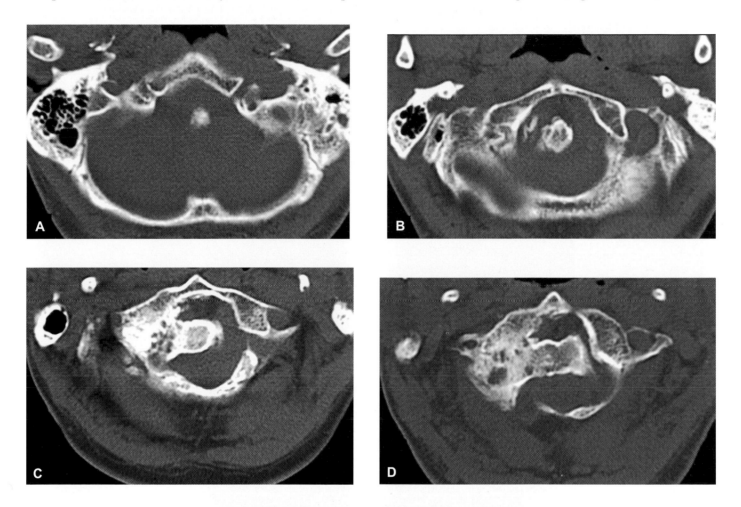

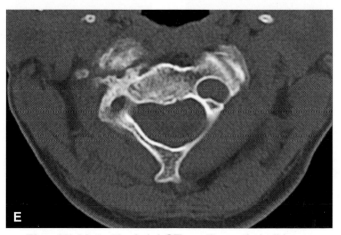

Figs 37.4A to E: Axial CT sections of skull base show occipitalization of atlas

37.5 Degenerated Disk with Vacuum Phenomenon (Figs 37.5A to D)

C5-C6 intervertebral disk shows reduced height and hypodense appearance.

Disk height is reduced because of degeneration and hypodense appearance is due to nitrous oxide gas which is released due to degeneration.

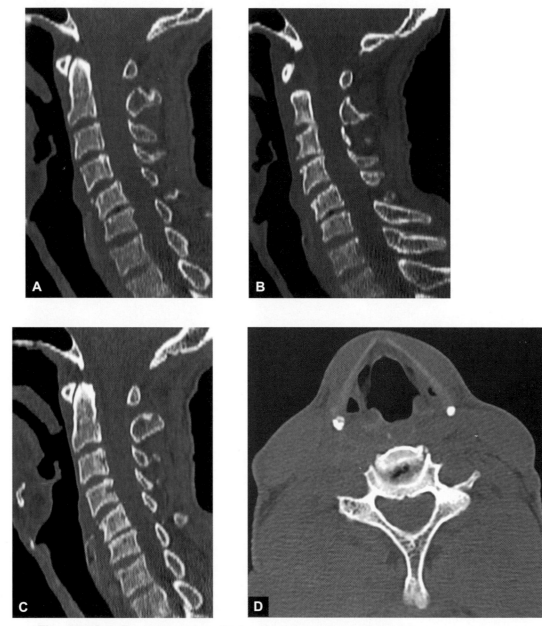

Figs 37.5A to D: Axial and sagittal recon images demonstrate the degenerated disk with vacuum phenomenon

Section 7

Head, Neck and Face

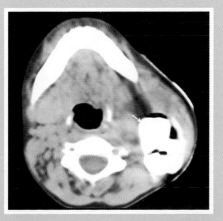
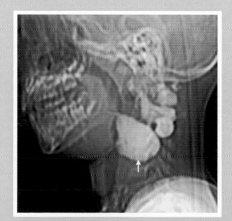
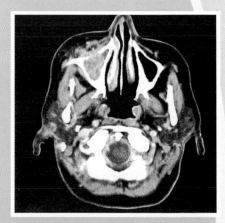

38. NORMAL ANATOMY HEAD, NECK AND FACE

38.1 Normal Anatomy Neck

Axial CT sections of neck are shown in Figures 38.1A to J.

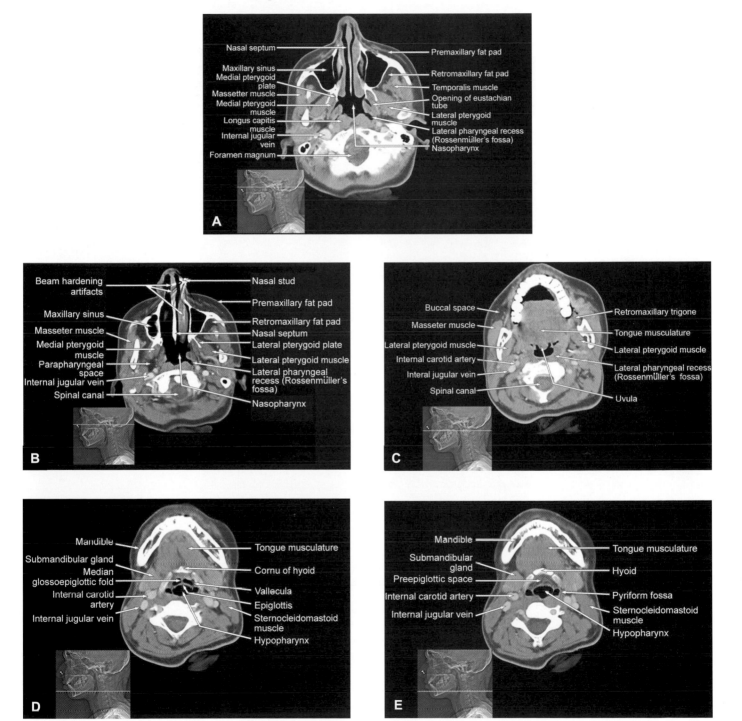

Figs 38.1A to E: Axial CT sections of neck

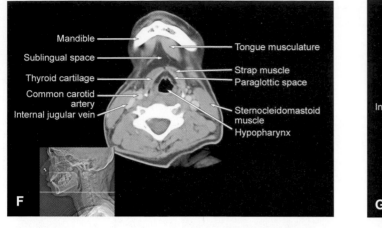

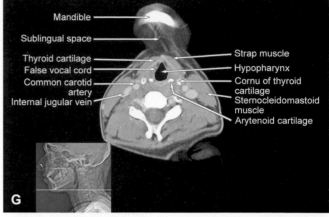

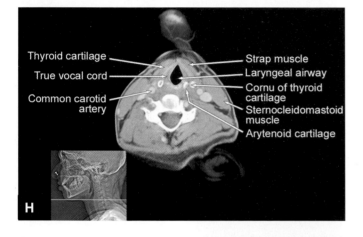

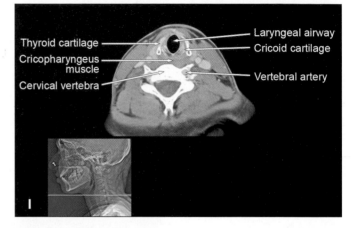

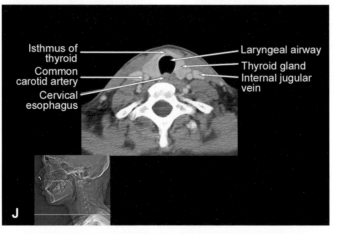

Figs 38.1F to J: Axial CT sections of neck

38.2 Normal Anatomy Paranasal Sinuses (Figs 38.2A to M)

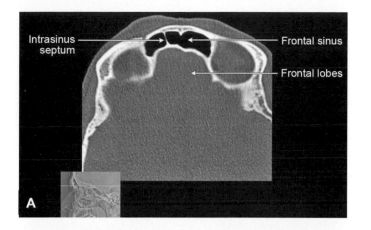

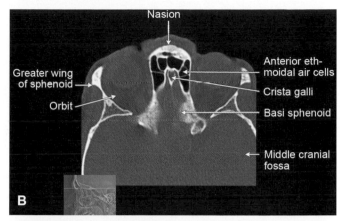

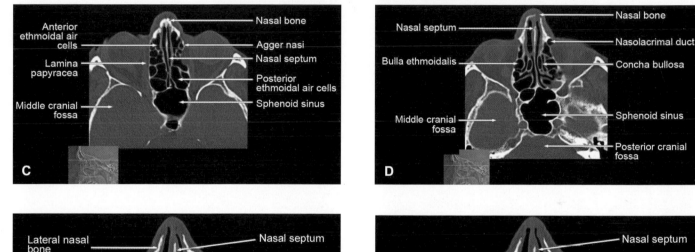

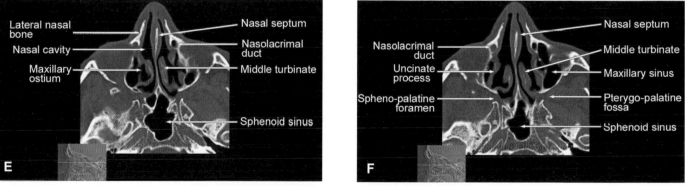

Figs 38.2A to F: Axial CT sections of paranasal sinuses

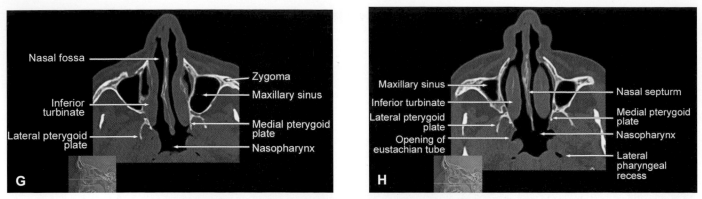

Figs 38.2G and H: Axial CT sections of paranasal sinuses

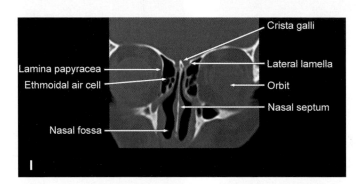

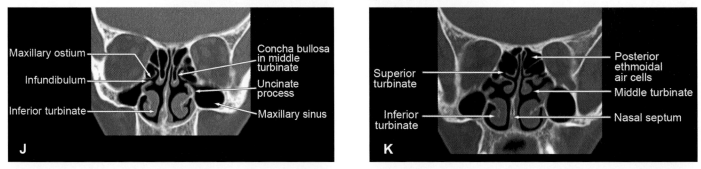

Figs 38.2I to K: Coronal CT reconstructions of paranasal sinuses

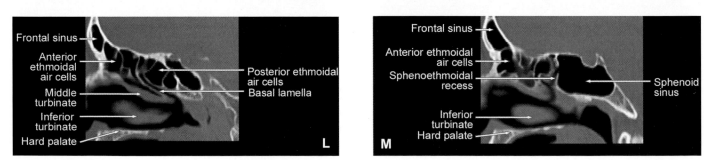

Figs 38.2L and M: Sagittal CT reconstructions of paranasal sinuses

38.3 Normal Anatomy Temporal Bone (Figs 38.3A to H)

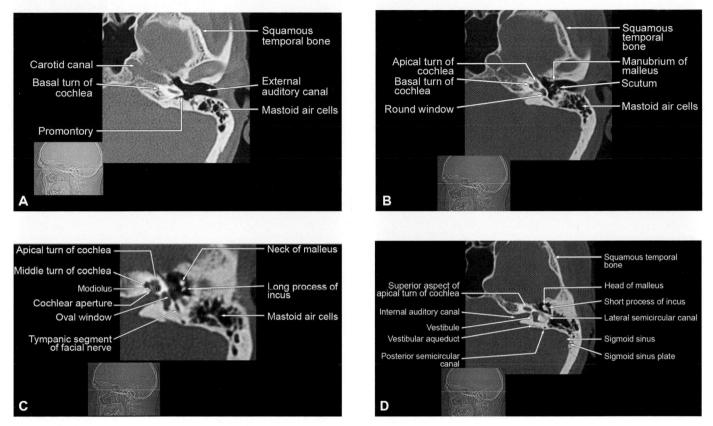

Figs 38.3A to D: Axial CT sections of temporal bone

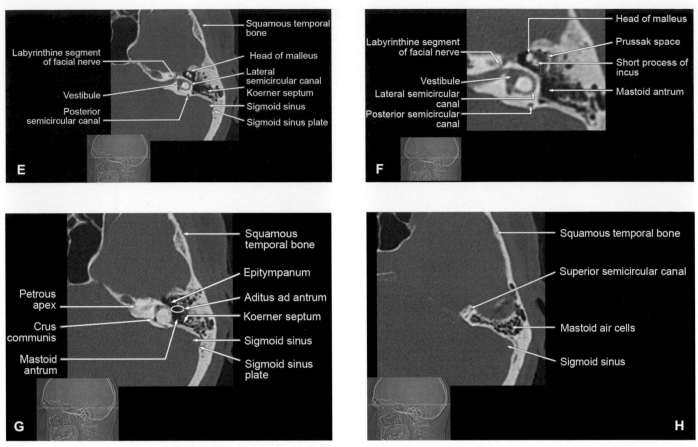

Figs 38.3E to H: Axial CT sections of temporal bone

39. CONGENITAL

39.1 Retention Cyst Epiglottis

Figures 39.1A and B, Axial, C (coronal) and D (sagittal) CT images show a cystic space occupying lesion arising from epiglottis which was confirmed as retention cyst.

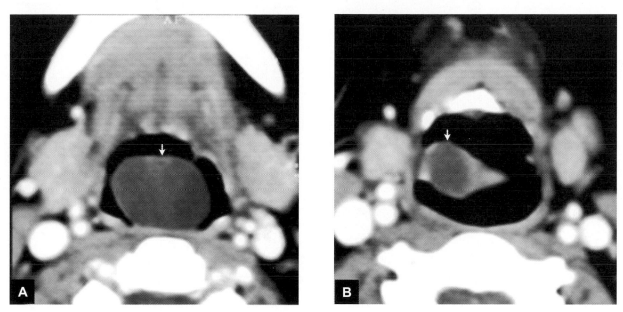

Figs 39.1A and B: Axial CT section shows retention cyst epiglottis

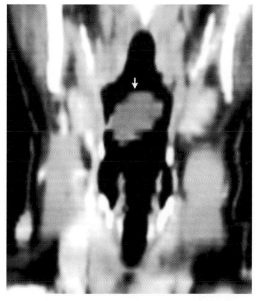

Fig. 39.1C: Coronal CT recon shows retention cyst epiglottis

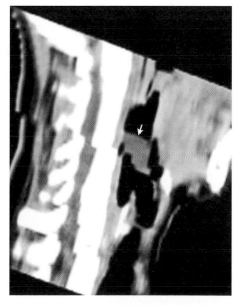

Fig. 39.1D: Sagittal CT recon shows retention cyst epiglottis

39.2 Unilateral Michel's Aplasia

HRCT temporal bone shows absence of inner ear structures on left side (Fig. 39.2A), jugular bulb is also absent on the left side (Fig. 39.2B).

Michel's aplasia is characterized by total absence of inner ear structures associated with other skull base anomalies including an abnormal course of the facial nerve and jugular veins.

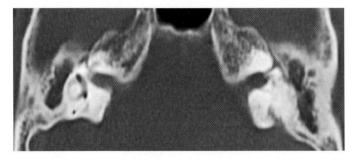

Fig. 39.2A: HRCT temporal bone shows absence of inner ear structures on left side

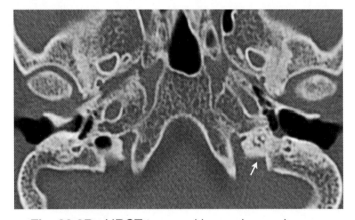

Fig. 39.2B: HRCT temporal bone shows absence of jugular bulb on left side

40. INFECTIVE-INFLAMMATORY

40.1 Eyelid Abscess

Figures 40.1A and B are CT images of a patient with right orbital swelling. Irregular enhancing orbital mass is seen which is an eyelid abscess.

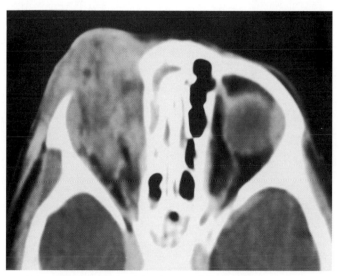

Fig. 40.1A: CT orbit shows right orbital swelling with irregular orbital mass

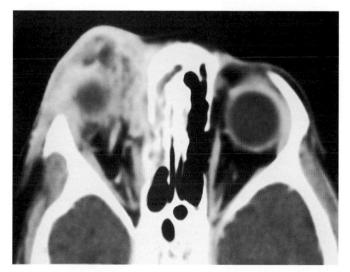

Fig. 40.1B: CT orbit shows enhancing irregular orbital mass

40.2 Antrochoanal Polyp 1

Coronal (Figs 40.2A and B) and axial (Figs 40.2C and D) CT images of paranasal sinuses shows soft tissue mass lesion extending from right maxillary sinus into the posterior nasal choanal space and extending to the nasopharynx. It also crosses the midline in posterior nasopharyngeal area. Left maxillary sinus also shows mucosal thickening.

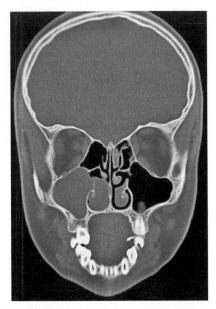

Fig. 40.2A: Coronal CT PNS shows soft tissue mass lesion extending from right maxillary sinus into the posterior nasal choanal space

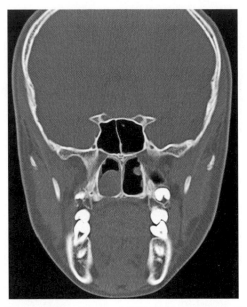

Fig. 40.2B: Coronal CT PNS shows soft tissue mass extending to the nasopharynx

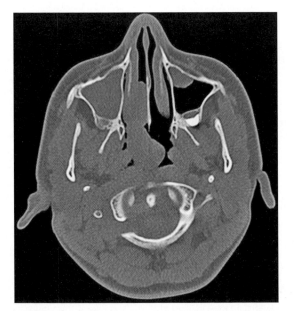

Fig. 40.2C: Axial CT PNS shows soft tissue mass lesion extending from right maxillary sinus to the posterior nasal choanal space and nasopharynx. It crosses the midline in posterior nasopharynx

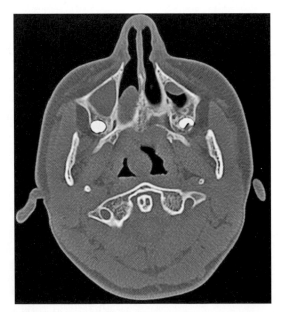

Fig. 40.2D: Axial CT PNS shows soft tissue mass lesion in right maxillary sinus into the posterior nasal choanal space and extending to the nasopharynx. Left maxillary sinus shows mucosal thickening

40.3 Antrochoanal Polyp 2

Axial (Figs 40.3A and B) and coronal (Figs 40.3C and D) HRCT PNS images show right antrochoanal polyp and left maxillary polyp.

Antrochoanal polyps are solitary polyps arising from the maxillary antrum. Allergy has been implicated as etiology. These polyps originate in the lining of the maxillary antrum and gradually prolapse through the natural or an accessory ostium into the nasal cavity and enlarge towards the posterior choana and nasopharynx. They cause nasal obstruction and serous otitis media if they occlude the eustachian tube.

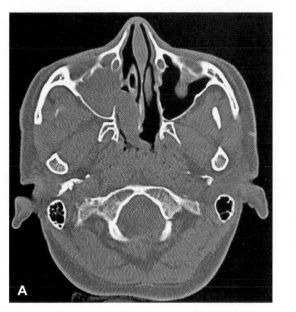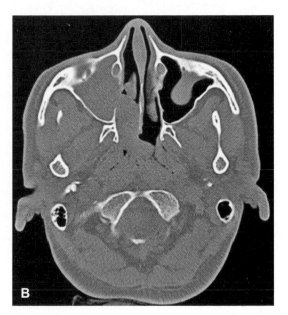

Figs 40.3A and B: Axial CT PNS shows right antrochoanal polyp and left maxillary polyp

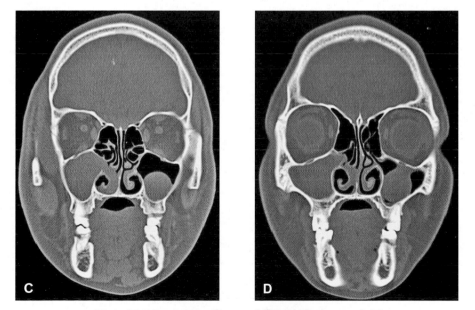

Figs 40.3C and D: Coronal CT PNS shows right antrochoanal polyp and left maxillary polyp

40.4 Maxillary Polyp

Plain CT shows a polypoidal soft tissue lesion in left maxillary sinus (Fig. 40.4).

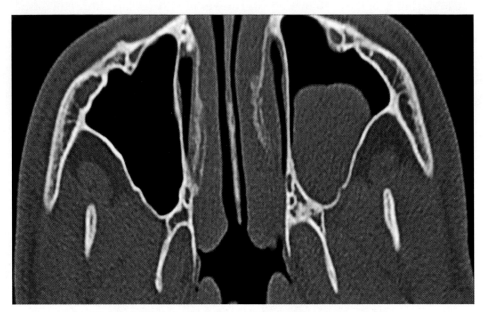

Fig. 40.4: Plain CT shows left maxillary sinus polyp

40.5 Sinonasal Polyposis

HRCT PNS image shows abnormal soft tissues occupying the left maxillary, ethmoid and frontal sinuses. There is erosion of left uncinate process, middle turbinate and few ethmoid air cells (Fig. 40.5). There is widening of left osteomeatal unit complex.

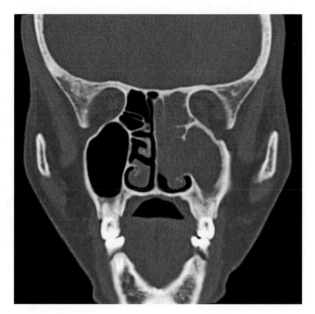

Fig. 40.5: HRCT PNS shows left maxillary, ethmoid and frontal sinuses polyposis with erosion of left uncinate process, middle turbinate and few ethmoid air cells

40.6 Sinonasal Polyposis with Dehiscence of Lamina Papyracea

Soft tissue mass lesions (polyposis) are seen to occupy and expand all the paranasal sinuses. There is dehiscence of lamina papyracea (Figs 40.6A to D).

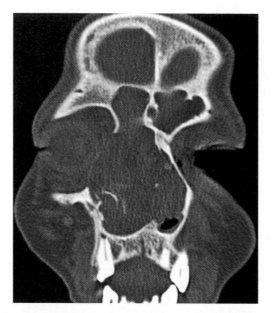

Fig. 40.6A: Coronal CT PNS shows polyposis occupying all paranasal sinuses with mass effect, there is dehiscence of lamina papyracea

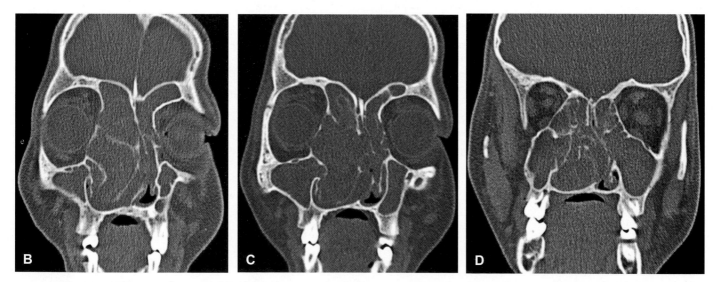

Figs 40.6B to D: Coronal CT PNS shows polyposis occupying all paranasal sinuses with mass effect

40.7 Cholesteatoma

CT images show soft tissue lesion in right mastoid cavity (Figs 40.7A and D). There is destruction of tympanic membrane (Fig. 40.7A), scutum and ossicles (Figs 40.7B and C). Sclerosis of mastoid air cells is seen. Erosion of anterior cortex of lateral semicircular and facial nerve canal (Fig. 40.7D) is also present.

Cholesteatoma is a collection of keratinizing squamous epithelium in the middle ear cleft associated with bone resorption. Treatment demands a surgical approach.

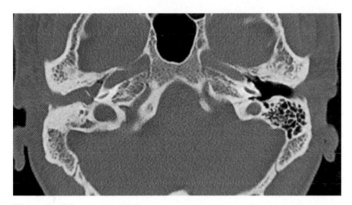

Fig. 40.7A: Axial CT temporal bones show soft tissue lesion in right mastoid cavity, external and internal auditory canal with partial destruction of tympanic membrane

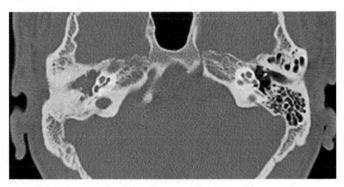

Fig. 40.7B: Axial CT temporal bones show soft tissue lesion in right mastoid cavity, here is destruction of scutum and ossicles

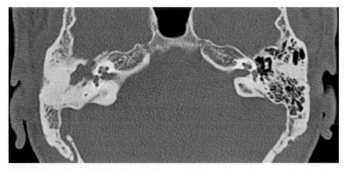

Fig. 40.7C: Axial CT temporal bones show soft tissue lesion with sclerosis in right mastoid cavity, here is destruction of scutum and ossicles

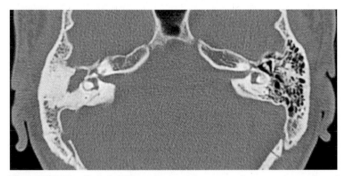

Fig. 40.7D: Axial CT temporal bones show sclerosis of mastoid air cells, there is erosion of anterior cortex of lateral semicircular and facial nerve canal

40.8 Recurrence Cholesteatoma

This 23 years male presented with pain in right ear. He was operated two years ago for right attic cholesteatoma.

Enhancing abnormal soft tissue is seen in right middle ear and mastoid cavity. Ossicles are destroyed (Figs 40.8A and B). Posterior wall of external ear and mastoid shows thinning and dehiscence (Figs 40.8C and D).

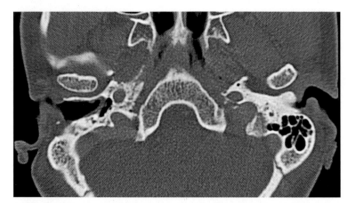

Fig. 40.8A: Axial CT temporal bones show abnormal soft tissue in right middle ear and mastoid cavity, ossicles are destroyed

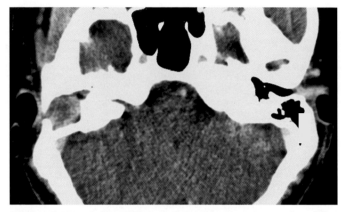

Fig. 40.8B: Axial CT temporal bones show abnormal enhancing soft tissue in right middle ear and mastoid cavity, ossicles are destroyed

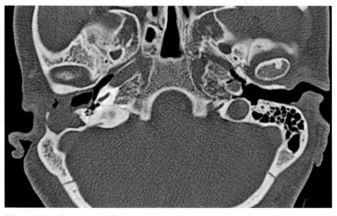

Fig. 40.8C: Axial CT temporal bones show abnormal soft tissue in right middle ear and mastoid cavity, ossicles are destroyed. Posterior wall of external ear and mastoid shows thinning and dehiscence

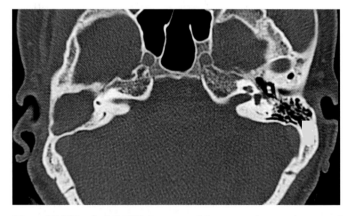

Fig. 40.8D: Axial CT temporal bones show abnormal enhancing soft tissue in right middle ear and mastoid cavity, ossicles are destroyed. Posterior wall of external ear and mastoid shows thinning and dehiscence

40.9 Parotid Abscess

Plain (Fig. 40.9A) and contrast (Fig. 40.9B) CT shows hypodense collection with thick irregular walls in the right parotid gland suggestive of abscess. Inflammatory mucosal thickening is seen in the right maxillary sinus.

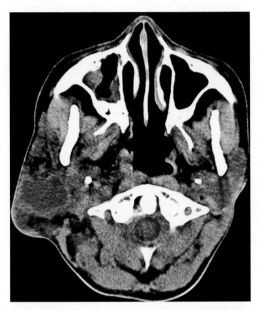

Fig. 40.9A: Plain CT shows parotid abscess

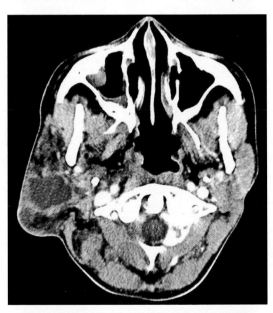

Fig. 40.9B: Contrast CT delineates the enhancing wall of parotid abscess

40.10 Cellulitis Neck after Shave

CT images show extensive soft tissue edema in the anterolateral aspect of the subcutaneous tissues of neck and thorax (Figs 40.10A to F). This extensive soft tissue edema developed within 3 days after neck injury by razor blade while shaving. Patient responded to broad spectrum antibiotics, analgesics and edema reducing agents.

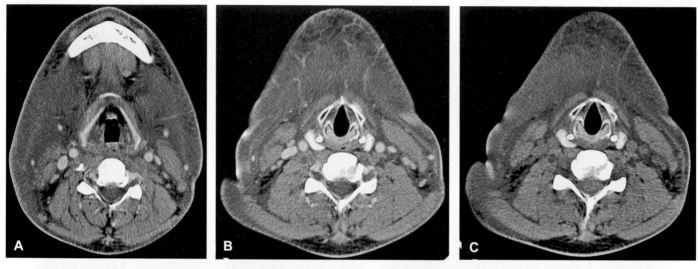

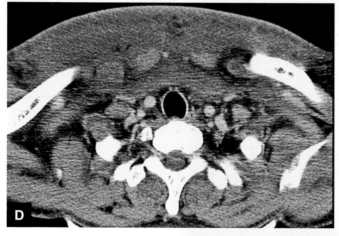
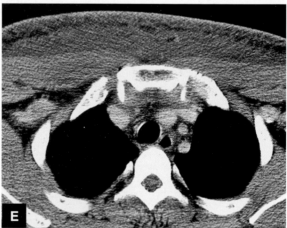

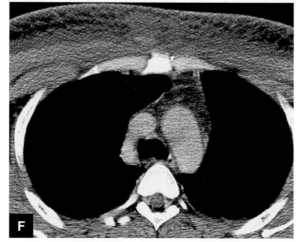

Figs 40.10A to F: Cellulitis neck

40.11 Ivory Osteoma Ethmoid Sinus (Figs 40.11A and B)

CT PNS shows an ivory osteoma as a hyperdense focus in ethmoidal sinus.

Paranasal sinus osteomas are slow-growing, encapsulated bony benign tumors that usually cause few symptoms. Most commonly seen in the frontal sinus, it is less common in the ethmoid and maxillary sinuses.

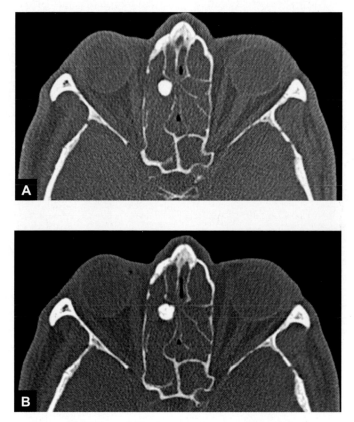

Figs 40.11A and B: Ivory osteoma ethmoid sinus

40.12 Ameloblastoma

Ameloblastoma of Mandible

- Pantomogram shows multiseptated expansile lucency involving the body of mandible on right side with loss of adjacent teeth (Fig. 40.12A).
- Contrast CT shows mildly enhancing soft tissue component (Fig. 40.12B).
- CT in bone window shows the expansile lucency with thinning of mandibular cortex (Figs 40.12C and D). A large left maxillary polyp is also present.

Ameloblastoma is a benign tumor of odontogenic epithelium (ameloblasts) more common in mandible than maxilla however most common site is posterior body and angle of the mandible. On X-ray it appears as a lucency in the bone of varying size often as a multiloculated "soap bubble" appearance.

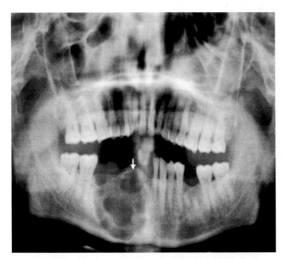

Fig. 40.12A: Pantomogram shows multi-septated expansile lucency in the mandible

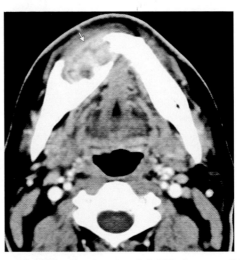

Fig. 40.12B: Contrast axial CT shows mildly enhancing soft tissue component

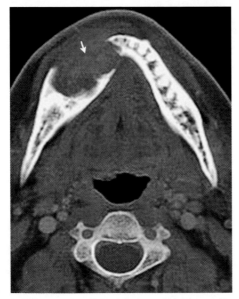

Fig. 40.12C: Axial CT in bone window shows the expansile lucency with thinning of mandibular cortex

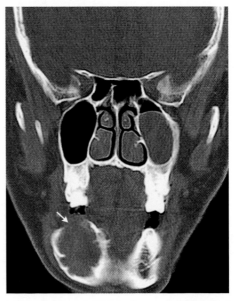

Fig. 40.12D: Coronal CT in bone window shows the expansile lucency with thinning of mandibular cortex. A large left maxillary polyp is also present

41. NEOPLASTIC

41.1 Carcinoma Gingivobuccal Space 1

Contrast CT shows a heterogeneously enhancing right gingivobuccal space mass involving entire right maxillary sinus with destruction of the walls (Fig. 41.1A). The mass has also spread into cheek involving the overlying skin and posteriorly into the infra-temporal fossa (Fig. 41.1B). On histopathology it was confirmed as invasive squamous cell carcinoma of right gingivo-buccal space.

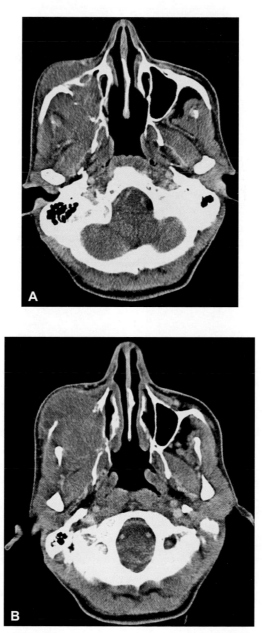

Figs 41.1A and B: Carcinoma of right gingivobuccal space

41.2 Carcinoma Gingivobuccal Space 2

Contrast CT shows a heterogeneously enhancing right gingivobuccal space mass involving entire right maxillary sinus (Figs 41.2A to D). Minimal early extension into fat plane of the cheek is seen. On histopathology it was confirmed as invasive squamous cell carcinoma of right gingivobuccal space.

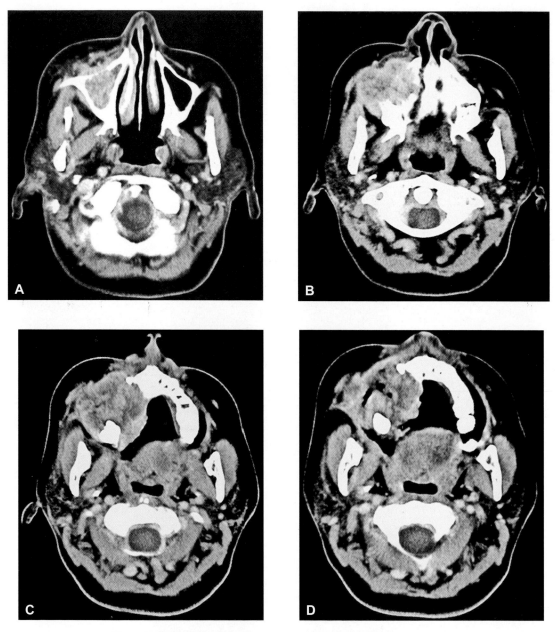

Figs 41.2A to D: Carcinoma of right gingivobuccal space

41.3 Carcinoma Tongue

- Contrast CT shows a hyperdense mass at base of tongue extending into the pre-epiglottic space (Figs 41.3A and B). This turned out to be a carcinoma of base of tongue.

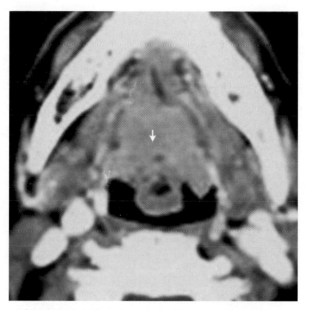

Fig. 41.3A: Carcinoma tongue presented as a hyperdense mass at base of tongue

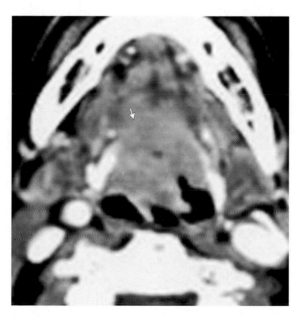

Fig. 41.3B: Carcinoma tongue, the hyperdense mass at base of tongue is extending into the pre-epiglottic space

41.4 Carcinoma Aerodigestive Tract (Figs 41.4A to F)

Circumferential soft tissue thickening of hypopharynx, cricophayrnx and upper esophagus is seen. Aryepiglottic folds are thickened. Thyroid is pushed anteriorly by the mass. The fat plane between the mass and posterior surface of left lobe of thyroid is lost. Anteriorly the mass is extending into the trachea and posteriorly extends to the vertebral bodies. Fat plane between the mass and neck vessels are preserved.

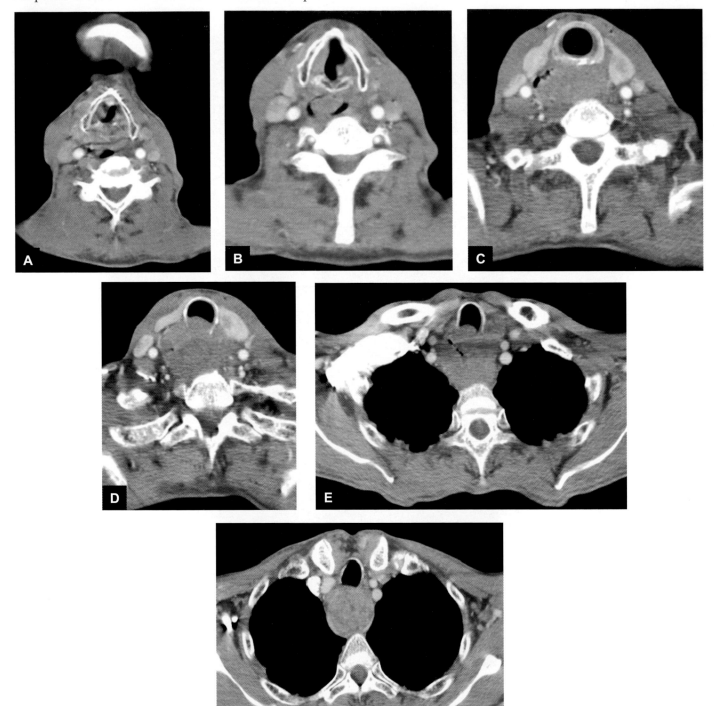

Figs 41.4A to F: Carcinoma aerodigestive tract

41.5 Carcinoma Nasopharynx

- CT shows vague enhancing mass in nasopharynx (Fig. 41.5A).
- Bilateral posterior cervical lymph nodes are enlarged (Fig. 41.5B).
  Confirmed as undifferentiated carcinoma of nasopharynx with cervical lymph node metastasis.

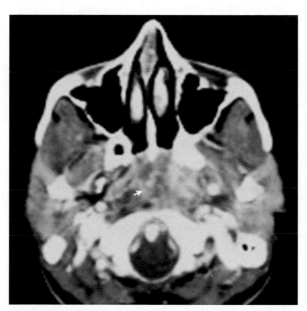

Fig. 41.5A: CT shows vague enhancing mass in nasopharynx

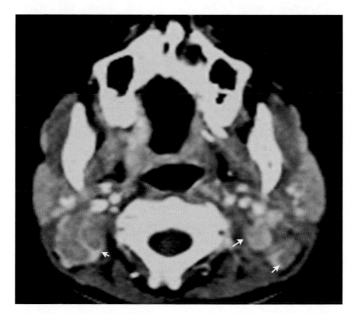

Fig. 41.5B: CT shows bilateral enlarged posterior cervical lymph nodes

41.6 Nasolacrimal Duct Adenocarcinoma

CT shows a round mass at the inner canthus of right eye entering into right nasolacrimal duct (Figs 41.6A and B). CECT shows enhancement of the mass with spread of tumor into the right nasolacrimal duct (Figs 41.6C to E). Histopathology proved it to be a nasolacrimal duct adenocarcinoma.

Primary adenocarcinoma of the lacrimal gland is much less common than in salivary glands. The invasive nature of the primary ductal adenocarcinoma of the lacrimal gland dictates aggressive therapy. Combination therapy of wide surgical excision, followed by radiation therapy.

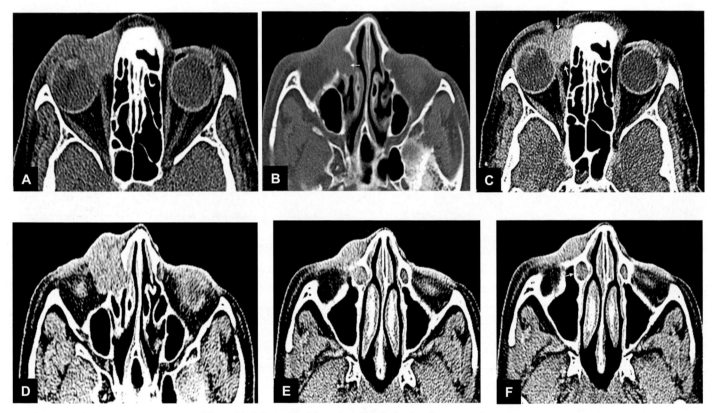

Figs 41.6A to F: Nasolacrimal duct adenocarcinoma

41.7 Juvenile Nasal Angiofibroma (JNAF)

Soft tissue mass is seen occupying the left maxillary sinus, nasopharynx, left nasal fossa and extending into infratemporal fossa and orbital floor. There is ballooning of nasal fossa, sinuses and their walls with bone damage at places (Figs 41.7A to F).

JNAF is usually found in adolescent boys. The tumor contains many blood vessels, spreads within the area in which it started (locally invasive) and can cause bone damage. Although not cancerous, angiofibromas may continue to grow. Some may disappear on their own. It is common for the tumor to return after surgery. Nasal mucosal biopsy can be very dangerous and should only be done after CT scan and angiogram.

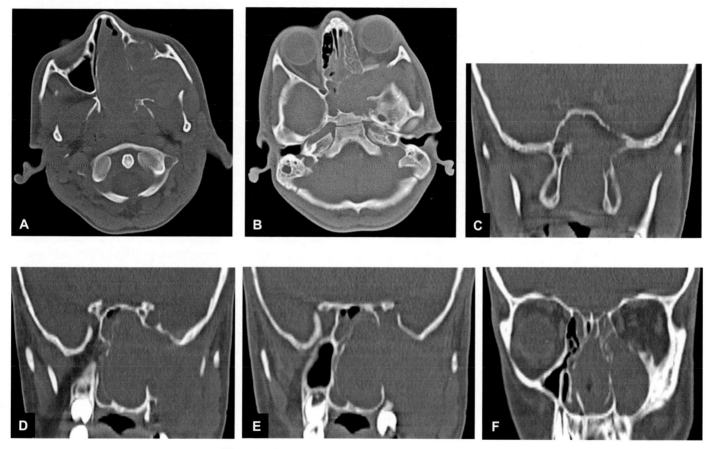

Figs 41.7A to F: Juvenile nasal angiofibroma

41.8 Carcinoma Larynx

Squamous cell carcinoma (SCC) of right pyriform fossa.
- Axial CT images show a right pyriform fossa mass with supraglottic and glottic involvement (Figs 41.8A to C).
- Coronal CT image shows the extent better (Fig. 41.8D).

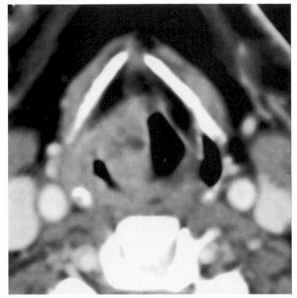

Fig. 41.8A: Axial CT shows right pyriform fossa mass

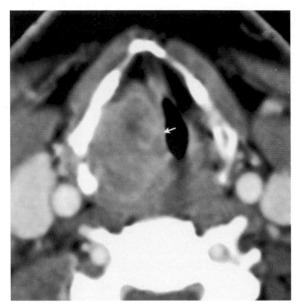

Fig. 41.8B: Axial CT shows right pyriform fossa

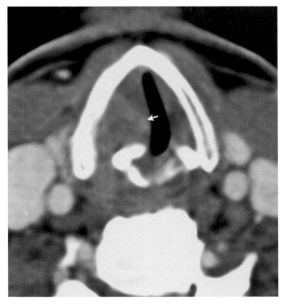

Fig. 41.8C: Axial CT shows right pyriform fossa mass with supraglottic and glottic involvement

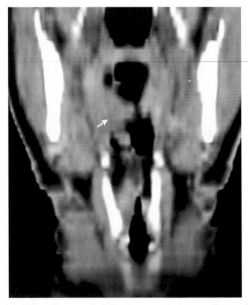

Fig. 41.8D: Coronal CT shows right pyriform fossa mass with supraglottic and glottic involvement

41.9 Carcinoma Larynx with Tracheostomy

Tracheostomy (Fig. 41.9C) in a case of inoperable carcinoma of larynx having glottic and supraglottic component (Figs 41.9A to C) with surgical emphysema (arrow) and pneumomediastinum (Figs 41.9C and D) secondary to tracheostomy.

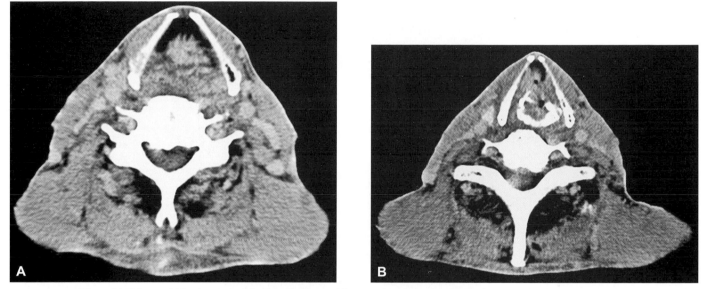

Figs 41.9A and B: Inoperable carcinoma of larynx having glottic and supraglottic component

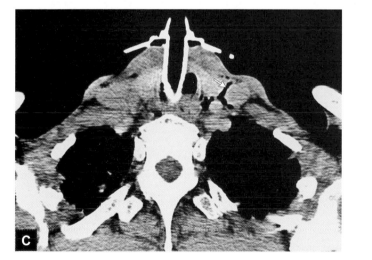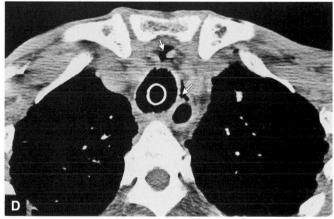

Figs 41.9C and D: Carcinoma larynx with tracheostomy tube *in situ*.
Surgical emphysema and pneumomediastinum secondary to tracheostomy

41.10 Recurrence Carcinoma Larynx

Post-radiotherapy carcinoma larynx with recurrent lesion in anterior commissure.
- Recurrent carcinoma in anterior commissure post radiotherapy (Fig. 41.10A).
- Increased thickening and density of the soft tissues of neck is seen following radiotherapy (Figs 41.10A and B).

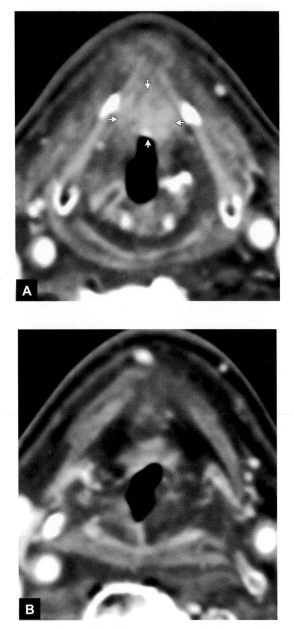

Figs 41.10A and B: Recurrence carcinoma of larynx

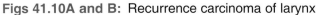

41.11 Rhabdomyosarcoma Maxilla

- Heterogenous soft tissue enhancement is seen in the region of right maxilla and infratemporal fossa (Figs 41.11A and B). Pterygoid plates are also involved by this mass.
- Coronal CT shows the infratemporal extension of this mass better (Fig. 41.11C). Note the loss of fat planes in between the adjacent muscle planes as shown by horizontal arrow. Vertical arrow shows erosion of skull base.
- Bone window shows involvement of pterygoid plates (Fig. 41.11D).

Rhabdomyosarcoma involving the right maxilla with infratemporal extension and erosion of skull base with remodeling of pterygoid plates.

Rhabdomyosarcoma is a malignant soft tissue tumor of unknown cause, found most often in children. The most common sites are the structures of the head and neck, the urogenital tract and the arms or legs. Diagnosis is often delayed because of lack of symptoms.

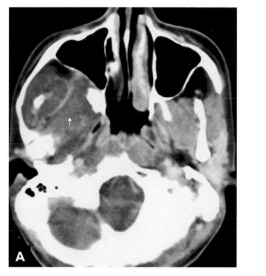 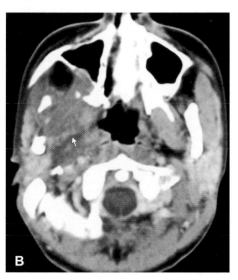

Figs 41.11A and B: Axial CT shows heterogenous soft tissue enhancement in the region of right maxilla and infratemporal fossa. Pterygoid plates are involved

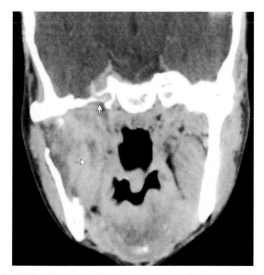 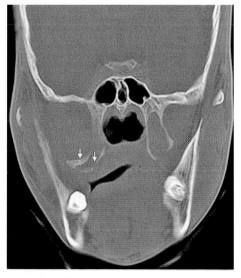

Fig. 41.11C: Coronal CT shows the infra-temporal extension of the mass, erosion of skull base and involvement of pterygoid plates

Fig. 41.11D: Coronal CT in bone window shows the mass with erosion of skull base and involvement of pterygoid plates

41.12 Parotid Tumor

Superficial as well as the deep lobes of parotid are enlarged and show avid contrast enhancement. No calcification or cysts are seen *in situ*. The left parapharyngeal airway and nasopharynx are slightly compressed (Figs 41.12A to D). No abnormal lymphadenopathy is seen. Histopathology confirmed it to be oxyphilic adenoma/oncocytoma with capsular invasion.

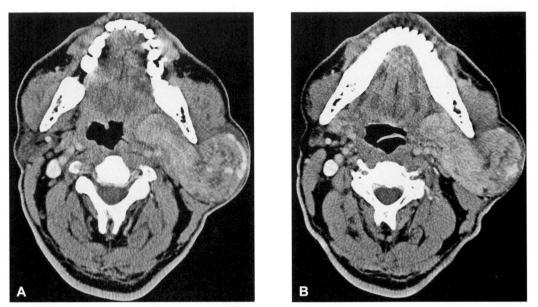

Figs 41.12A and B: Parotid tumor involving superficial as well as the deep lobes of parotid with avid contrast enhancement. The left parapharyngeal airway and nasopharynx are compressed

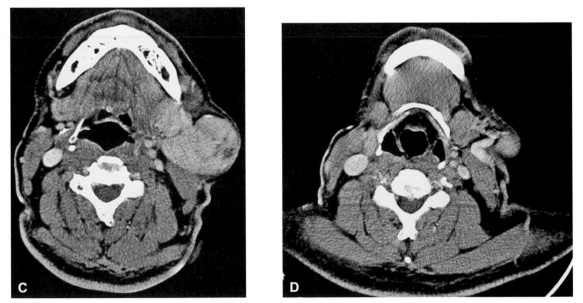

Figs 41.12C and D: Parotid tumor involving superficial as well as the deep lobes of parotid with avid contrast enhancement

41.13 Parotid Lymphoma

Plain and contrast CT images show diffuse enlargement of superficial as well as deep lobes of right parotid gland (Figs 41.13A to D). There is homogenous enhancement of the gland parenchyma. Retromandibular vein is encased. Cervical lymph nodes are enlarged. Biopsy proved it to be a lymphoma.

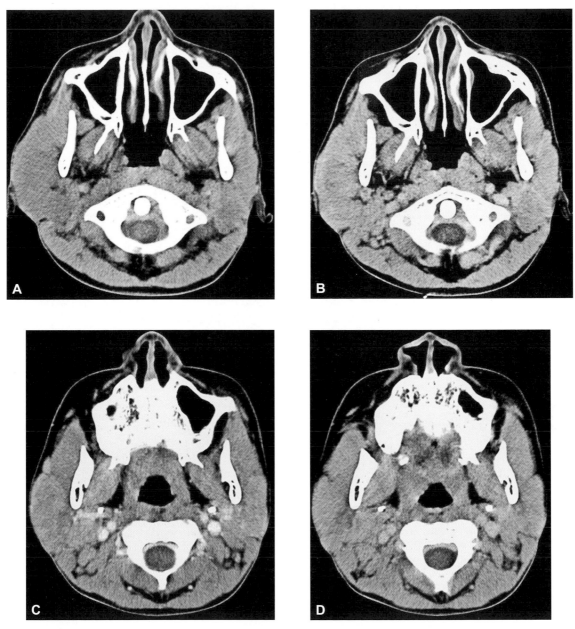

Figs 41.13A to D: Parotid lymphoma

41.14 Pleomorphic Adenoma Parotid

Enhancing mass seen in the deep lobe of left parotid gland. Left parapharyngeal space is partially effaced (Fig. 41.14). This proved out to be mixed pleomorphic adenoma from left parotid gland.

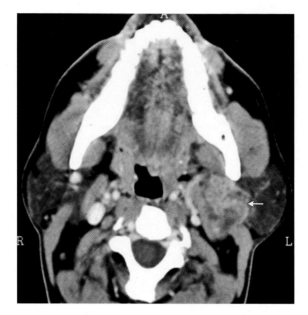

Fig. 41.14: Axial CT shows enhancing mass in deep lobe of left parotid gland. Left parapharyngeal space effaced

41.15 Glomus Tympanicum

50 years old female had decreased hearing, tinnitus and giddiness for the past one year. Left ear showed a bulging red mass classical of a glomus tumor (Figs 41.15A and B). Post-contrast HRCT temporal bone showed abnormal enhancing soft tissue lesion in left middle ear and extending into the promontory.

Glomus tympanicum is the most common primary neoplasm of the middle ear. Although histologically benign, glomus tympanicum is slow growing, locally destructive, spreading along paths of least resistance. The most common presenting symptoms are conductive hearing loss and pulsatile tinnitus.

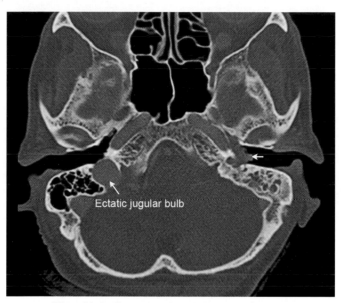

Ectatic jugular bulb

Fig. 41.15A: Axial CT shows enhancing soft tissue lesion in left middle ear

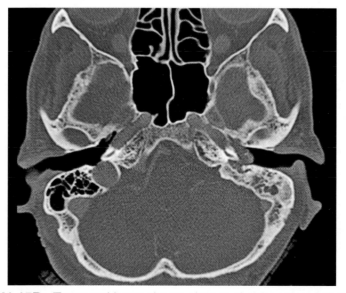

Fig. 41.15B: Temporal bone shows abnormal enhancing soft tissue lesion in left middle ear extending into the promontory

41.16 Giant Cell Granuloma

Plain (Figs 41.16A and B) and post-contrast (Figs 41.16C and D) CT images show moderately enhancing expansile lytic lesion of angle of mandible with fluid-fluid levels within. This is typical of an aneurysmal bone cyst in this 7 years old male with non tender gradually increasing swelling. Biopsy proved this to be a giant cell granuloma. Aneurysmal bone cyst of mandible and ameloblastoma are the other radiological differentials.

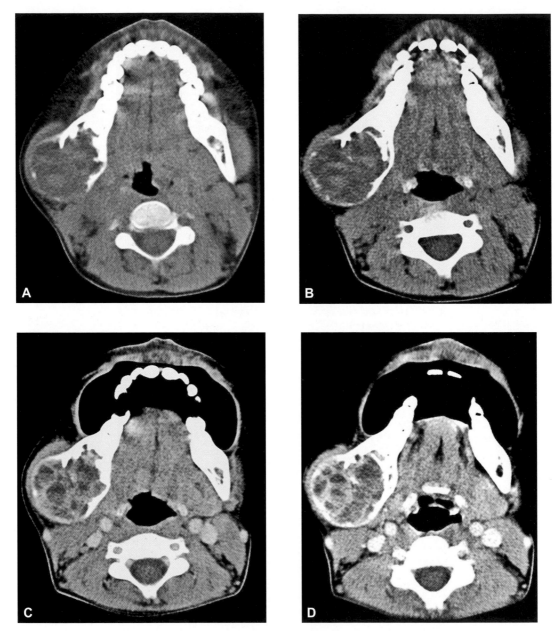

Figs 41.16A to D: Axial plain and contrast CT sections show giant cell granuloma

41.17 Malignant Mass Submandibular Region

Heterogeneously enhancing mass showing ulceration is seen to occupy left side of neck region with destruction of mandible, invasion of submandibular gland and adjacent neck muscles. Extensive necrotic malignant cervical lymphadenopathy is seen at levels I, II and III (Figs 41.17A to D).

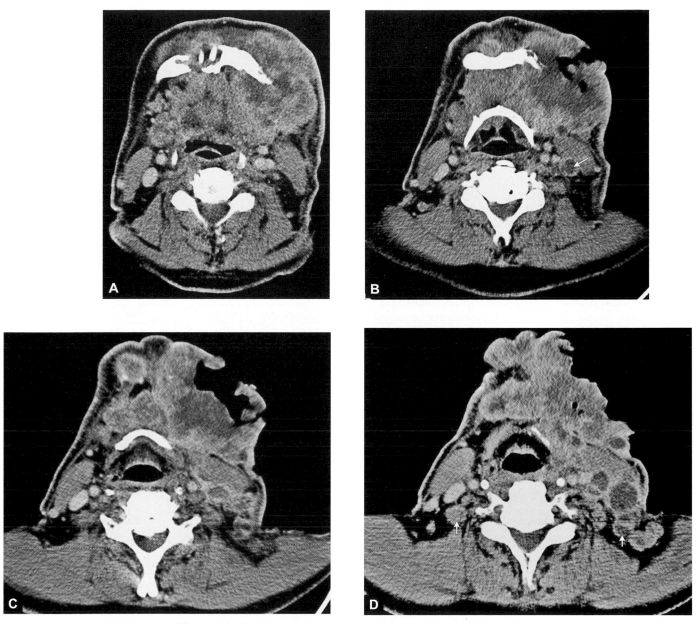

Figs 41.17A to D: Axial CT images show malignant mass submandibular region with cervical lymphadenopathy

41.18 Carcinoma Thyroid

CT images show a moderately enhancing solid mass arising from right lobe of thyroid extending below up to the suprasternal notch (Figs 41.18A to D). No retrosternal extension is seen.

The simplest way to find out if a thyroid lump or nodule is cancerous is with a fine needle aspiration (FNA) of the thyroid nodule.

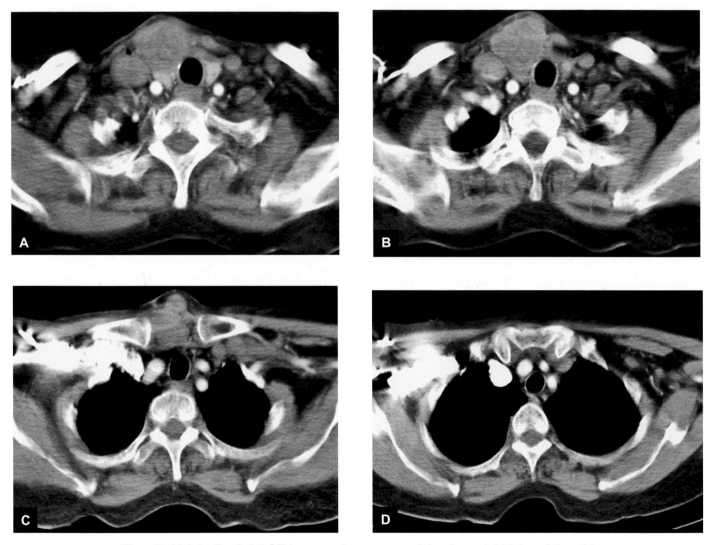

Figs 41.18A to D: Axial CT images show mass arising from right lobe of thyroid

41.19 Toxic Multinodular Goiter

Enlarged thyroid gland shows multiple nodules more in the right lobe with retrosternal extension (Fig. 41.19D). Scattered punctuate calcifications are seen in both the lobes. Trachea is compressed and pushed towards the left by the mass (Figs 41.19A to D).

Toxic multinodular goiter is a form of hyperthyroidism - where there is excess production of thyroid hormones. It emerges insidiously from nontoxic multinodular goiter. It is the second most common cause of hyperthyroidism after Graves disease.

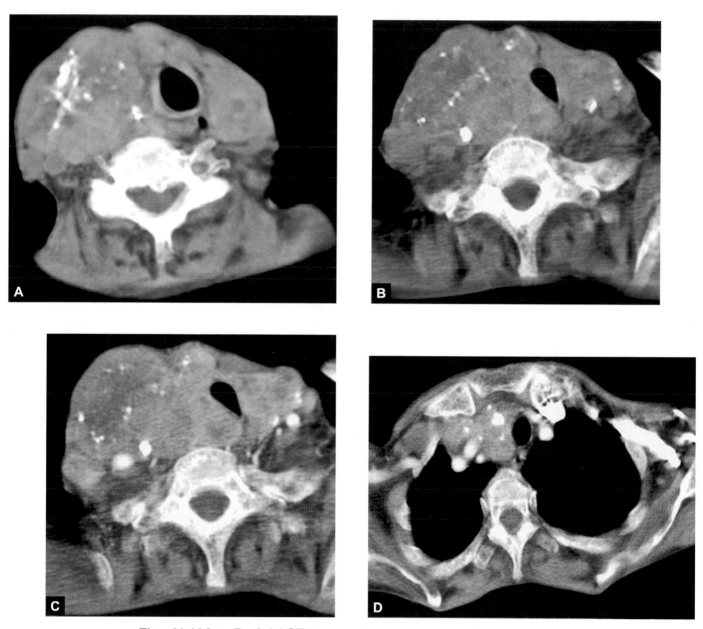

Figs 41.19A to D: Axial CT images show enlarged thyroid gland having multiple nodules with retrosternal extension

42. MISCELLANEOUS

42.1 Polyp and Granulation Tissue Temporal Bone

HRCT Temporal Bone

17 years male was operated one year ago for bilateral chronic suppurative otitis media (CSOM).

A soft tissue density polyp is seen in right external auditory canal (Fig. 42.1A).

CT images show mastoidectomy cavity on both sides. Recurrent granulation tissue is seen as soft tissues in the middle ear cavity and mastoidectomy cavity on either side (Figs 42.1B to D).

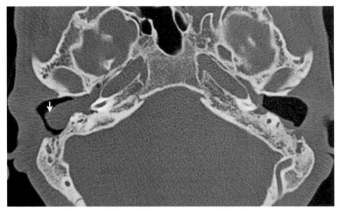

Fig. 42.1A: Axial CT shows a soft tissue density polyp in right external auditory canal

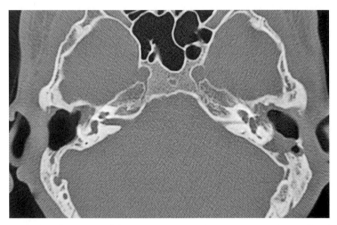

Fig. 42.1B: Axial CT shows mastoidectomy cavity on both sides and granulation tissue is seen as soft tissues in the middle ear cavity extending below up to the suprasternal notch

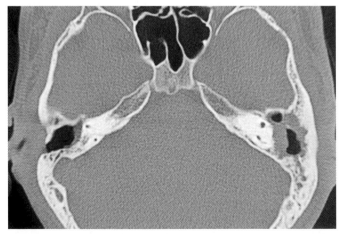

Fig. 42.1C: Axial CT shows mastoidectomy cavity on both sides and granulation tissue is seen as soft tissues in the middle ear cavity

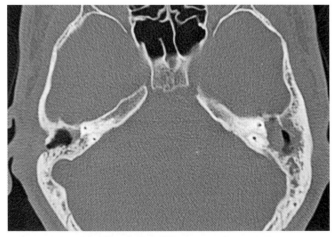

Fig. 42.1D: Axial CT shows granulation tissue in the middle ear cavity

42.2 Inverted Papilloma (Figs 42.2A to F)

Plain and contrast CT in 55 years female shows the histopathologically proven inverted papilloma as an enhancing mass with craniofacial extension up to the right cavernous sinus with proptosis of right eyeball.

Inverted papilloma is a benign neoplasm originating from the schneiderian membrane of nose and paranasal sinus cavities. These are true epithelial neoplasms characterised by hyperplastic epithelium inverting itself into the underlying stroma. Its potential for malignant transformation is (7.7 %) quite high.

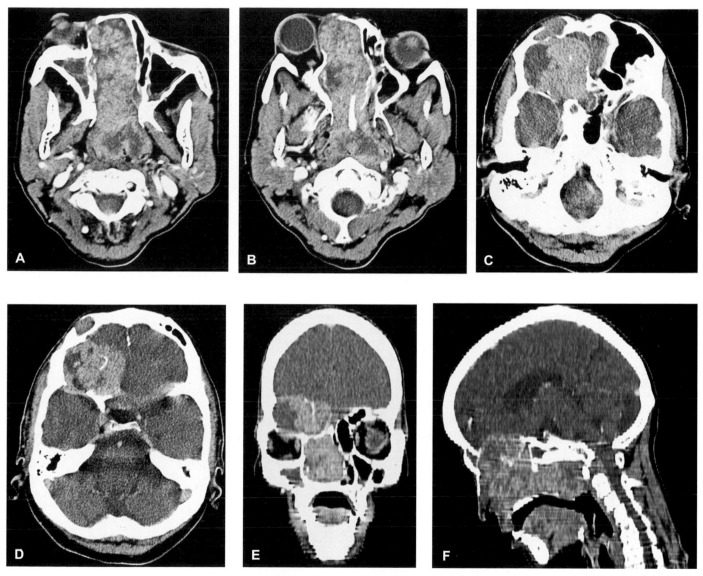

Figs 42.2A to F: Inverted papilloma

42.3 PNS Post FESS

Post FESS (Functional Endoscopic Sinus Surgery) HRCT images.

Bony defect is seen in inferolateral wall of maxillary sinus with fluid collection seen in right maxillary sinus as an air-fluid level (Figs 42.3A to D). Post-surgery uncinate process of right maxillary sinus is not visualized and the aditus to right osteo-meatal unit is widened.

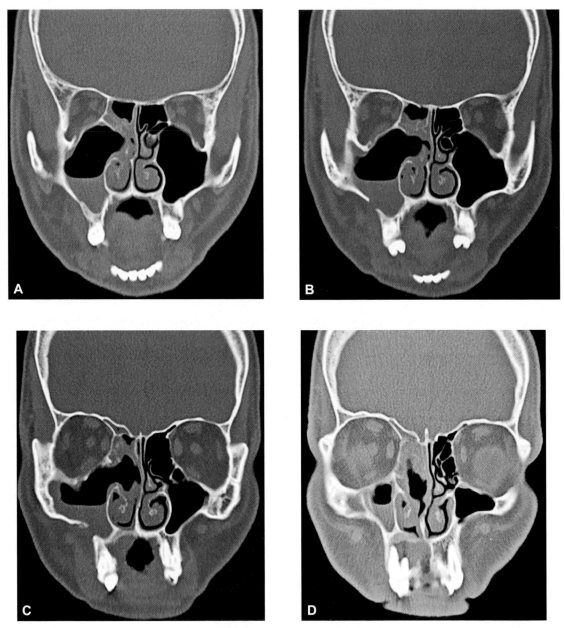

Figs 42.3A to D: Post FESS PNS

42.4 Laryngeal Cyst

- Plain CT neck shows round hypodense lesion occupying the left pyriform fossa and extending into the left aryepiglottic fold (Fig. 42.4A).
- Post contrast CT shows enhancement of the walls of the lesion (Fig. 42.4B). The center remains hypodense there by confirming it to be a cyst. On surgery it was found to be a saccular cyst of larynx also known as internal type of laryngocele.
- Reconstructed coronal CT image shows the location and extent better (Fig. 42.4C).

  Laryngeal cysts are rare, generally benign and can affect all age groups. Mucous glands line all other surfaces of the larynx, except the free edge of the true vocal cord.

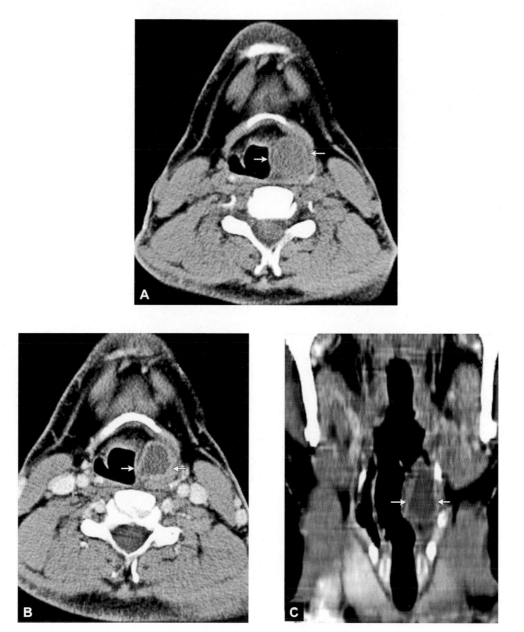

Figs 42.4A to C: Laryngeal cyst

42.5 Colloid Cyst Thyroid (Figs 42.5A and B)

Contrast CT neck shows hypodense non enhancing lesions in right as well as left lobe. No enhancing mural nodule or solid components or calcifications are seen.

Colloid cysts of thyroid are often incidental benign lesions but can appear as a mass to be distinguished from possible carcinoma. They contain gelatinous material with high protein content. Most thyroid cysts originate from cystic degeneration of adenomas.

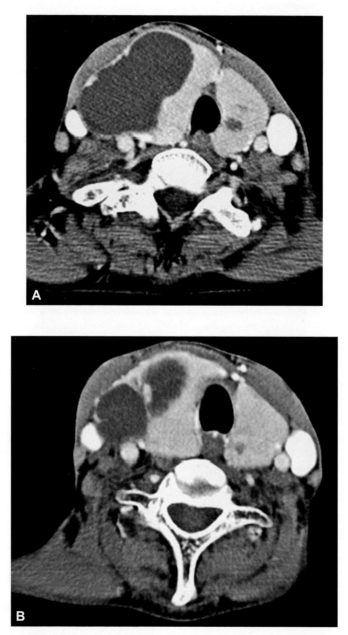

Figs 42.5A and B: Colloid cyst of thyroid gland

42.6 Cystic Hygroma 1

- Hypodense fluid filled mass is seen insinuating in the right retropharyngeal and parapharyngeal spaces, displacing the carotid space laterally (Fig. 42.6A).
- Cyst shows internal septae but no solid component (Fig. 42.6B).

A cystic hygroma is benign, congenital multiloculated lymphatic lesion that can arise anywhere, but is classically found in the left posterior triangle of the neck. It can be disfiguring.

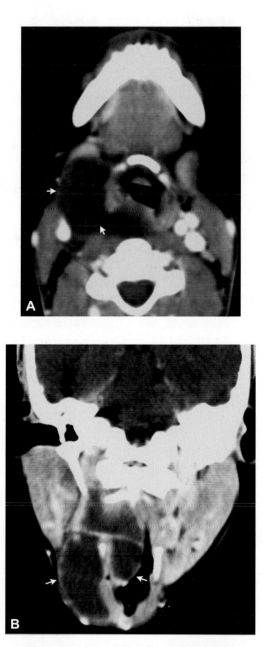

Figs 42.6A and B: Cystic hygroma

42.7 Cystic Hygroma 2

- CT neck shows a cystic hygroma characterized by multiloculated fluid filled cavities on left side of neck (Fig. 42.7A).
- CT guided sclerotherapy with sodium tetradecyl sulphate (shown by vertical arrow). Site of injection is shown by horizontal arrow (Fig. 42.7B).
- Sclerosant is seen filling almost entire lesion (Fig. 42.7C).
- Scout image shows complete extent of the spread of sclerosant (Fig. 42.7D).

Cystic hygroma is a lymphangioma developing in the connective tissues.
CT guided sclerotherapy with sodium tetradecyl sulphate is found to be effective.

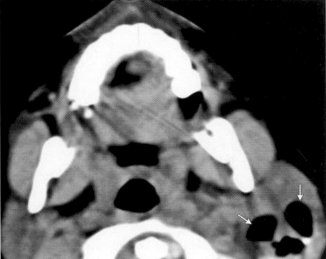

Fig. 42.7A: CT neck shows multiloculated fluid filled cavities on left side of neck

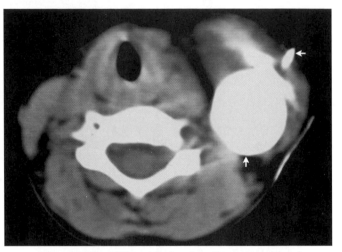

Fig. 42.7B: CT guided sclerotherapy, site of injection is shown by horizontal arrow

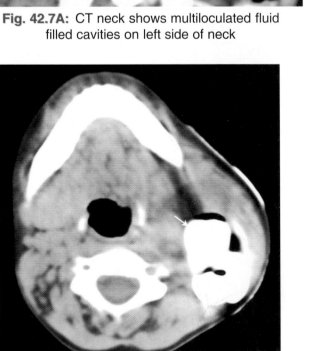

Fig. 42.7C: Sclerosant is seen filling almost entire lesion

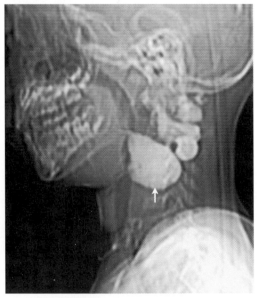

Fig. 42.7D: Scout image shows spread of sclerosant

42.8 Dentigerous Cyst

Well defined expansile cystic non enhancing lesion is seen located in alveolar process of maxilla on left side associated with the unerupted tooth (Figs 42.8A to D).

   A dentigerous cyst is an odontogenic cyst associated with the crown of an unerupted tooth. It is thought to be of developmental origin. Some authors have suggested that periapical inflammation of non-vital deciduous teeth in proximity to the follicles of unerupted permanent successors may be a factor for triggering this type of cyst formation. The cyst cavity is lined by epithelial cells derived from the reduced enamel epithelium of the tooth forming organ. Regarding its pathogenesis, it has been suggested that the pressure exerted by an erupting tooth on the follicle may obstruct venous flow inducing accumulation of exudate between the reduced enamel epithelium and the tooth crown.

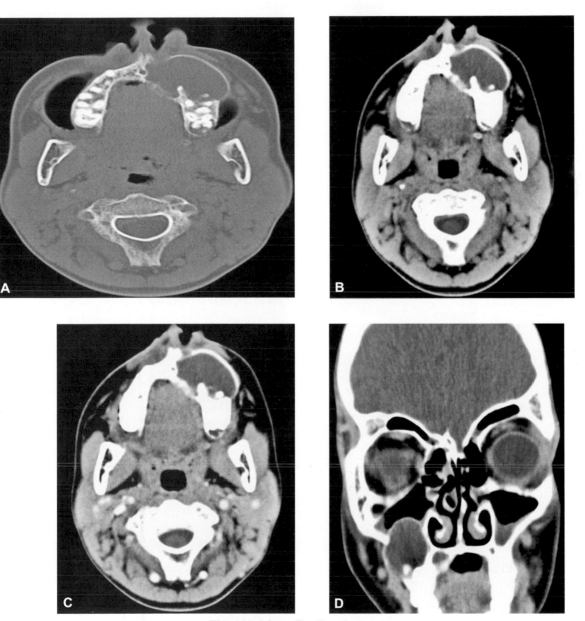

Figs 42.8A to D: Dentigerous cyst

42.9 Phlebectasia Internal Jugular Vein

- Swelling in the neck seen only while coughing (Fig. 42.9A).
- CT scan at the level of thyroid shows gross dilatation of the right internal jugular vein (arrow) as compared to that on the left (Fig. 42.9B). Diagnosis is internal jugular phlebectasia.

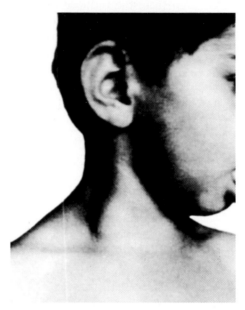

Fig. 42.9A: Swelling in the neck seen only while coughing

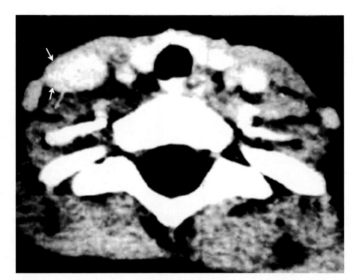

Fig. 42.9B: Axial CT at the level of thyroid shows gross dilatation of the right internal jugular vein as compared to that on the left

Section 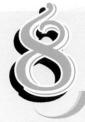 8

Miscellaneous

- ✍ **Artifacts**
- ✍ **Xenon CT**
- ✍ **Unknown Primary**

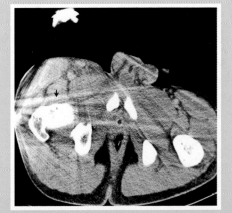 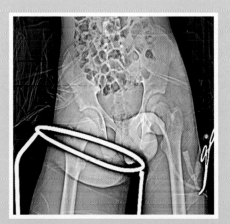 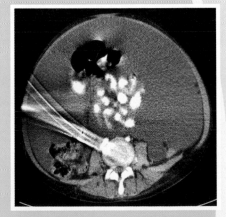

43. ARTIFACTS

43.1 Artifact

An artifact is an abnormal looking/appearing false finding in an image and is unrelated to the patient. It is thus a ghost appearance and in reality it does not exist.

Motion artifacts occur due to patient's motion, implants or ornaments and give rise to streak artifacts or beam hardening artifacts due to which adjacent structural details are obscured. Ring artifacts occur due to problems in detectors. When a partial volume is sampled or included in the field of view of imaging it gives rise to partial volume artifact.

- Angulation artifact seen as the asymmetric appearance of frontal horns of lateral ventricles as head was not symmetrically positioned. In reality, both ventricles are equal in size and are symmetrical (Fig. 43.1A).
- Ring artifacts occur as a result of detector malfunction which could either be due to improper calibration or due to detector-data ring mismatch. The center of the detector arc is the most sensitive region where ring artifacts can occur (Fig. 43.1B).
- Motion artifact due to accidental motion of right hand by patient (Fig. 43.1C).
- Streak artifacts due to metallic implant in tibia (Fig. 43.1D).

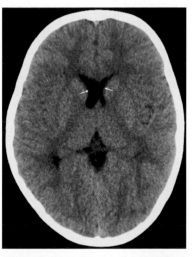

Fig. 43.1A: Angulation artifact

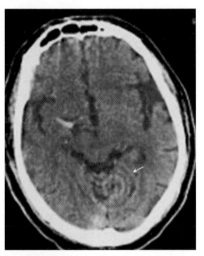

Fig. 43.1B: Ring artifact

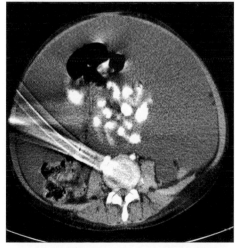

Fig. 43.1C: Motion artifact

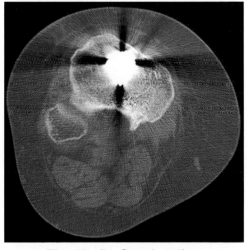

Fig. 43.1D: Streak artifact

43.2 Extrinsic Artifact

- Scout image shows right thigh in Thomas splint (Fig. 43.2A).
- Axial image shows hyperdense streaks on the pelvic structures due to reverberation artifacts from proximity of metallic Thomas splint (Fig. 43.2B).

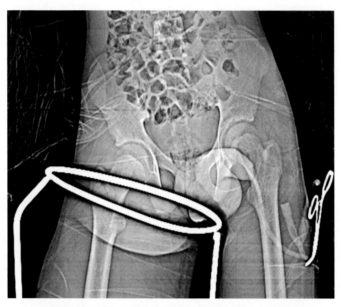

Fig. 43.2A: Right thigh in Thomas splint

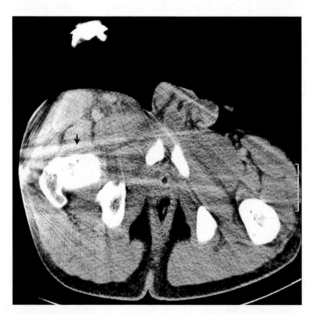

Fig. 43.2B: Streak artifact seen as hyperdense streaks due to reverberation from metallic thomas splint

43.3 Partial Volume Artifact

Symmetric hyperdensities seen in the frontal region are due to partial volume of the bone (Figs 43.3A and B).

Partial volume artifacts seen when tissues with different absorption properties occupy the same voxel, the beam is attenuated on basis of average of attenuation values of all those tissues. This volume averaging leads to partial volume artifacts. Common sites are posterior fossa and lung diaphragm interface.

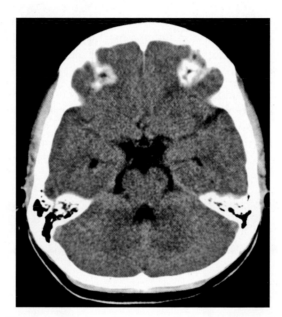

Fig. 43.3A: Hyperdensities seen in the frontal region are due to partial volume of the bone

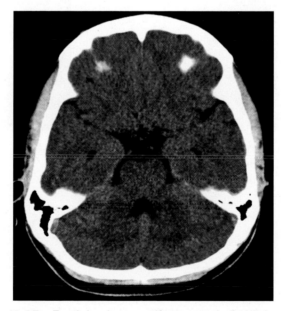

Fig. 43.3B: Partial volume artifact seen in frontal region

44. XENON CT

Xenon-CT is a noninvasive technique for measuring blood flow by xenon-enhanced CT scan. For this non radioactive xenon gas is inhaled, and the enhancement so produced is measured by sequential CT imaging. Time dependent concentration of xenon in various tissue is used to provide blood flow data which is mapped.

Cerebral blood flow (CBF) is important to the neurosurgeons, neurologists and psychiatrists. Xenon-CT is effectively used to provide CBF in cerebovascular diseases, tumors, head injury, neuropsychiatric disorders and in brain death.

Normal CBF in cortical gray matter is about 80 ml/100 g/min, white matter has mean CBF of about 20 ml/100 g/min and areas containing both gray and white matter have a mean flow of 40–60 ml/100 g/min.

The range of blood perfusion in renal cortex is between 150 to 280 ml/100 cc/min and hepatic tissue perfusion blood flow is from 80 to 120 ml/100 cc/ min.

- Axial CT (Fig. 44.1A) of a 67-year old male presented with cognition and behavior dysfunction, dyspraxia and loss of short-term memory. Neurological investigations including CT scan were normal
- Axial xenon-enhanced CT (Fig. 44.1B) shows reduced cerebral blood flow in the right posterior temporal lobe (arrows) consistent with the patient's dysfunctions. The color scale represents cerebral blood flow.

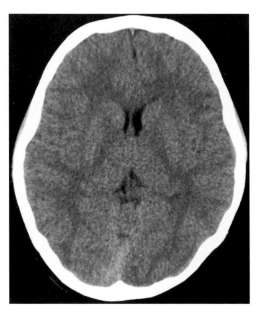

Fig. 44.1A: Axial CT head

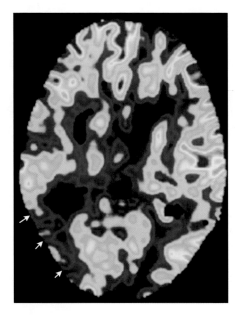

Fig. 44.1B: Axial xenon-enhanced CT

45. UNKNOWN PRIMARY

Metastatic right supraclavicular node (Fig. 45.1A), pre and para tracheal nodes (Figs 45.1B and C) and left adrenal deposit (Fig. 45.1D). Suspicious lesions are seen in the right lung (Figs 45.1E and F), but the primary tumor remained elusive.

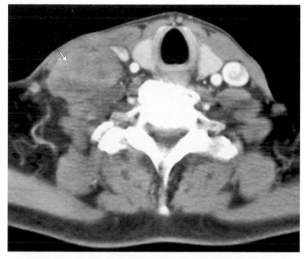

Fig. 45.1A: Metastatic right supraclavicular node

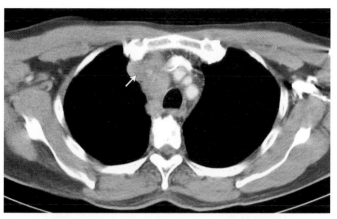

Fig. 45.1B: Metastatic pre and para tracheal nodes

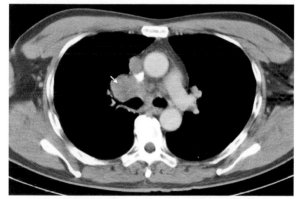

Fig. 45.1C: Metastatic Tracheaobronchial nodes

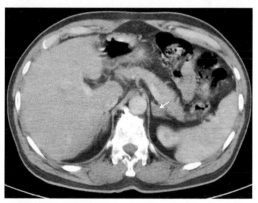

Fig. 45.1D: Metastatic deposit left adrenal gland

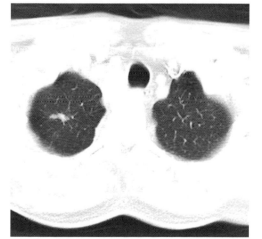

Fig. 45.1E: Suspicious pulmonary deposit

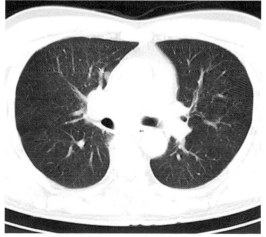

Fig. 45.1F: Suspicious pulmonary deposits

Section 9

Quiz

- Osteomyelitis Skull
- Vocal Cord Palsy
- Ossifying Fibroma
- Carcinoma Lung with Bronchoceles
- Allergic Bronchopulmonary Aspergillosis
- Mucinous Cystadenoma of Pancreas
- Wilm's Tumor
- Metastatic Endometrial Carcinoma
- Heterotopic Ossification
- Macrodystrophia Lipomatosa
- Branchial Cleft Cyst
- Osteoid Osteoma
- Retinoblastoma
- Ossifying Epidural Hematoma
- Multiple Myeloma

- Percheron Infarct
- Ethmoidal Mucocele
- Intraspinal Dermoid
- Parathyroid Adenoma
- Pulmonary Koch's
- Orbital Hemangioma
- Sclerosing Cholangitis
- Giant Osteoma of Mandible
- Open Lip Schizencephaly
- Tuberous Sclerosis
- Cold Abscess
- Subdural Hematoma
- Pachydermoperiostosis
- Hepatoblastoma
- Pan Sinusitis and Orbital Pseudotumor
- Fetus-in-fetu

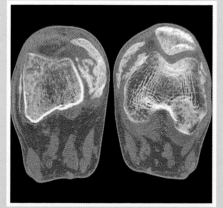
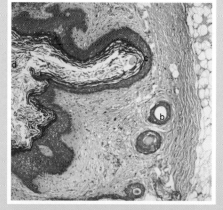
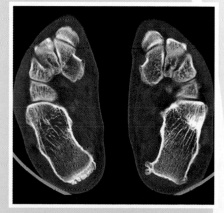

46. QUIZ

Quiz No: 46.1

An elderly diabetic whose complaint was dysphagia, left ear discharge and left hemi facial numbness since 6 months.

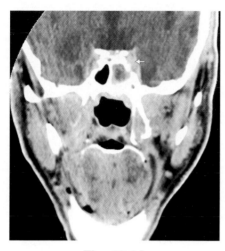

Fig. 46.1A

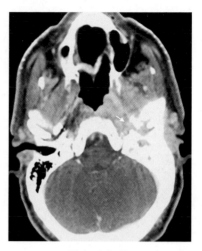

Fig. 46.1B

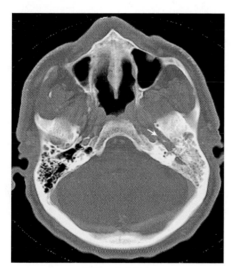

Fig. 46.1C

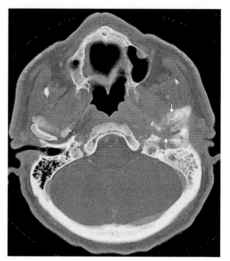

Fig. 46.1D

Answer

Osteomyelitis of skull base secondary to sphenoid sinusitis and otitis media causing cranial nerve palsy.

- Left sphenoid sinusitis with focal dehiscence of lateral wall of left sphenoid sinus (Fig. 46.1A).
- Permeative destruction of floor of middle cranial fossa in the region of cranial nerve foramina with enhancing soft tissue in infratemporal fossa. Also there is soft tissue in left middle ear cavity and mastoid air cells suggesting otomastoiditis (Fig. 46.1B).
- Bone window images show permeative destruction of floor of middle cranial fossa in the region of cranial nerve foramina with left pharyngeal wall deviation suggesting cranial nerve palsy (Figs 46.1C and D).

Quiz No: 46.2

Gradually progressive hoarseness of voice in a middle aged female.

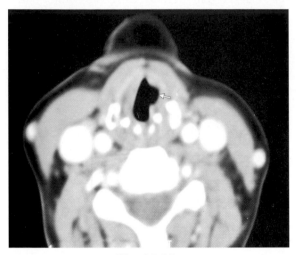

Fig. 46.2A

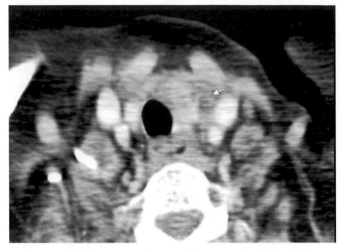

Fig. 46.2B

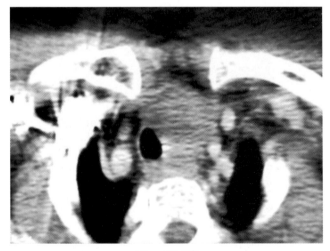

Fig. 46.2C

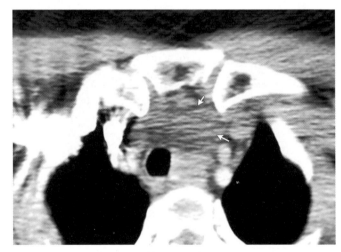

Fig. 46.2D

Answer

Left vocal cord palsy secondary to retrosternal goiter.
- CT neck shows left vocal cord palsy (Fig. 46.2A).
- Post-contrast CT scan shows left hemithyroid goiter with retrosternal extension causing compression on left recurrent laryngeal nerve leading to vocal cord palsy (Figs 46.2B to D).

Quiz No: 46.3

Gradually progressive swelling right cheek.

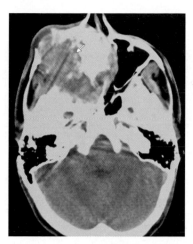
Fig. 46.3A

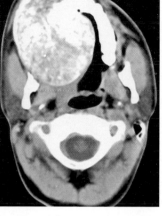
Fig. 46.3B

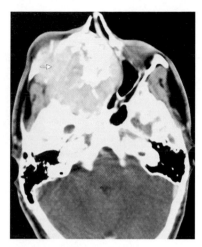
Fig. 46.3C

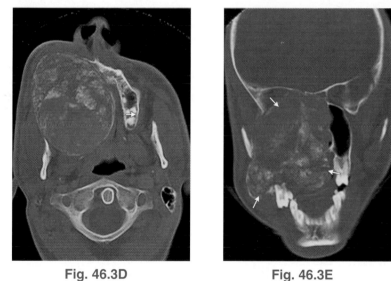

Fig. 46.3D   Fig. 46.3E

Answer

Ossifying fibroma of right maxilla.
- Plain axial CT sections showing a mass with diffuse calcification involving the maxillary alveolar ridge, occupying and expanding the right maxillary sinus and involving the ipsilateral hard palate, projecting into the right nasal cavity (Figs 46.3A and B).
- Post-contrast axial CT sections show that the mass is poorly enhancing (Fig. 46.3C).
- Axial (Fig. 46.3D) and coronal (Fig. 46.3E) sections in bone window show the extent and nature of mass better.

Differential diagnosis includes:
1. Ossifying fibroma
2. Cemento-ossifying fibroma
3. Osteosarcoma
4. Chondrosarcoma

Quiz No: 46.4

Elderly male with history of productive cough, anorexia, weakness and weight loss.
- CT Chest mediastinal window (Figs 46.4A to C) and (Fig. 46.4D) in lung window.

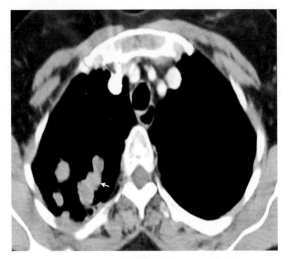

Fig. 46.4A

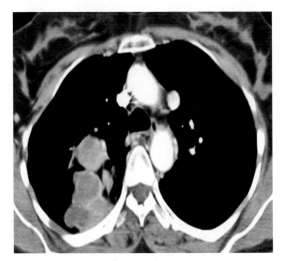

Fig. 46.4B

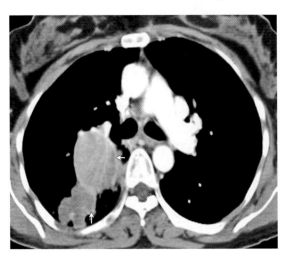

Fig. 46.4C

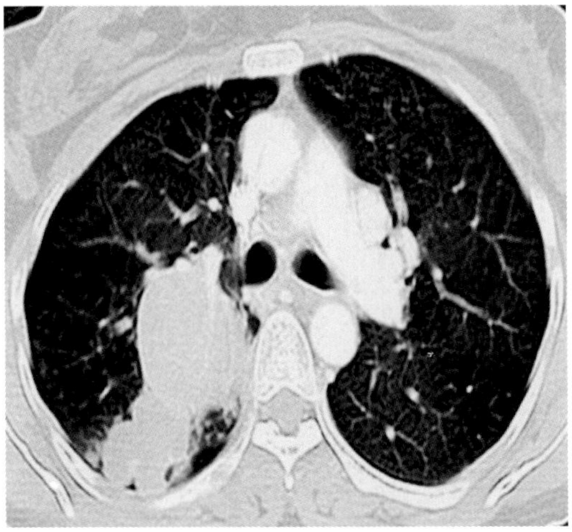

Fig. 46.4D

Answer

Carcinoma lung with bronchoceles
Non small cell lung carcinoma (NSCLC)
- CT shows dilated fluid filled bronchi (bronchoceles) (Figs 46.4A and B).
- Mediastinal window (Fig. 46.4C) and lung window (Fig. 46.4D) setting CT shows an enhancing solid mass shown by horizontal arrow and distal bronchoceles by vertical arrow.

Quiz No: 46.5

A male farmer, 25 years age suffered from breathlessness on and off. Clinically he had asthma and blood counts showed eosinophilia.
- Chest radiograph PA view (Fig. 46.5A).
- CT chest in lung window (Figs 46.5B to D).

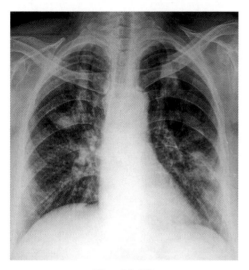

Fig. 46.5A

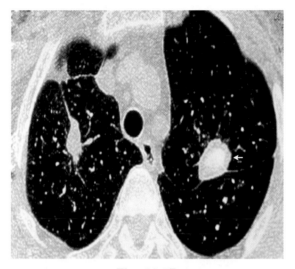

Fig. 46.5B

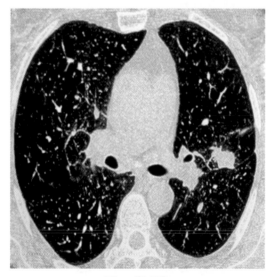

Fig. 46.5C

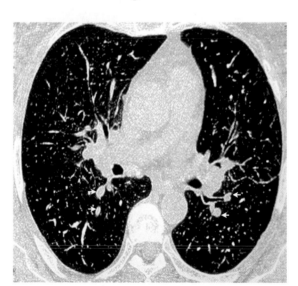

Fig. 46.5D

Answer

Allergic bronchopulmonary aspergillosis.
- Radiograph of chest shows gloved finger opacities (Figs 46.5A and B).
- Lung window CT shows mucoid impaction in the dilated bronchioles and air trapping (Figs 46.5B to D). This type of lung infiltrates and finger-in-glove appearance of bronchioles is diagnostic of allergic bronchopulmonary aspergillosis.

Quiz No: 46.6

Adult female patient presented with recurrent dull abdominal pain of 6 months duration, was subjected to CT abdomen and pelvis.

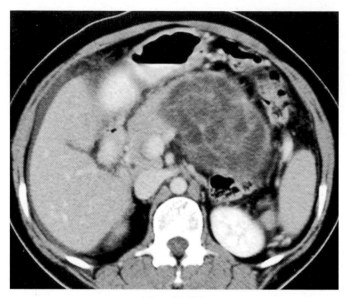

Fig. 46.6A

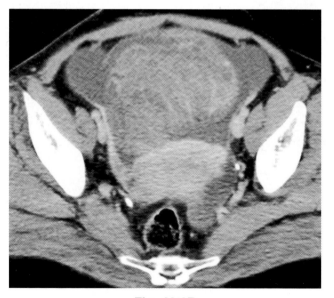

Fig. 46.6B

Answer

Mucinous cystadenocarcinoma of pancreas with ovarian metastases.
- Multiseptated cystic mass in the body and tail of pancreas (Fig. 46.6A).
- Similar morphology mass arising from the pelvis of ovarian origin. Ascites is also present (Fig. 46.6B).
  FNAC of pelvic mass suggested metastases from mucinous cystadenocarcinoma of pancreas.

Quiz No: 46.7

Six years old male child presented with gradually increasing lump abdomen.

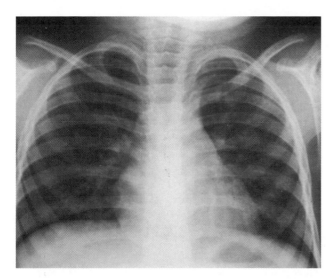

Fig. 46.7A

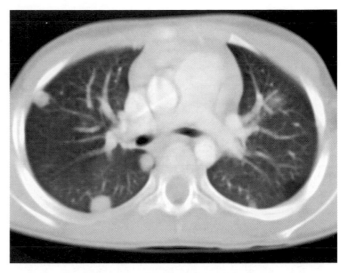

Fig. 46.7B

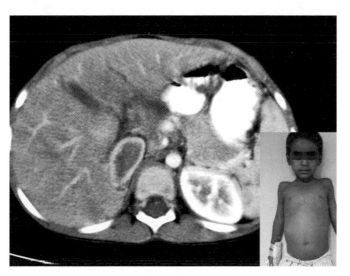

Fig. 46.7C

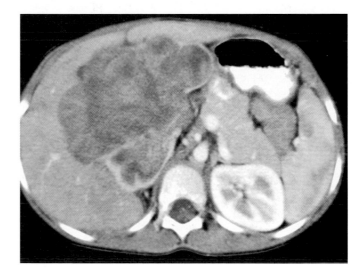

Fig. 46.7D

Answer

Wilm's tumor (nephroblastoma) with hepatic and pulmonary metastases (Figs 46.7A to H).
Large well defined enhancing mass lesion 9 × 10 cm with few areas of necrosis, involving the right kidney, sparing its upper pole. Medially the lesion is seen to displace the pancreas and great vessels to left side with compression of IVC. Cranially the lesion is seen to abutt the inferior surface of liver and inferiorly extend up to iliac crest.

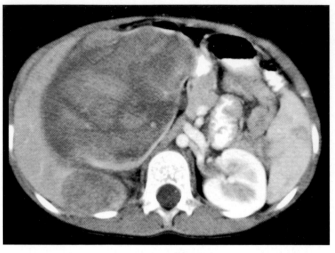

Fig. 46.7E

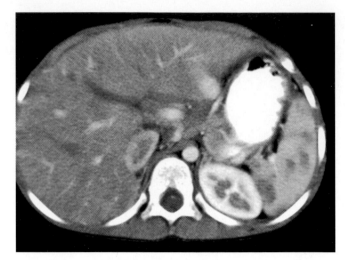

Fig. 46.7F

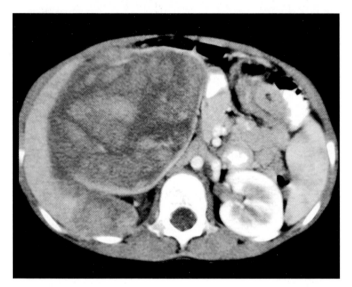

Fig. 46.7G

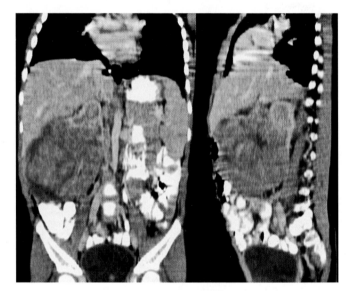

Fig. 46.7H

Another 3 × 2.4 cm heterogenously enhancing lesion is seen in posteroinferior segment of right lobe of liver is metastases.

Multiple well defined metastatic lesions are seen in the lungs.

Quiz No: 46.8

An elderly female presented with post menopausal bleed subjected to CT abdomen and pelvis.

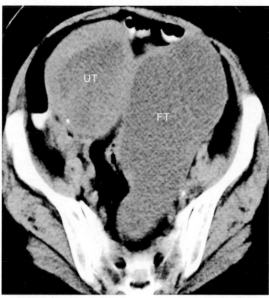

Fig. 46.8A

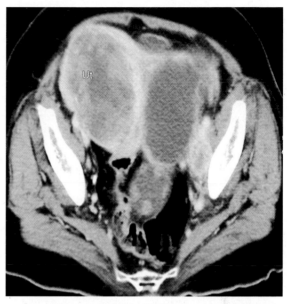

Fig. 46.8B

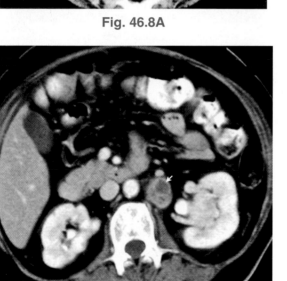

Fig. 46.8C

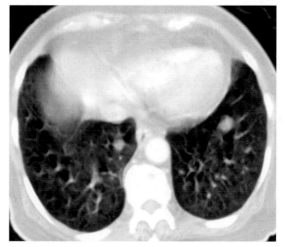

Fig. 46.8D

Answer

Metastatic endometrial carcinoma.
A diagnosed case of endometrial carcinoma with myometrial invasion.
Left renal and pulmonary metastases with metastatic para-aortic adenopathy.
- CT shows enlarged uterus and cystic structure in left adnexa (Fig. 46.8A).
- Contrast CT shows heterogenous enhancement of uterus. No distinction is seen between myometrium and endometrium. Tubular fluid collection seen in the left adnexa (Fig. 46.8B).
- Contrast CT shows a mass in left kidney. Left paraaortic nodes are enlarged (Fig. 46.8C).
- HRCT Thorax shows metastatic lesions in lungs (Fig. 46.8D).

Quiz No: 46.9

32 years old male had intracranial right ganglio-capsular hematoma. He was in coma for a month but eventually recovered. 6 months later he developed difficulty in walking and had reduced range of movement at knee joints. Following are the images at 6 months stage.

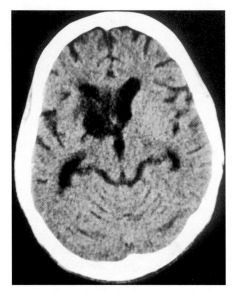

Fig. 46.9A

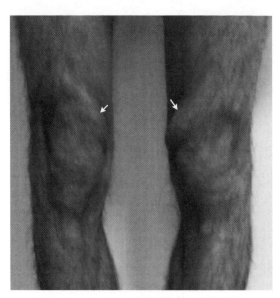

Fig. 46.9B

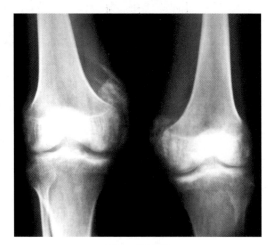

Fig. 46.9C

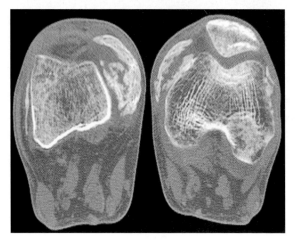

Fig. 46.9D

Answer

Heterotopic ossification.

- CT Brain shows residual gliotic changes in right gangliocapsular region indicating old CNS insult (Fig. 46.9A).
- Photograph of knees show swelling in the supero-medial aspect of both knee joints (Fig. 46.9B).
- Plain radiograph shows ossification in soft tissues near distal ends of femur. Separate line of demarcation from femur is not seen (Fig. 46.9C).
- CT scan shows the juxta articular new bone (heterotopic ossification) formation separate from femur (Fig. 46.9D). Heterotopic ossification around knees as a sequela of old CNS insult.

Quiz No: 46.10

Radiograph of right hand shows gigantic enlargement of both soft tissues and osseous parts of ring and middle finger with syndactyly.

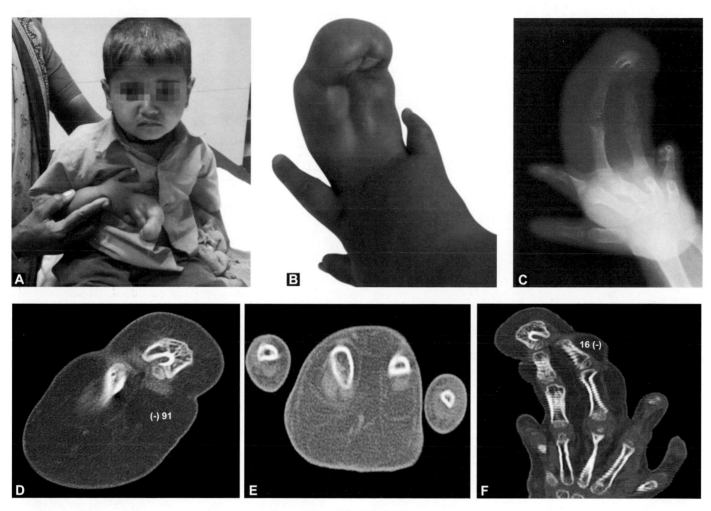

Figs 46.10A to F

Answer

Macrodystrophia lipomatosa (Figs 46.10A to F).
The distal end of terminal phalanges are fused in an arched manner.

Axial CT confirms the enlargement of both soft tissues and bones of ring and middle finger with syndactyly. The gigantic soft tissue component is essentially fat.

Paraxial recon of CT images confirm the X-ray findings. The CT value of the gigantic soft tissue lies between (-)87 to (-)110 HU confirming it to be fat.

Quiz No: 46.11

16 years male with painless cystic swelling on left side of neck.

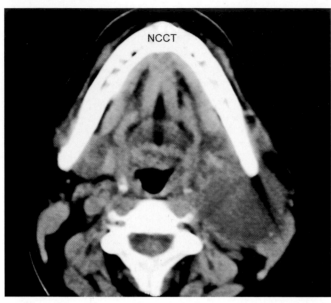

Fig. 46.11A

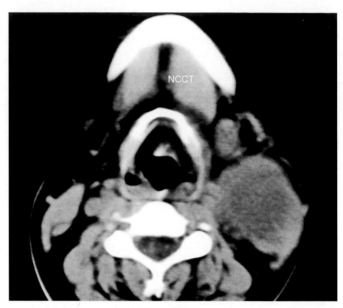

Fig. 46.11B

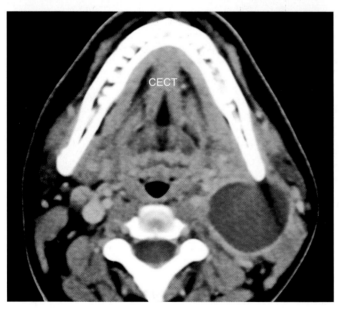

Fig. 46.11C

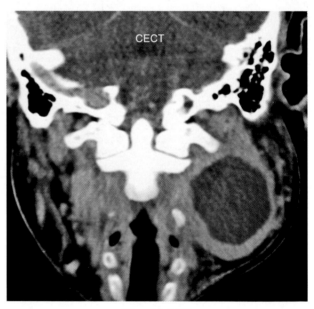

Fig. 46.11D

Answer

Second branchial cleft cyst (Figs 46.11A to D).
Branchial cleft cysts are most common cysts to arise in the neck and the most common congenital masses of the lateral neck. Others masses include thyroglossal duct cyst, ectopic thymic cyst, lymphangioma, dermoid and epidermoid cysts. Cross-sectional imaging is the mainstay of diagnosis for these lesions.

Quiz No: 46.12

20 years male with left heel pain relieved with NSAIDS. Plain radiograph (Fig. 46.12A) and CT (Fig. 46.12B).

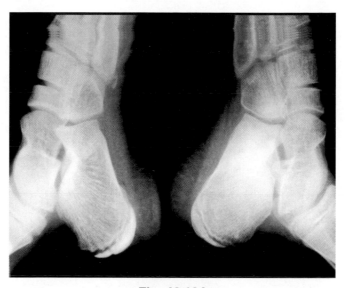

Fig. 46.12A

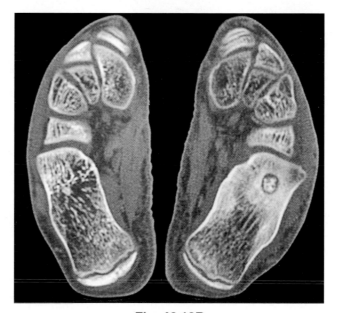

Fig. 46.12B

Answer

Osteoid osteoma in left calcaneum.

Suspicion of an osteoid osteoma should arise when young people present with subtalar pain that does not respond to the usual treatment. CT sections of the tarsal bones reveal the lesion. MRI usually does not trace the tumor in the early stage.

Subtle nature of radiographic findings in patients with juxtaarticular lesions may lead to long delays in diagnosis and treatment.

A double-ring sign in a bone scan is highly indicative of osteoid osteoma.

Quiz No: 46.13

2 years old boy with proptosis of left eyeball.

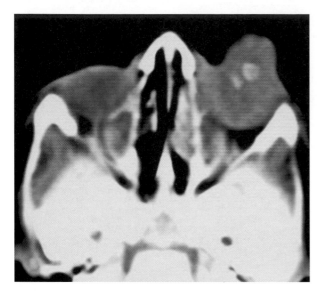

Fig. 46.13A

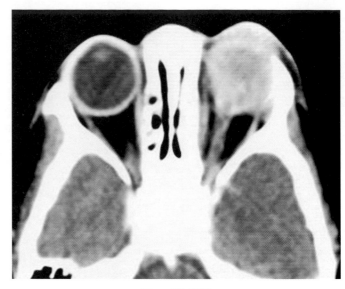

Fig. 46.13B

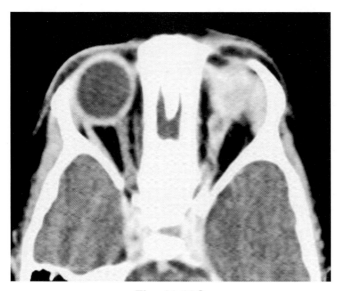

Fig. 46.13C

Fig. 46.13D

Answer

Retinoblastoma left eye
- CT orbits show calcification in the retinal soft tissue mass (Figs 46.13A and B).
- Contrast CT shows enhancing retinal soft tissue mass (Figs 46.13C and D).

It arises from primitive neuroectodermal cells in retina. It may be hereditary or sporadic and may be bilateral. Over 80% of retinoblastoma show evidence of calcification on CT scan. In patients under three years of age in whom a retinoblastoma is suspected, the presence of calcification on CT scan is virtually diagnostic.

Quiz No: 46.14

A case of epidural hematoma managed conservatively. X-ray and CT scan performed after 4 weeks. Figures 46.14A and B are the skull radiographs and Figures 46.14C and D are CT images.

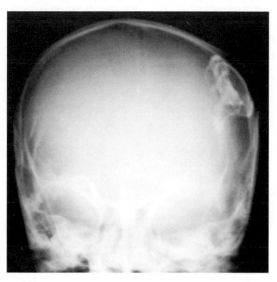

Fig. 46.14A

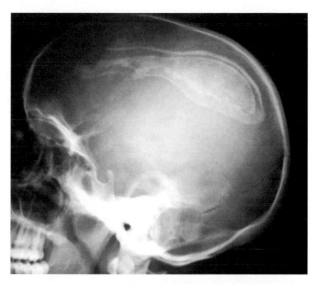

Fig. 46.14B

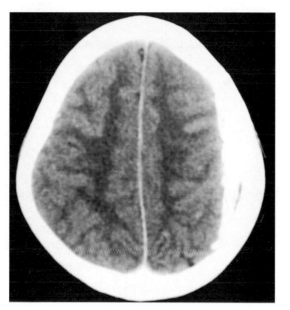

Fig. 46.14C

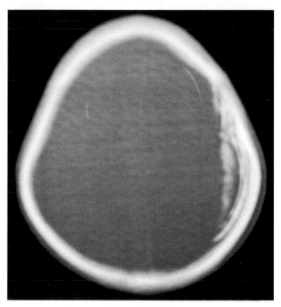

Fig. 46.14D

Answer

Ossifying epidural hematoma.

An epidural hematoma with mild symptoms treated conservatively and not naturally absorbed carries the risk of calcification and ossification in 10 days to 10 weeks period.

Quiz No: 46.15

Figure 46.15A is lateral radiograph and Figures 46.15B to D are CT images of 68 years male giving history of weight loss.

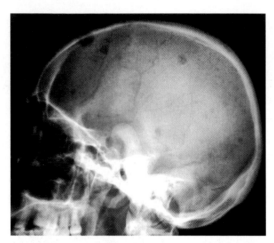

Fig. 46.15A

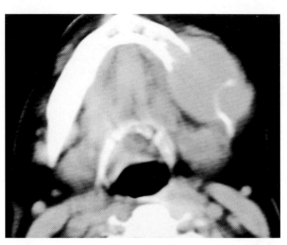

Fig. 46.15B

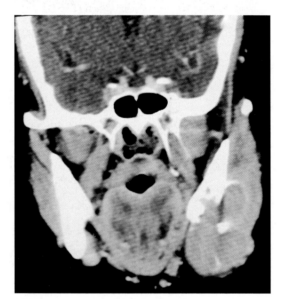

Fig. 46.15C

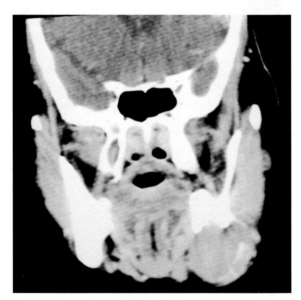

Fig. 46.15D

Answer

Multiple myeloma.

Multiple myeloma or plasma cell myeloma also known as Kahler's disease is a cancer of the white blood cells known as plasma cells, which produce antibodies. Many organs can be affected by myeloma, there by the symptoms and signs vary greatly. Presence of Bence Jones proteins in urine establishes the diagnosis and helps to monitor the disease. The workup of suspected multiple myeloma includes a skeletal survey. Myeloma activity appears as lytic lesions and on the skull X-ray as "punched-out lesions" (pepper pot skull). CT scan is performed to show the exact size and extent of soft tissue plasmacytomas. Bone scans are not of any additional value.

Quiz No: 46.16

Plain (Fig. 46.16A) and contrast (Fig. 46.16B) CT brain in an elderly male who was brought in coma from which he eventually recovered but had vertical gaze paresis, altered behavior and excess sleep.

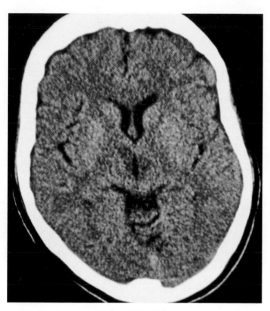

Fig. 46.16A

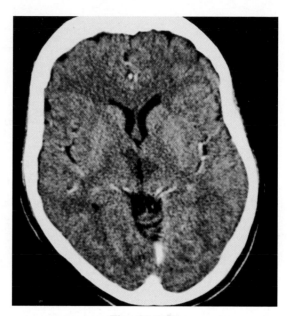

Fig. 46.16B

Answer

Percheron infarct (bilateral median thalamic infarct).

Percheron infarct as a result of bilateral infarct of paramedian artery supplying the thalamus. This is possible because the vessels of both sides can originate from a single trunk. Many times these infarcts also extend to the territory of polar arteries.

Damage to mammillo-thalamic tract is responsible for memory disorders which include impaired vigilance, amnesia and delusions. Mood changes, bulimia and vertical gaze paresis also complicate the picture.

Quiz No: 46.17

Adult male presented with proptosis.

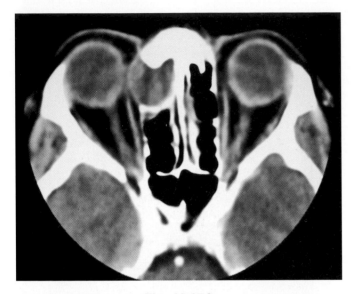

Fig. 46.17A

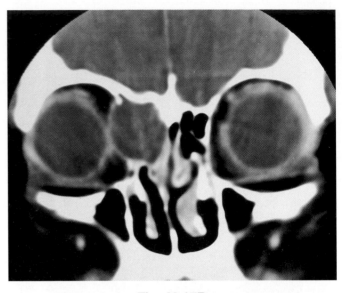

Fig. 46.17B

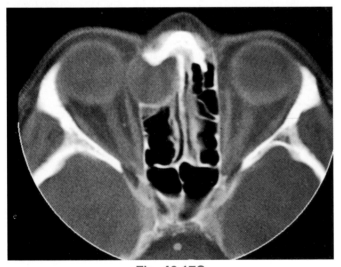

Fig. 46.17C

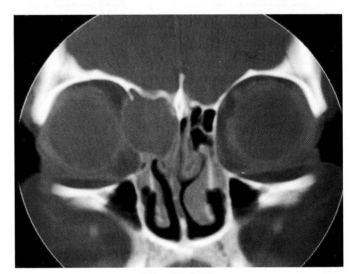

Fig. 46.17D

Answer

Mucocele right anterior ethmoidal sinus (Figs 46.17A to D).

    Mucoceles are benign mucus-filled lesions, the cause has not been clearly determined and are lined with columnar or cuboidal epithelium. They are most frequently found in the frontal and ethmoid sinuses causing expansion of the paranasal sinuses. The typical radiographic appearance of mucoceles is a fully opacified sinus with evidence of rounded or ovoid expansion and bone erosion.

Quiz No: 46.18

21 years female presented with weakness in both lower limbs since 3 years and difficulty in passing urine since one year. She was subjected to CT scan spine.

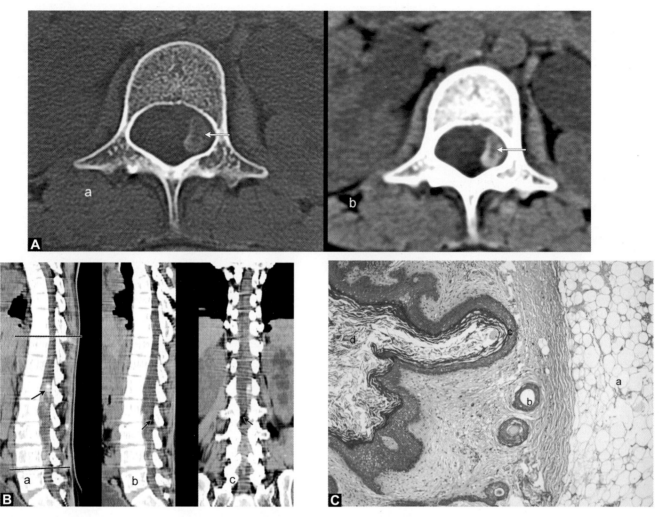

Figs 46.18A to C

Answer

Intraspinal dermoid.
- CT scan of spine bone window (a) and soft tissue window (b) reveal widening of spinal canal with areas of calcification (arrow) (Fig. 46.18A).
- Reformatted sagittal (a, b) and coronal (c) CT images of spine reveals calcification (black arrow), fat (white arrow) and shows the lesion extending from D11-12 to L4-5 level with widening of the bony spinal canal (Fig. 46.18B).
- Photomicrograph reveals cyst containing keratinized material lined by stratified squamous epithelial with skin adnexal structures. a-fat, b-hair follicle, c-stratified squamous epithelial and d- keratin (Fig. 46.18C).

CT spine with sagittal and coronal reformations showed a mass lesion with presence of fat and calcification. Likely diagnosis is intraspinal dermoid. Confirmed on histopathology.

Spinal dermoid is a rare, benign, slow-growing tumor arising from primitive germ cell layers. It is commonly intradural in location. Imaging demonstrates areas of fat and calcification within it and helps in giving definite diagnosis.

Quiz No: 46.19

Patient presented with history of weakness and tiredness with neck pain was subjected to radiograph of skull and CT neck and chest.

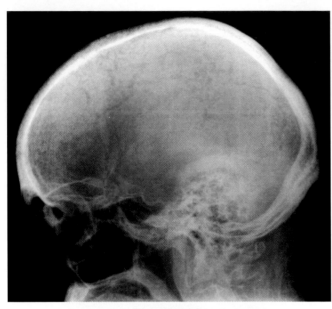

Fig. 46.19A

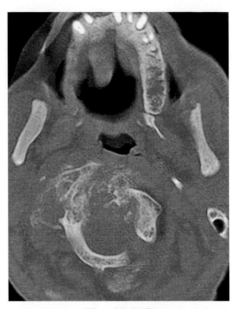

Fig. 46.19B

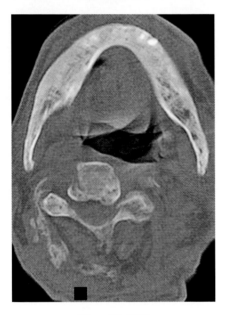

Fig. 46.19C

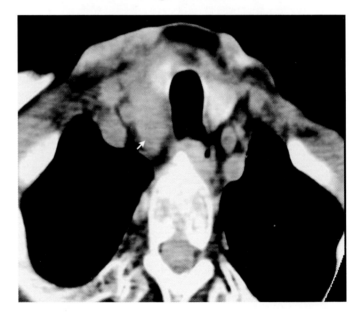

Fig. 46.19D

Answer

Parathyroid adenoma with caries spine (Figs 46.19A to D).

Skull shows ground glass pattern, granular salt and pepper appearance and there is loss of distinction between inner and outer skull tables. Osteosclerosis in mandible, metastatic soft tissue calcification near C1 and C2 with vertebral bodies already destroyed by Koch's and diffuse enlargement of parathyroid glands seen here are features of secondary hyperparathyroidism.

Quiz No: 46.20

Patient with persistent productive cough. No resolution even after multiple courses of routine antibiotics. HRCT chest was done.

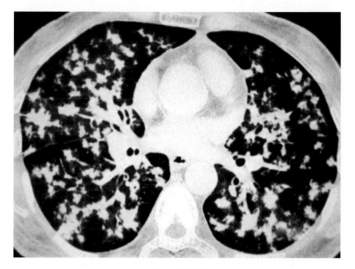

Fig. 46.20

Answer

Centrilobular opacities in pulomary Koch's (Fig. 46.20).

On CT chest pulmonary tuberculosis can manifest in following ways – tuberculoma, miliary form, cavitary form and endobronchial/acinar form in which active bacilli spread along the airway and appear on HRCT as centrilobular opacities which is diagnostic.

Quiz No: 46.21

27 years old male presented with complaints of diplopia.

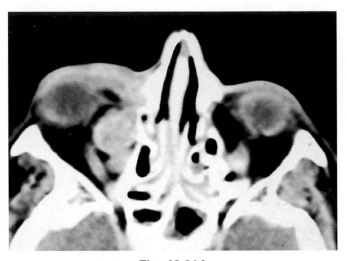

Fig. 46.21A

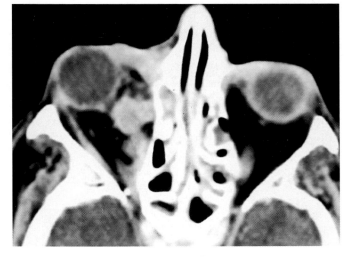

Fig. 46.21B

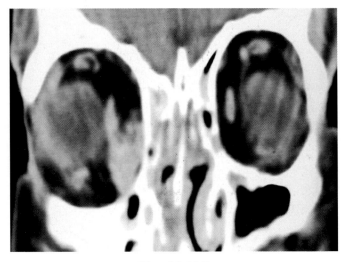

Fig. 46.21C

Answer

Orbital hemangioma (Figs 46.21A to C).
Post-contrast CT images show an enhancing intraconal mass on inferomedial aspect of orbit causing displacement of optic nerve to the right.

Cavernous hemangioma is the benign orbital tumor and most common vascular tumor of the orbit (intraconal) in adults. Affected patients present with slowly progressive unilateral proptosis, diplopia or decreased visual acuity. CT scan shows a well-demarcated homogenous intraconal mass, rarely associated with bone expansion or erosion.

Quiz No: 46.22

CT images in a 20 years female with recurrent right upper quadrant pain.

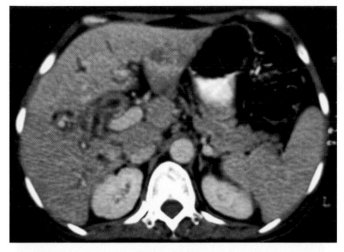

Fig. 46.22A

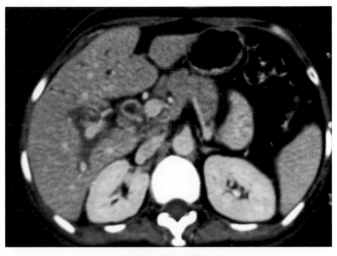

Fig. 46.22B

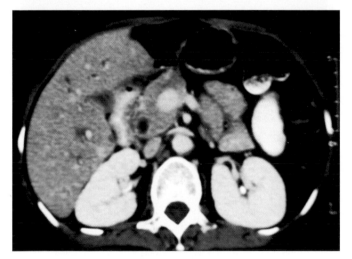

Fig. 46.22C

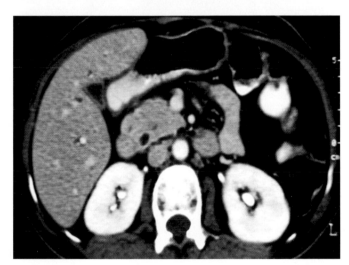

Fig. 46.22D

Answer

Sclerosing cholangitis (Figs 46.22A to D).

Sclerosing cholangitis is chronic inflammation of the bile ducts without a known cause. In this condition, the bile ducts inside and outside the liver become narrowed and scarred. The diagnosis is arrived at by ruling out other diseases. On CT scan mural contrast enhancement of the extra hepatic ducts in seen, along with dilatation, stenosis, wall thickening and nodularity. Dilatation, stenosis, pruning and beading of intrahepatic bile ducts can be appreciated. Nodes in the porta hepatitis may be present.

Quiz No: 46.23

A 50 years old female presented with painless slowly progressive swelling in the right submandibular region with resultant cosmetic disfigurement over last 15 years. Subjected to X-rays, panoramic view and CT.

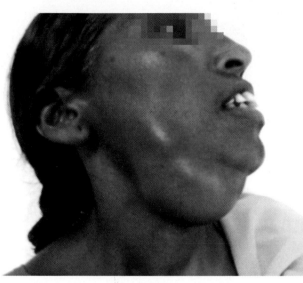

Fig. 46.23A

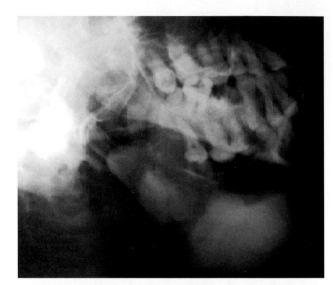

Fig. 46.23B

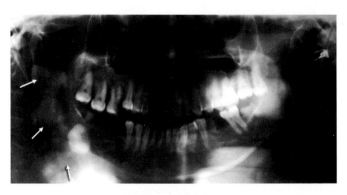

Fig. 46.23C

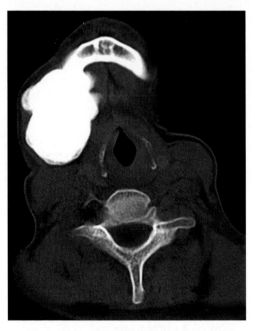

Fig. 46.23D

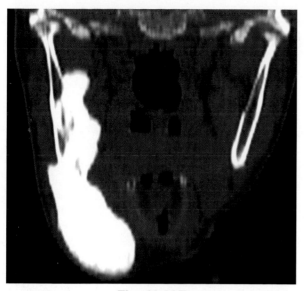

Fig. 46.23E

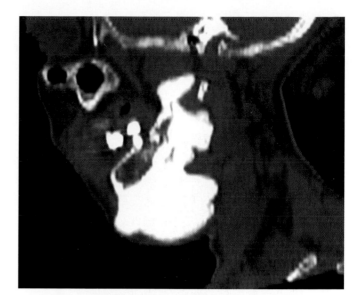

Fig. 46.23F

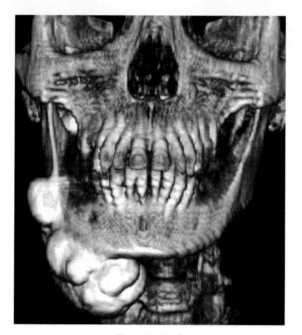

Fig. 46.23G

Answer

Giant peripheral osteoma of mandible (Figs 46.23A to G).
Imaging showed a giant exophytic radiodense peripheral osteoma involving buccal and lingual surface of the body, ramus, angle and inferior border of right side of mandible.

Quiz No: 46.24

40 years old male presented with history of seizures of long duration.

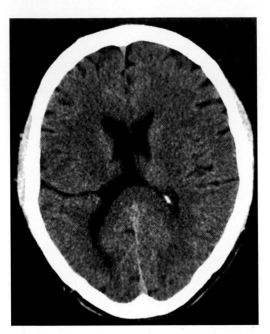

Fig. 46.24A

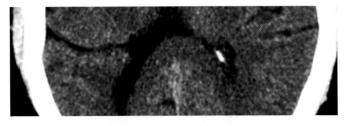

Fig. 46.24B

Answer

Open lip schizencephaly.

Plain CT Brain shows a linear CSF density extending from cerebral surface up to the ventricle. This CSF density is lined by gray matter (Fig. 46.24A).

Magnified view shows gray matter lining CSF density (Fig. 46.24B).

Schizencephalies are migrational disorders of brain which are characterized by grey matter lined cleft that extends from the ependymal surface of the brain through white matter to pia matter. Grey matter is dysplastic and heterotopic. The margins of the clefts may be either widely separated by interposing cerebrospinal fluid space (open lip form) or opposed to one another (closed lip form).

Quiz No: 46.25

Three year old female born of nonconsanguineous marriage presented with delayed language development skills and was able to speak only few familiar words. She had two episodes of seizures in infancy. She presented with intermittent hematuria of 15 days duration.

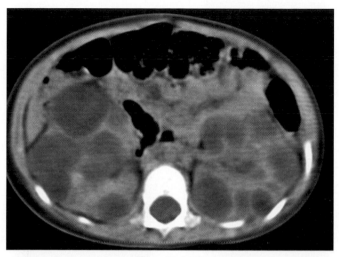

Fig. 46.25A

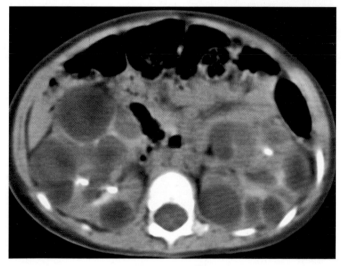

Fig. 46.25B

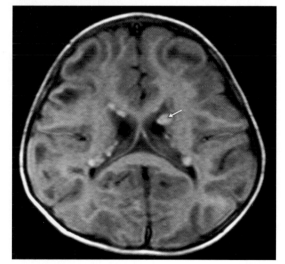

Fig. 46.25C

Answer

Tuberous sclerosis with polycystic renal disease.

CT abdomen shows bilateral renomegaly with multiple cysts in both kidneys causing severe parenchymal thinning (Fig. 46.25A). CECT shows minimal enhancement of renal parenchyma and delayed excretion of contrast (Fig. 46.25B) consistent with bilateral polycystic kidneys. Post contrast MRI brain (Fig. 46.25C) shows intensely enhancing subependymal tubers (arrow).

Findings suggest tuberous sclerosis.

Tuberous sclerosis is a multi-system, congenital disorder of autosomal dominant variety that causes benign tumors to grow in the brain and other vital organs such as the kidneys, heart, eyes, lungs and skin. Kidney findings include polycystic kidney disease and angiomyolipomas, which can cause hypertension.

Quiz No: 46.26

Seven months female child was brought with history of fever, pain and gradual distension of left side of abdomen extending to left thigh.

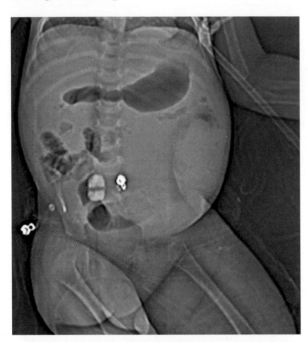

Fig. 46.26A

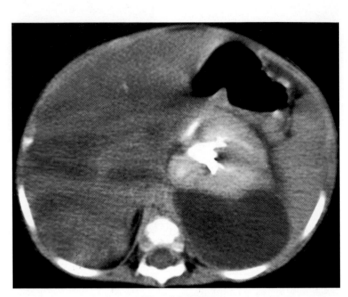

Fig. 46.26B

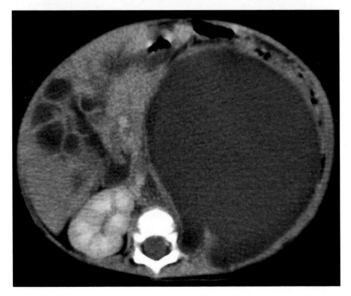

Fig. 46.26C

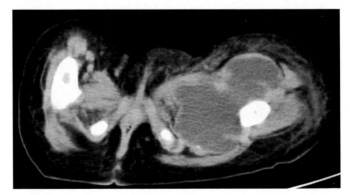

Fig. 46.26D

Answer

Large cold abscess.
CT images show a large hypodense collection in left ilio-psoas compartment pushing the left kidney anteriorly and bowel loops to the right (Figs 46.26A to D). The lesion has mildly enhancing walls. The collection is seen to track into the left thigh. This is the cause of fixed flexion deformity of left leg.

Quiz No: 46.27

70 years old male presented with chronic headache and sudden weakness in left upper and lower limbs.

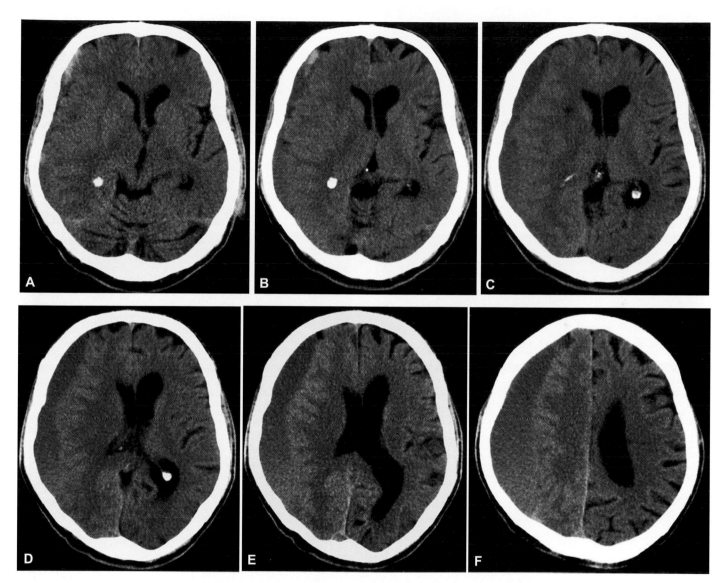

Figs 46.27A to F

Answer

Large right subacute subdural hematoma with lacunar infarct (Figs 46.27A to F).

Large right subacute subdural hematoma causing mass effect in the form of compression of right lateral ventricle and shift of midline structures to the contralateral side. A small fresh bleed (hyperdensity) is seen anterior to the large subacute subdural hematoma. Acute lacunar infarct is seen in anterior limb of right internal capsule.

Quiz No: 46.28

25 years male presented with intermittent pain and swelling of both the ankle and knee joints for last 7 years. Clinically patient had clubbing of nails of both extremities. It was present since childhood and was progressively increasing in severity.

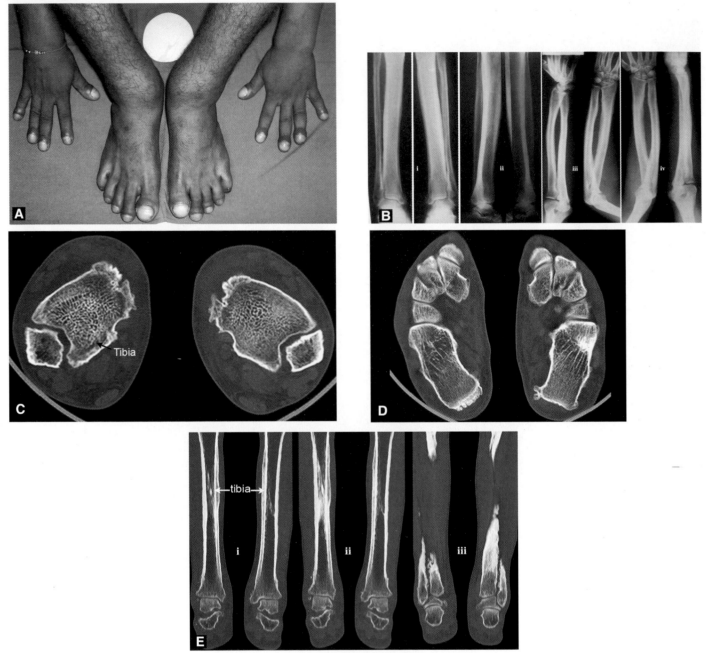

Figs 46.28A to E

Answer

Pachydermoperiostosis (Figs 46.28A).

X-ray and CT scan showed shaggy irregular periosteal reaction involving diaphysis, metaphysis and epiphysis of tibia, fibula, radius, and ulna (Figs 46.28B to E). There was cortical thickening of shaft of tibia in diphyseal region. It was diagnosed as pachydermoperiostosis, which is relatively rare. Diagnosis is by exclusion as no confirmatory gold standard test is available.

Quiz No: 46.29

12 years male with pain in abdomen and fever since 20 days.

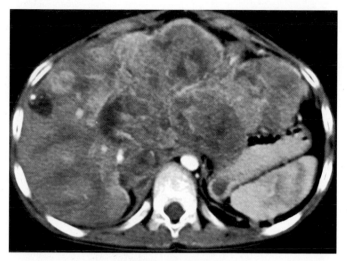

Fig. 46.29A

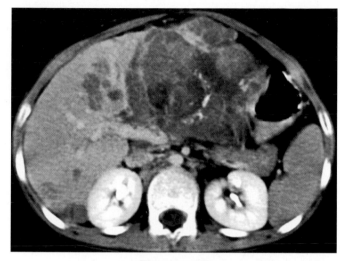

Fig. 46.29B

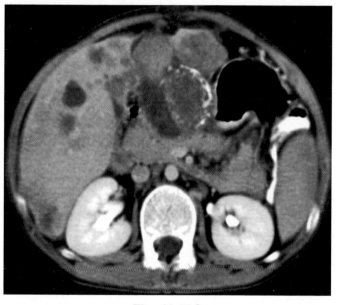

Fig. 46.29C

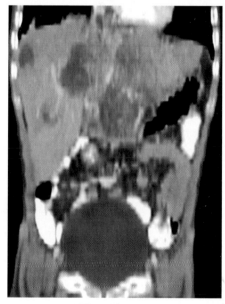

Fig. 46.29D

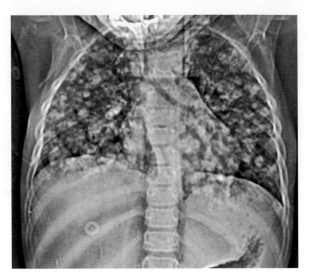

Fig. 46.29E

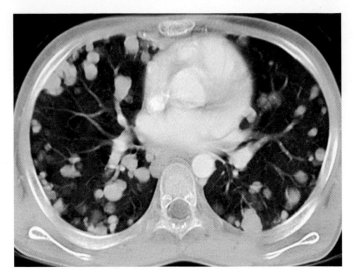

Fig. 46.29F

Answer

Hepatoblastoma with pulmonary metastases (Figs 46.29A to F).

Hepatoblastoma is the most common primary liver tumor in children, accounting for 79% of pediatric liver malignancies in children younger than 15 years.

Quiz No: 46.30

55 years female with persistent headache.
- Plain CT images (Figs 46.30A and B).
- Post-contrast CT images (Figs 46.30C and D).

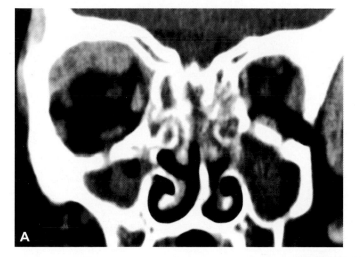
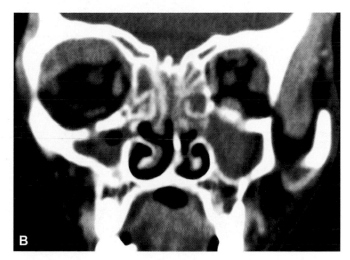

Figs 46.30A and B

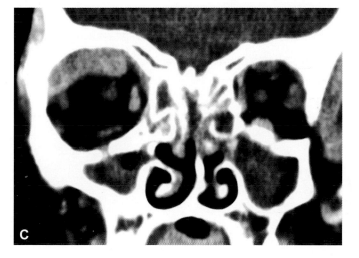
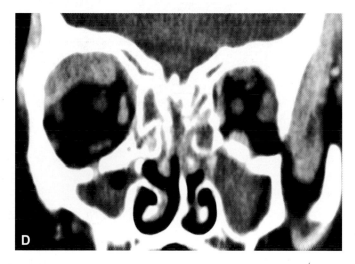

Figs 46.30C and D

Answer

Pan sinusitis and orbital pseudotumor.
Orbital pseudotumor is a nongranulomatous inflammatory process affecting orbital soft tissues. Minimal enhancement is seen in post contrast study. Clinically characterized by painful ophthalmoplegia and has dramatic response to steroids and antibiotics.

Quiz No: 46.31

5 year's male presented with a palpable mass in upper abdomen since birth (Fig. 46.31A).

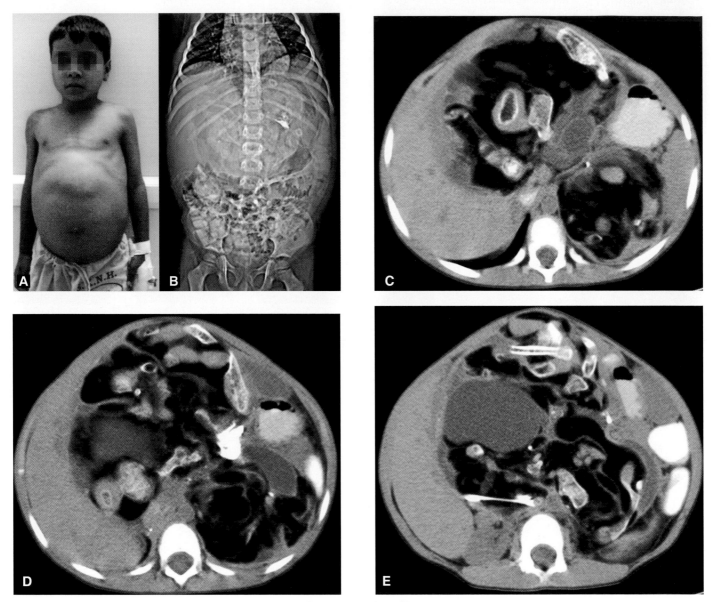

Figs 46.31A to E

Answer

Fetus-in-fetu

CT images show a large heterogeneous density mass lesion in the peritoneal cavity containing solid, cystic, fatty and osseous components (Figs 46.31B to E). Few well formed tubular bones and joints are seen. The fat plane between the lesion and adjacent abdominal structures is well defined, however the normal structures are displaced.

Complete surgical excision of the lesion was performed (Figs 46.31F and G) and the diagnosis was confirmed histopathologically.

Fetus-in-fetu is an uncommon developmental anomaly in which an abnormal fetus is enclosed within the abdomen of a normally developing fetus.

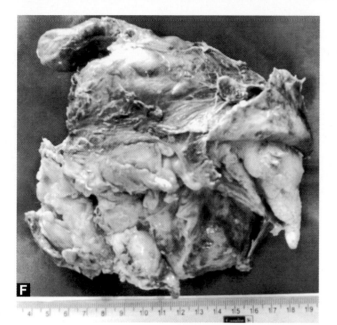

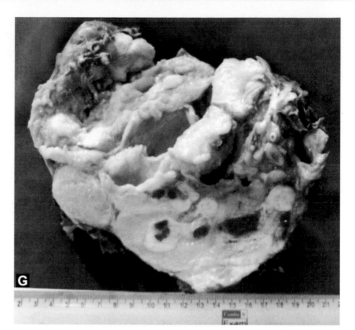

Figs 46.31F and G

Section 10

PET-CT

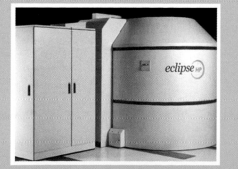
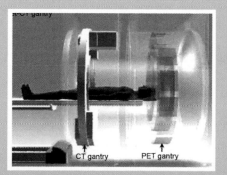
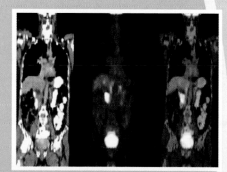

47. PET-CT

Positron emission tomography – computed tomography (PET-CT) has revolutionized field of medical diagnosis, PET alone lacked anatomic localization and CT lacked functional aspect of imaging. PET-CT has the advantages of both modalities, i.e. PET and CT. Patient is subjected to both the modalities in the same session and images are acquired. The system combines the images into superimposed images. In this way, functional imaging obtained by PET, which depicts the distribution of metabolic or biochemical activity in the body is aligned to the anatomic image obtained by CT.

PET-CT is used for early diagnosis of malignant diseases, its staging and follow up, surgical planning and radiation therapy and response to treatment. It determines the location and extent of cancer indicating spread to other areas of the body such as lymph nodes, liver, bones or brain in the form of metastatic disease. It distinguishes between malignant and benign tumors and recurrent cancer from scar tissue or fibrosis.

PET-CT is also used to study brain function in epilepsy, diagnosing Alzheimer's disease and other types of dementia, evaluating viability of heart muscle and study of coronary artery disease.

2-Deoxy-2-(18f), fluoro-deoxy-glucose or 18F-FDG, is a radioactive form of glucose and is the most common radiopharmaceutical used in PET. 18F-FDG has a half-life of approximately 110 minutes, so it is quickly expelled from the body. It is produced by cyclotron. Other radioisotope-positron emitters which can be used are carbon-11, nitrogen-13 and oxygen-15, having much shorter half life.

Patient is kept fasting for atleast 4 hours prior to scan. 10 mCi (370 MBq) of 18F-FDG is injected and imaging is done after one hour. Normal PET image shows more uptake in brain and cardiac muscles where there is increased metabolism. Pelvicalyceal system and urinary bladder show high uptake due to excretion.

Standardized uptake value (SUV) enables comparison within and between different patients and diseases.

$$SUV = \frac{\text{Radionuclide distribution in region of interest}}{\text{Radionuclide dose injected}/\text{Patient's weight in Kg}}$$

Sr. No.	Region	SUV
1	Soft tissue	0.6-0.8
2	Liver	2.2 -2.5
3	Kidneys	3.3- 3.5
4	Neoplasm	5.0-20.0

47.1 PET-CT Gantry (Fig. 47.1)

First the patient is put through CT gantry and CT scan is done and patient is shifted further into the PET gantry. Thus first the CT images are acquired followed by PET images and these images are then fused by software resulting in PET-CT images.

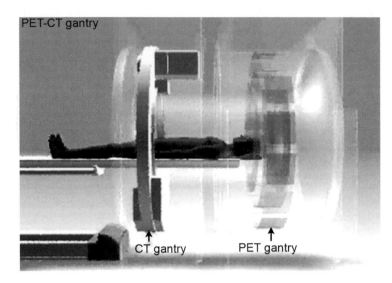

Fig. 47.1: PET-CT gantry

47.2 Cyclotron (Fig. 47.2)

Cyclotron is the equipment with the help of which 18F-FDG glucose is prepared in 5 hours. FDG glucose is tagged to fluorine molecule resulting in 18F-FDG glucose molecule used for PET imaging.

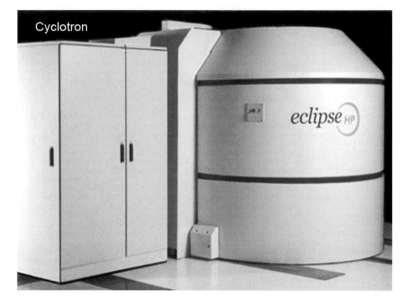

Fig. 47.2: Cyclotron

47.3 Normal PET Images

Normal PET images showing more uptake in brain and cardiac muscles where there is increased metabolism (Fig. 47.3). Pelvicalyceal system and urinary bladder show high uptake due to excretion of 18F-FDG.

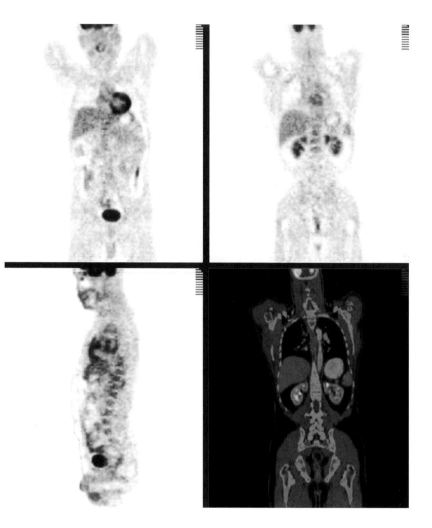

Fig. 47.3: Normal PET images

47.4 Lung Metastasis (Fig. 47.4)

Postoperative case of carcinoma of anal canal. CT scan shows a small nodule in left upper lobe of lung. Corresponding PET image shows increased uptake with a SUV of 8, confirming it to be a malignant nodule.

SUV is standardized uptake value of tissue. Higher the SUV value, more is the tissue metabolism and higher are the chances of it being malignant.

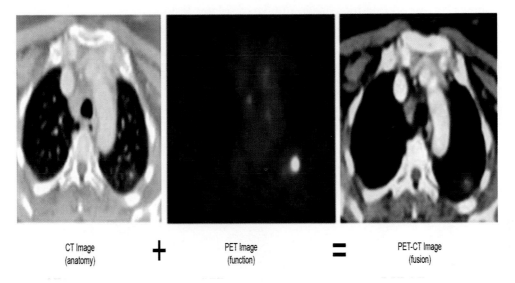

CT Image   +   PET Image   =   PET-CT Image
(anatomy)   (function)   (fusion)

Fig. 47.4: Lung metastasis

47.5 Splenic Metastases in Endometrial Carcinoma

47 years old suffering from menorrhagia since last 2 months.

USG showed endometrial thickening, proven as carcinoma of endometrium on histopathology.

PET-CT for Staging

CT axial section shows small multiple hypodense non-enhancing lesions in the spleen.

PET-CT image shows corresponding increase in uptake of splenic lesions suggesting malignancy (Fig. 47.5).

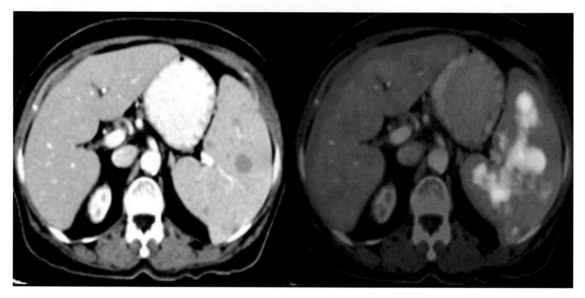

Fig. 47.5: PET-CT image shows increase uptake by splenic lesions

47.6 Peritoneal Metastases in Ovarian Carcinoma (Fig. 47.6)

59 years old, a postoperative case of carcinoma ovary for PET-CT.

PET-CT for Restaging

CT shows diffuse peritoneal thickening.

PET images show nonspecific increase in uptake.

PET-CT image shows increased uptake corresponding to peritoneal thickening on CT image suggestive of metastasis.

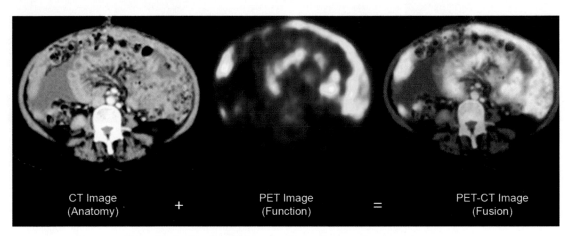

Fig. 47.6: Peritoneal metastases in ovarian carcinoma

47.7 Klatskin's Tumor

Intrahepatic central cholangiocarcinoma occurring at the confluence of hepatic ducts is known as Klatskin's tumor.

A case of Klatskin's tumor with multiple peritoneal nodules is shown here. They may sometimes be missed as unopacified bowel loops. CT shows multiple nodules with corresponding increased uptake on PET (Fig. 47.7).

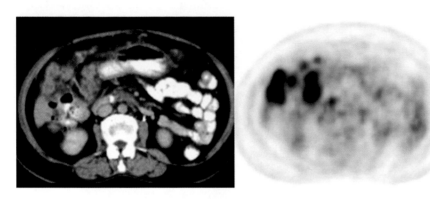 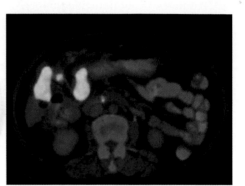

Fig. 47.7: Klatskin's tumor

47.8 Umbilical Hernia

PET-CT image of umbilical hernia with mild uptake in bowel loops (Fig. 47.8). Bowel activity should be ruled out by CT with oral and intravenous contrast media. PET is nonspecific for bowel wall pathologies where CT is more sensitive.

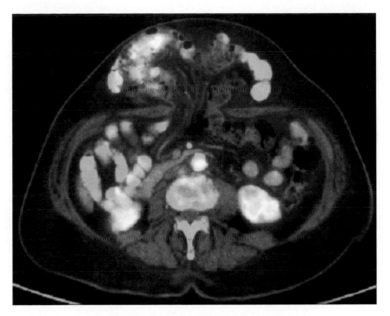

Fig. 47.8: Umbilical hernia

47.9 Wilm's Tumor (Fig. 47.9)

8 years male with urinary symptoms.

Limited PET-CT abdomen done to avoid more radiation.

CT shows mass in upper pole of right kidney.

PET image shows increase uptake but can be mistaken for pelvicalyceal system so CT scan is mandatory in renal pathologies.

PET-CT image shows increased uptake with void in central area corresponding to the necrosis on CT.

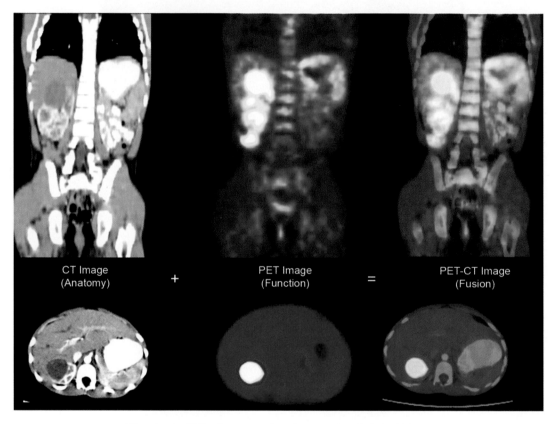

Fig. 47.9: Wilm's tumor in upper pole of right kidney

47.10 Renal Cell Carcinoma (Fig. 47.10)

64 years old male with right flank pain, came for master health check.

Axial CT images show heterogenous right upper pole mass categorized as a renal cell carcinoma on histopathology.

PET-CT image shows corresponding increased uptake. No renal vein or IVC involvement noted.

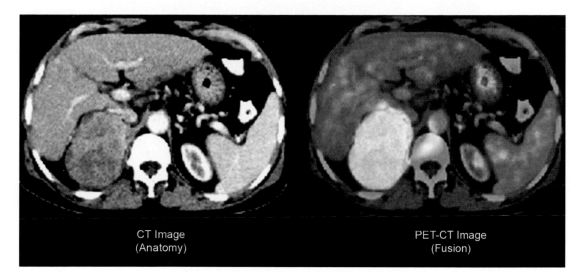

Fig. 47.10: Right renal cell carcinoma

47.11 Carcinoma Pancreas (Fig. 47.11)

Coronal CT image shows bulky pancreatic head infiltrating into adjacent duodenum. Corresponding PET image shows increased uptake. Fused images showing exact anatomy and increased uptake.

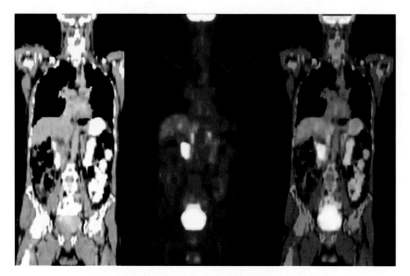

Fig. 47.11: Carcinoma head pancreas

47.12 Lymphoma

PET image of pre and post treatment in a case of lymphoma showing complete response (Fig. 47.12). Increased focal uptake in post therapy images is seen in region of heart due to higher metabolism and in the region of urinary bladder due to excretion.

Increased uptake seen in liver and intrabdominal lesions of lymphoma in pre-therapy images is not seen in post therapy images indicating good response.

PET can thus be used for monitoring response to treatment in cases of malignancy as it shows changes at metabolic level. It is more sensitive and specific than CT scan.

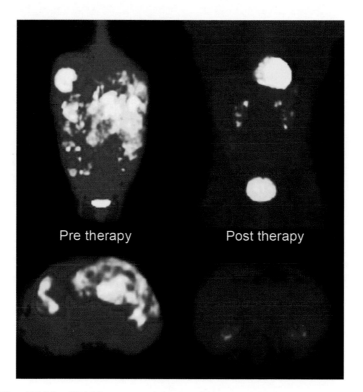

Fig. 47.12: PET images of pre and post treatment in a case of lymphoma shows complete response

47.13 Rectal Melanoma

45 years male presented with constipation on and off, progressing since 3 months.

CT shows diffuse circumferential anorectal wall thickening that was confirmed as melanocytic melanoma on histopathology.

PET shows corresponding increase uptake.

PET-CT fused image shows rectal thickening with corresponding increase uptake suggesting rectal malignancy (Fig. 47.13).

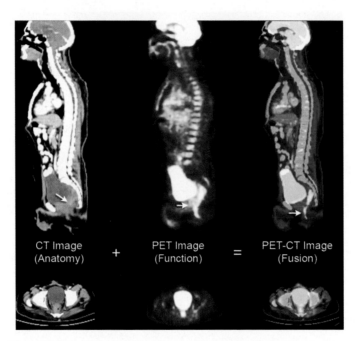

Fig. 47.13: PET-CT shows rectal thickening with increase uptake suggesting rectal malignancy

47.14 Carcinoma Prostate (Fig. 47.14)

CT pelvis in 64 years old patient shows enlarged prostate with patchy area of enhancement with calcific focus. PET-CT shows small focus of avid uptake by prostate suggesting malignancy, confirmed on biopsy.

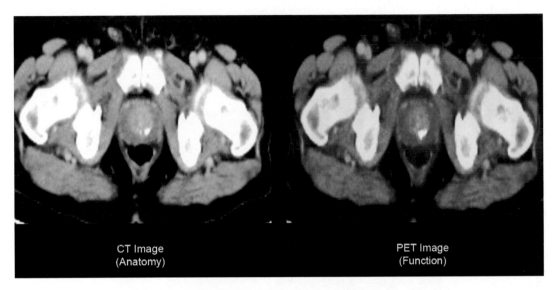

Fig. 47.14: Carcinoma prostate

47.15 Soft Tissue Sarcoma (Fig. 47.15)

34 years male with dull pain in left thigh gradually progressing with tenderness and swelling.

PET-CT for staging

CT shows illdefined soft tissue lesion in medial compartment of the left thigh with necrotic areas and was confirmed as soft tissue sarcoma on histopathology.

PET shows very high uptake with clear delineation of extent of tumor.

PET-CT image shows corresponding increase uptake with void area in the center corresponding to the necrotic area on CT.

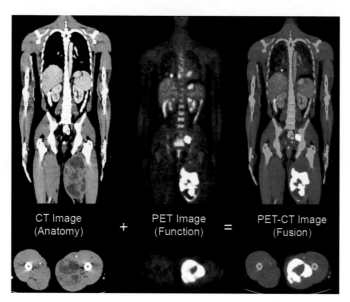

Fig. 47.15: Soft tissue sarcoma left thigh

47.16 Non-Hodgkin's Lymphoma

51 years male presented with pain in left hip rapidly progressing in nature.

CT shows destructive left femoral lesion with large soft tissue component which was diagnosed as Non Hodgkin's lymphoma on histopathology.

PET-CT was performed for staging which showed corresponding increase in uptake in left thigh corresponding to lesion on CT (Fig. 47.16).

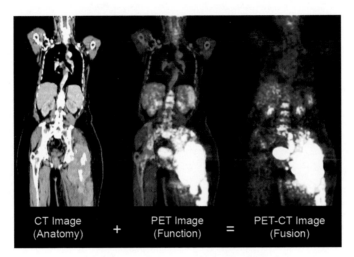

CT Image   PET Image   PET-CT Image
(Anatomy)   +   (Function)   =   (Fusion)

Fig. 47.16: PET-CT shows increase uptake in left thigh in Non-Hodgkin's lymphoma

Section 11

Radiation Safety Measures

48. RADIATION SAFETY MEASURES

Radiation is a form of energy which can travel from one place to another even in vacuum. Radiation hazards are the harmful effects that can occur to our body due to radiations.

Heat and light are the form of radiations that can be felt by our senses. Although X-rays are ionizing radiations, they cannot be felt by our skin. Hence it is important to be aware of radiation hazards and radiation protection.

Natural sources of radiation are radon and cosmic rays. Artificial sources of radiation are a) diagnostic radiation in the form of radiography, CT scan, PET scan and nuclear scan. b) therapeautic radiation in the form of brachytherapy and teletherapy.

Units of Radiation

As per the International System of units, dose of ionizing radiation is measured in unit called as gray (Gy). One Gy is defined as that quantity of radiation which results in energy deposition of one joule per kilogram in the irradiated tissue. Gray has replaced the earlier unit known as the rad. 1Gy is equal to 100 rad.

Effective dose of radiation is different for different tissues and is measured in terms of a unit called as Sieverts (Sv). This depends on the quality factor (Q) of the tissue which permits passage of energy. Dose equivalent (Sv) = Quality factor (Q) × Dose (Gy).

Effects of Radiation

Stochastic effects of radiation are the ones whose probability of occurrence increases with increase in dose and include cancer and genetic effects.

Deterministic effects are the ones which increase in severity with increase in dose and include cataract, blood dyscrasias and impaired fertility.

Irradiation *in utero* can lead to developmental abnormalities (8-25 weeks), cancer which can be expressed in childhood or in adults due to DNA damage by radiation.

Preconception maternal irradiation in therapeutic doses gives rise to defects in 1 out of 10 exposed children. Non urgent radiological testing should not be done between 8-17 weeks of gestation, which is the most sensitive period for organogenesis.

Children are 10 times more sensitive for hazards of radiations than adults. Hence radiography with high kV and low mAs technique is recommended in children.

Acute radiation syndrome is said to occur when high doses kill so many cells that tissues and organs are damaged immediately. The higher the radiation dose, the sooner the effects of radiation will appear and higher will be the probability of death. This was seen in atomic bomb survivors in 1945 and emergency workers responding to the 1986 Chernobyl nuclear power plant accident who received radiation to the tune of 800 to 16,000 mSv.

Acute radiation at doses in excess of 100 Gy to the total body, usually result in death within 24 to 48 hrs from neurological and cardiovascular failure. This is known as the cerebrovascular syndrome.

Chronic radiation causes radiation pneumonitis and even permanent scarring that results in respiratory compromise.

Average Effective Dose in mSv

- X-ray Chest - 0.02
- CT Orbits - 0.8
- CT Temporal bone - 1.0
- CT Head - 2.0

- CT Spine - 3.0
- CT Chest - 8.0
- CT Abdomen - 10.0
- CT Pelvis - 10.0

The International Commission of Radiation Protection (ICRP) was formed in 1928 on the recommendation of the first International Congress of Radiology in 1925 which formed the International Commission on Radiation Units (ICRU). The National Commission for Radiation Protection (NCRP) in America and the Atomic Energy Regulatory Board (AERB) in India are the regulatory bodies that recommend norms for permissible doses of radiation for radiation workers and for the general public.

Atomic Energy Regulatory Board (AERB) which is the Indian regulatory board was constituted on November 15, 1983 by the President of India by exercising the powers conferred by Section 27 of the Atomic Energy Act, 1962. The regulatory authority of AERB is derived from the rules and notifications promulgated under the Atomic Energy Act, 1962 and the Environmental (Protection) Act, 1986. Radiation safety in handling of radiation generating equipment is governed by Section 17 of The Atomic Energy Act, 1962 and the Radiation Protection Rules 1971 issued under the Act.

The overall objective of radiation protection is to provide an appropriate standard of protection for man without unduly limiting the beneficial practices giving rise to radiation exposure.

Atomic Energy Regulatory Board (AERB) recommends and lays down guidelines regarding the specifications of medical X-ray equipment, for the room layout of X-ray installation, regarding the work practices in X-ray department, the protective devices and also the responsibilities of the radiation personnel, employer and Radiation Safety Officer (RSO). It is the authority in India which exercises a regulatory control and has the power to decommissioning X-ray installations and also for imposing penalties on any person contravening these rules.

Benefit Risk Analysis

Since radiation exposure entails inherent risks of radiation effects, no decision to expose an individual can be undertaken without weighing benefits of exposure against potential risks, that is, making a benefit risk analysis.

Principles of Radiation Protection

    (a) Justification of a practice
    (b) Optimized protection
    (c) Dose limitation

Radiation Protection Actions

The triad of radiation protection actions comprise of "time-distance-shielding". Reduction of exposure time, increasing distance from source, and shielding of patients and occupational workers have proven to be of great importance.

Shielding

Shielding implies that certain materials (concrete, lead) will attenuate radiation (reduce its intensity) when they are placed between the source of radiation and the exposed individual.

Source Shielding

X-ray tube housing is lined with thin sheets of lead because X-rays produced in the tube are scattered in all directions, to protect both patients and personnel from leakage radiation. AERB recommends a maximum allowable leakage radiation from tube housing not greater than 1mGy per hour per 100 cm^2.

Structural Shielding

The lead lined walls of radiology department are referred to as protective barriers because they are designed to protect individuals located outside the X-ray rooms from unwanted radiation.

(a) Primary barrier is one which is directly struck by the primary or the useful beam.

(b) Secondary barrier is one which is exposed to secondary radiation either by leakage from X-ray tube or by scattered radiation from the patient.

The room housing X-ray unit is not less than 18 m² for general purpose radiography and conventional fluoroscopy equipment and that of the CT room housing the gantry of the CT unit should not be less than 25 m².

Wall of the X-ray rooms on which primary X-ray beam falls is not less than 35 cm thick brick or equivalent. Walls of the X-ray room on which scattered X-rays fall is not less than 23 cm thick brick or equivalent. The walls and viewing window of the control booth should have material of 1.5 mm lead equivalent.

Personnel Shielding

Shielding apparel should be used as and when necessary which comprise of lead aprons, eye glasses with side shields, hand gloves and thyroid shields. The minimum thickness of lead equivalent in the protective apparel should be 0.5 mm. These are classified as a secondary barrier to the effects of ionizing radiation as they protect an individual only from secondary (scattered) radiation and not the primary beam.

Patient Shielding

Thyroid, breast and gonads are shielded to protect these organs especially in children and young adults.

The responsibility for establishing a radiation protection programme rests with the hospital administration/owners of the X-ray facility. The administration is expected to appoint a Radiation Safety Committee (RSC) and a Radiation Safety Officer (RSO).

Every radiation worker prior to commencing radiation work and at subsequent intervals not exceeding 12 months shall be subjected to the medical examinations. Radiation Safety Officer (RSO) should be an individual with extensive training and education in areas such as radiation protection, radiation physics, radiation biology, instrumentation, dosimetry and shielding design. Duties include assisting the employer in meeting the relevant regulatory requirements applicable to the X-ray installation and ensuring that all radiation measuring and monitoring instruments under custody are properly calibrated and maintained in good condition.

Recommended Dose Limits

Once pregnancy is established the dose equivalent to the surface of pregnant woman's abdomen should not exceed 2 mSv for the remainder of the pregnancy. Ten Day Rule states that all females of reproductive age who need an X-ray examination should get it done within first 10 days of menses to avoid irradiation to possible conception.

As a general principle radiation exposure should be less than 20 mSv/year for radiation workers and less than 1 mSv/year for general public.

Optimization of protection can be achieved by optimizing the procedure to administer a radiation dose which is as low as reasonably achievable (ALARA), so as to derive maximum diagnostic information with minimum discomfort to the patient.

Detection of Radiation

Following methods of detecting radiation based on physical and chemical effects produced by radiation exposure are available:

1. Ionization-The ability of radiation to produce ionization in air is the basis for radiation detection by the ionization chamber.
2. Photographic effect-The ability of radiation to blacken photographic films, is the basis of detectors that use film.
3. Luminescence-When radiation strikes certain materials they emit light that is proportional to the radiation intensity.
4. Scintillation-Here radiation is converted into light, which is then directed to a photomultiplier tube, which then converts the light into an electrical pulse.

Personnel dosimetry is the monitoring of individuals who are exposed to radiation during the course of their work. It is accomplished through the use of devices such as the pocket dosimeter, the film badge or the thermoluminescent dosimeter (TLD). The dose is subsequently stated as an estimate of the effective dose equivalent to the whole body in mSv for the reporting period. Dosimeters used for personnel monitoring have dose measurement limit of 0.1-0.2 mSv (10-20 mrem).

TLD can measure exposures as low as $1.3\mu C/kg$ (5 mR) and the pocket dosimeter can measure up to $50\mu C/kg$ (200 mR). The film badge however cannot measure exposures < $2.6 \mu C/kg$ (10 mR). TLD can withstand a certain degree of heat, humidity, and pressure; their crystals are reusable; and instantaneous readings are possible if the department has a TLD analyzer. The greatest disadvantage of a TLD is its cost.

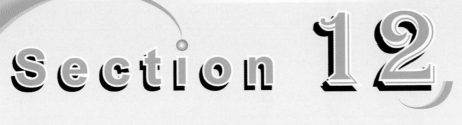

Section 12

CT Contrast Media

49. CT CONTRAST MEDIA

I. Iodinated Intravascular Agents

Intravascular radiological contrast media are iodine containing chemicals which add to the details from any given CT scan study and thereby aid in the diagnosis. They were first introduced by Moses Swick. Iodine (atomic weight 127) is an ideal choice element for X-ray absorption because the k shell binding energy of iodine (33.7) is nearest to the mean energy used in diagnostic radiography and thus maximum photoelectric interactions can be obtained which are a must for best image quality.

These compounds after intravascular injection are rapidly distributed by capillary permeability into extravascular extra-cellular space and almost 90% is excreted via glomerular filtration by kidneys within 12 hours.

Following iodinated contrast media are available:
1. Ionic monomers, e.g. Diatrizoate, Iothamalate, Metrizoate.
2. Non-ionic monomers, e.g. Iohexol, Iopamidol, Iomeron.
3. Ionic dimer, e.g. Ioxaglate.
4. Non-ionic dimer, e.g. Iodixanol, Iotrolan.

The amount of contrast required is usually 1-2 ml/kg body weight.

Normal osmolality of human scrum is 290 mOsm/kg. Ionic contrast media have much higher osmolality than normal human serum and are known as High Osmolar Contrast Media (HOCM), while non-ionic contrast media have lower osmolality than normal human serum and are known as Low Osmolar Contrast Media (LOCM).

Side effects or adverse reactions to contrast media are divided as:
1. Idiosyncratic anaphylactoid reactions.
2. Non-idiosyncratic reactions like nephrotoxicity and cardio-toxicity.

Adverse reactions are more with HOCM than LOCM. So LOCM are preferred.

Delayed adverse reactions although very rare are, however, more common with LOCM and include iodide mumps, systemic lupus erythematosus (SLE) and Stevens-Johnson syndrome.

Principles of treatment of adverse reaction involves mainly five basic steps: ABCDE

A – Maintain proper airway

B – Breathing – Support for adequate breathing

C – Maintain adequate circulation. Obtain an IV access.

D – Use of appropriate drugs like antihistaminics for urticaria, atropine for vasovagal hypotension and bradycardia, beta agonists for bronchospasm, hydrocortisone etc.

E – Always have emergency back up ready including ICU care.

II. Barium Sulphate

Barium sulphate preparations are used for evaluating gastrointestinal tract. Barium (atomic weight 137) is an ideal choice element for X-ray absorption because the k shell binding energy of barium (37) is near to the mean energy used in diagnostic radiography and thus maximum photoelectric interactions can be obtained which are a must for best image quality. Moreover, barium sulphate is non-absorbable, non-toxic and can be prepared into a stable suspension.

For CT scan of abdomen, 1000-1500 ml of 1-5% w/vol barium sulphate suspension can be used.

Severe adverse reactions are rare. Rarely mediastinal leakage can lead to fibrosing mediastinitis while peritoneal leakage can cause adhesive peritonitis.

III. Oral Iodinated Agents

Iodine containing contrast agents like Gastrograffin and Trazograf are given orally for evaluating gastrointestinal tract on CT scan.

IV. Carbon Dioxide

Rarely carbon dioxide is used for infradiaphragmatic CT angiography in patients who are sensitive to iodinated contrast.

Index